P9-CSA-260

Language Perspectives

# Language Perspectives

## Acquisition, Retardation, and Intervention

SECOND EDITION

EDITED BY
RICHARD L. SCHIEFELBUSCH
AND
LYLE L. LLOYD

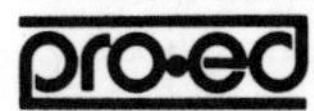

5341 Industrial Oaks Boulevard
Austin, Texas 78735

Copyright © 1988 by PRO-ED, Inc.

All rights reserved. No part of this book may be reproduced
in any form or by any means without
the prior written permission of the publisher.

Printed in the United States of America

**Library of Congress Cataloging-in-Publication Data**

Language perspectives.

Bibliography: p.
Includes index.
1. Language acquisition—Congresses.
2. Psycholinguistics—Congresses.
3. Nonverbal communication in children—
Congresses. 4. Mentally handicapped children—
Language—Congresses. 5. Language disorders
in children—Congresses. I. Schiefelbusch,
Richard L. II. Lloyd, Lyle L.
P118.L375 1988 401'.9 87-2375
ISBN 0-89079-148-1

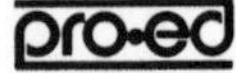

5341 Industrial Oaks Boulevard
Austin, Texas 78735

*10 9 8 7 6 5 4 3 2 1 88 89 90 91 92*

# *Contents*

# Contributors

**Terry Kit-fong Au, PhD**
Department of Psychology
Stanford University
Stanford, California

**Christiane A. M. Baltaxe, PhD**
Department of Psychiatry
Neuropsychiatric Institute
University of California–Los Angeles
Los Angeles, California

**Marion Blank, PhD**
Children's Hearing Institute
Manhattan Eye, Ear, and Throat Hospital
New York, New York

**Patricia A. Broen, PhD**
Department of Communication Disorders
University of Minnesota
Minneapolis, Minnesota

**Richard F. Cromer, PhD**
Medical Research Council
Cognitive Development Unit
London, England

**Barbara Harris Fiese**
Institute for the Study of Developmental Disabilities
University of Illinois at Chicago
Chicago, Illinois

**Ann P. Kaiser, PhD**
Department of Special Education
George Peabody College
Vanderbilt University
Nashville, Tennessee

**George Karlan, PhD**
Special Education Section
Purdue University
West Lafayette, Indiana

**Stan Kuczaj II, PhD**
Department of Psychology
Southern Methodist University
Dallas, Texas

**Laurence B. Leonard, PhD**
Audiology and Speech Sciences
Purdue University
West Lafayette, Indiana

**Lyle L. Lloyd, PhD**
Chairman, Special Education Section
Purdue University
West Lafayette, Indiana

**James E. McLean, PhD**
Senior Scientist
Parsons Research Center
Bureau of Child Research
University of Kansas
Lawrence, Kansas

**Dolores Perin, PhD**
Center for Advanced Study in Education
City University of New York, Graduate School
New York, New York

**Joe Reichle, PhD**
Department of Communication Disorders
University of Minnesota
Minneapolis, Minnesota

**Larry G. Richards, PhD**
Center for Computer Aided Engineering
University of Virginia
Charlottesville, Virginia

**Meredith Martin Richards, PhD**
Department of Psychology
University of Louisville
Louisville, Kentucky

**Mary Ann Romski, PhD**
Department of Psychology
Language Research Center
Georgia State University
Atlanta, Georgia

**Arnold J. Sameroff, PhD**
Bradley Research Center
Emma Pendleton Bradley Hospital
East Providence, Rhode Island

**Richard R. Schiefelbusch, PhD**
Director
Bureau of Child Research
University of Kansas
Lawrence, Kansas

**Rose A. Sevcik, MA**
Department of Psychology
Language Research Center
Georgia State University
Atlanta, Georgia

**Gerald M. Siegel, PhD**
Department of Communication Disorders
University of Minnesota
Minneapolis, Minnesota

**Jan Silverstein, PhD**
Department of Speech Pathology and Audiology
University of Denver
Denver, Colorado

**James Q. Simmons III, MD**
Department of Psychiatry and Behavioral Sciences
School of Medicine
University of California–Los Angeles
Los Angeles, California

**Margaret Snowling, PhD**
National Hospitals
College of Speech Sciences
London, England

**Lynn S. Snyder, PhD**
Department of Communication
University of Denver
Denver, Colorado

**Lee Snyder-McLean, PhD**
Parsons Research Center
Bureau of Child Research
University of Kansas
Lawrence, Kansas

**Steven F. Warren, PhD**
Department of Special Education
George Peabody College
Vanderbilt University
Nashville, Tennessee

# *Preface*

This second edition of *Language Perspectives: Acquisition, Retardation, and Intervention* is a lengthy effort by several collaborators to update and extend the original book published in 1974. Because the field the book addresses is changing, the current publication is essentially a new book. Consequently, this book is related to the original publication only in regard to descriptions of critical issues. The closest content match comes in nonspeech communication (augmentative and alternative systems) and thought and language (language and cognitive development).

This edition of *Language Perspectives* retains a strong emphasis on intervention and on efforts to integrate theoretical positions while introducing a number of areas not covered in the first volume. These additions emphasize developments during the past 14 years and thus provide a current perspective for 1988, much as the first volume did for 1974.

The reader should realize that neither volume was prepared as a comprehensive analysis of language acquisition as it applies to normal and handicapped children, nor as a comprehensive analysis of intervention. The books, consequently, reflect the view of the planners as to the critical issues of the time. For instance, in 1974 there was a range of speculation about infants, especially infants' perception of human speech. We also were concerned about but not fully able to place infants into our language intervention plans. The spirit of the current scene is different. We now have an infant-at-risk field of strategic planning leading to infant intervention, usually with accompanying parental training.

Another area of great change appears in language intervention. In 1974 there were formal training designs for teaching language as a system of symbols. We were keying on language rules and relating language to cognitive development. In the current volume the emphasis has shifted to communicative competence. During the past 12 years the issues of generalization and functional language have gained prominence. Also, we now see language in relation to cultural issues, while in 1974 culture was virtually ignored. Although the current edition was not developed as a systematically updated volume, the reader is invited to use the two editions to analyze the 14 years of progress that are reflected. Even if no comparisons are made, there is enough emerging information to warrant our questioning where we are today and where we may be going. If the reader does wish to compare the two time-related orientations, the introduction to this volume provides a number of suggestions.

The current book was initiated by Janet Hankin, Lyle Lloyd, and Dick Schiefelbusch, who assembled a small committee of editors including Craig Ramey, Stan Kuczaj, Jim McLean, Richard Cromer, Jerry Siegel, and Mabel Rice. The committee planned the sections and selected the authors.

The committee agreed to use the format of the first perspectives (i.e., consisting of sections under which more than one chapter appears). However, instead of discussion summaries, the current book has section editors who helped authors provide an editorial balance. Consequently, each section can stand as an analysis of a critical area of the current field of language acquisition and intervention.

The book provides an up-to-date look at a rapidly changing field. Both clinicians and applied scientists will find the content useful in determining areas of strength and weakness. In addition, the book addresses current controversies. Finally, the authors suggest ways to further integrate the work of several relevant sectors of language research.

The editors wish to thank Janet Hankin, who guided the early development of the book. Most of all we wish to thank the section editors and authors whose patience was an essential condition for the final submission.

*Richard L. Schiefelbusch*
*Lyle L. Lloyd*

# Introduction

Richard L. Schiefelbusch

In 1973 several planners at the University of Kansas were encouraged by Dr. Lyle L. Lloyd (then a staff member at the National Institute of Child Health and Human Development) to organize a conference on language of the mentally retarded that would reflect recent developments in theory and practice. Seven converging themes were selected to represent important, but controversial, areas that could be studied by a group of scientists from several relevant disciplines.

The participants agreed to prepare manuscripts to be discussed at the conference and then revised for published proceedings. The resulting book—*Language Perspectives: Acquisition, Retardation, and Intervention*—became a widely circulated work about language acquisition and intervention. The book highlighted a number of issues in child language.

First, the conference, under the sponsorship of the National Institute of Child Health and Human Development, brought psycholinguists together with cognitive, behavioral, and developmental psychologists and speech pathologists and special educators. They found that they could communicate effectively and that they could respect one another's work. Consequently, the project reflected a condition that previously had not existed, a condition that could be called a search for synthesis among theories and methods of research. Prior to that time the various groups of researchers in child language had worked separately and often within theoretical frames that were oppositional.

Second, the group sought to update a converging set of themes, each of which was instrumental to the analysis of language acquisition and intervention. The updating was not done exclusively by individual authors who submitted finalized statements on the subject but also included suggestions, corrections, additions, and deletions resulting from open discussions by conference participants.

Third, the group did not seek to develop justifications for any approach to language acquisition and intervention, but sought rather to establish the existing knowledge base from which further work could be planned and promoted. This open-minded approach was maintained during the conference and the time required for the preparation of the book.

In addition to these apparent perspectives, several subtle beginnings can be traced back to the 1974 *Language Perspectives* project. One beginning was the delineation of a remedial (Guess, Sailor, & Baer, Chapter 21) and a developmental (Miller & Yoder, Chapter 20) approach to language intervention. Another was the identification of a nonspeech language and communication approach (Premack & Premack, Chapter 14; Moores, Chapter 15) for severely and multiply handicapped children. Still another was the emphasis on parents as language trainers (Horton, Chapter 18) and the importance of early beginnings (Bricker & Bricker, Chapter 17) in language stimulation. Also emerging from the publication are the importance of training receptive as well as expressive functions (Bloom, Chapter 11; Ingram, Chapter 12; Chapman, Chapter 13), training for uses in "ever widening contexts," and the process of mapping cognitive functions onto a formal language system (Clark, Chapter 4; Morehead & Morehead, Chapter 5; Bowerman, Chapter 7).

Although the 1974 publication was, by most standards, a reflection of the state of the field at that time, it omitted several critical areas that are important today. Chief among the omissions is the area of pragmatics (which was an active but small initiative at that time). Also largely omitted was a cross-cultural emphasis. Language assessment also was given short shrift in the publication.

The current publication includes emphases that were little known in 1974 such as generalization, early mother-child interaction, augmentative and alternative symbol systems, and *communicative competence* as a theoretical orientation.

The remainder of this introductory statement focuses on three issues: substantive shifts, theoretical shifts, and application (intervention) shifts. Each issue should spark interest in the exciting, rapidly changing language perspectives described in this volume.

## SUBSTANTIVE SHIFTS

McLean and Snyder-McLean (Chapter 10 of this volume) have observed that the dominant theoretical models of human language have shifted from those focused on idealized systems to those focused on the relationship between the language and the user in the environment. They further see pragmatics as an indication that language has been "returned to its human users." This view is consistent with views expressed throughout the book. For instance, there is a shift from the formal system of symbol processing to creativity, innovation, and discovery (Chapter 3) and to the acquisition and use of words (Chapter 4). Likewise, language and cognition are delineated in regard to language of the mentally retarded (Chapter 5) and to written language (Chapter 7).

Sections II and III describe an extensive functional shift in lexical and semantic topics in ways that scientists and practitioners alike can adapt to a range of users (i.e., mentally retarded, Chapter 5; readers, Chapter 7; the language impaired, Chapter 4; the emotionally disturbed, Chapter 9; and the severely and multiply handicapped, Chapters 10 and 13). This shift, of course, has also supported the work of scientists and clinicians who are adapting augmentative and alternative symbol systems (Chapters 13 and 14).

Another way to describe this functional shift is to say that we now tend to study language as the communicative competence of language users. Section IV deals extensively with communicative functions. In Chapter 9 it is explained that pragmatics has evolved from the work of social anthropologists, sociolinguists, and psycholinguists interested in social development. This approach attends to those social aspects that interact with language in communication.

This emphasis shift has led to a greater reliance on the "natural environment" as a locus for intervention planning and also on incidental or other milieu strategies for home-based or school-based language teaching programs (see Chapters 15 and 16).

## THEORETICAL SHIFTS

In 1974 theories were oriented to a structural system of language based primarily on Chomsky's theory of transformational grammar. This work previously had had more impact on studies of language acquisition of normal preschool children than on the study of impaired language development or language intervention.

However, a rereading of the 1974 book, with special reference to the last two summarizing chapters written by Staats and Schiefelbusch, respectively, conveys a strong continuing preoccupation with behavioral and cognitive theories. Staats (Chapter 24) was especially cogent about a rapprochement between behavioral and cognitive theoretical systems leading to a "neopsycholinguistic" proposal.

Staats's recommendations focused on "the importance of learning in the child's development of language and the child's interaction with his parents and others." He also recommended that we focus on "the context and functions of language for the individual." His recommendations seem to have presaged much of the social emphasis that is so apparent today.

Nevertheless, for the most part the book appeared during a period of strong structural emphasis, both linguistic and cognitive. The current emphasis, in contrast, is on social or communicative competence. This broadened analysis of communicative competence now includes knowledge about form, function, and use in context. The additional knowledge domains have been firmly labeled as semantics and pragmatics. Each area is regarded as a prominent part of a total concept of competence. A number of psycholinguists have analyzed this enlarged concept of competence to show the interrelationships and the specifics of each (Schiefelbusch, 1986; Schiefelbusch & Pickar, 1984). We can now describe communicative competence as the totality of experience-derived knowledge and skill that enables speakers to communicate effectively and appropriately in transactional contexts.

The key elements of this definition are knowledge (rules of syntax, semantics, and usage functions) and skill (effectiveness and appropriateness) in transactional contexts. (See Chapter 11 for a discussion of knowledge and skill.) The above definition, with its strongly inferred issues, is generally supported throughout the book.

What we have now is a broader theoretical frame of reference than we had in 1974, but one that includes previous emphases that are still instrumental—primarily grammar, semantics, and pragmatics. However, missing from this statement is the ostensible behavioral emphasis. Even though there is no section or chapter devoted to behavioral issues per se, there is still a measure of credibility in the acquisition literature for a behavioral explanation of language and, even more, for a behavioral tactic in intervention. It appears especially in studies regarding generalization, incidental teaching, teaching functional language, transactional assessment, and mand modeling.

Possibly, too, the current emphasis on usage contexts will emphasize further the contingent variables, including those expressed as semantic, role, register, or pragmatic counterfactuals (see Dore, 1986). As we attempt to address the social variables in communicative contexts, however, we may need a substantially more elaborated paradigm, one that is a combination of cognitive and behavioral theories. However, that might not surprise those who read Staats's (1974) prediction of a rapprochement between the two domains.

## INTERVENTION SHIFTS

Language intervention as an organized professional field has existed for only two decades, but children have been learning and using functional language for at least 40 thousand years (see Sameroff & Fiese, Chapter 1 of this volume). We are probably safe in estimating that mankind has had spoken languages for as long as tribal members have had something to convey to each other that could not be communicated by signs and other visual and auditory cues. Language emerged as a means for conveying information among and between members of tribal groups that had settled into increasingly stable relationships requiring codified information. Such information enabled the groups to establish rules, denote customs, and carry out agreements.

We know very little about how primitive languages were learned or taught. However, we do have ethnographic studies of primitive cultures that exist today or have existed in recent times (Schieffelin & Eisenberg, 1984). Well-formed languages that have a grammar, both in spoken and written form, and a designated cultural lexicon are limited to the last few thousand years. In light of man's history, then, refined, complete languages have existed for a relatively brief time. Nevertheless, languages have been learned in culturally organized environments by natural means far longer than our historical records reveal. Such learning took place long before academic language analyses were made and before linguistic theories emerged.

What is significant about recent language studies is that we can describe the lawful features of languages so that we can determine what constitutes a language, how languages are used, and how a language is possibly learned. A key question (in our curiosity about how languages are learned) might be, "How can we teach a language to a child who does not learn it in the natural social contexts of the home and cultural environment?"

There are several complicating features of this language intervention question. One feature is that the effort takes us out of (and perhaps beyond) the anthropological progressions human languages have achieved. There are several other ways to express this aspect of human language. For instance, if a child with a disability does not learn a language in the manner that children normally learn, then what makes us—whether we are psycholinguists, speech/language pathologists, or logopaedists—think we can design a training procedure that will result in the desired learning?

There can be no way to answer this question unless we know a great deal about the child who does not learn the language and the environment in which the child does not learn it. Also, there must be procedures to gain information about both. And we must make some theoretical assumptions about how language is learned and how we might facilitate learning for children who seem not to flourish in "natural" environments.

Under conditions of family and community life, most children learn a complete language. However, a significant number do not. The study of these children led to the field of speech and language pathology and the practice of language intervention. Both the 1974 and the 1988 *Language Perspectives* books are part of a search for the premises and the basic issues that characterize this work. Premises can also be called theories, intervention models, or simply approaches. In any event, we are seeking to formulate an organizing frame of reference for guiding our efforts. These assumptions must pertain to what we teach (the language) and how to teach (the training methods). These *what* and *how* questions must be adapted to fit the children to *whom* they apply. In addition, we must ask *why* the language is needed and used and *where* and *with whom*. These obvious questions lead to a comprehensive view of language as a functional part of the life experiences of children. Consequently, language cannot be simply an abstract system of rules, and the child cannot be a standard acquisition agent plugged into either an informal or formal training program.

The most logical generalization might be the following: If children have significant developmental disabilities, perhaps the environmental conditions that are adequate for most children will not work effectively for them. In other words, multiply handicapped children may fail to interact with their environments the way normal children do and for this reason may have drastically altered learning experiences. The challenge the interventionist faces is to create a prosthetic environment that works for the developmentally delayed child somewhat as a "natural" environment works for a "normal" child.

This possibility has led to several approaches to environmental designing. However, intervention procedures are not limited to the alterations of environmental variables. There are other strategies to consider, such as when to intervene, why to intervene, and how to intervene (transact) with the language delayed child.

During the past 14 years of language intervention experiences, several strategies have emerged. Principal among them are (a) early strategies (Schiefelbusch & Bricker, 1981), (b) augmentation strategies (Schiefelbusch, 1980), (c) pragmatic strategies (Schiefelbusch, 1986; Schiefelbusch & Pickar, 1984), and (d) generalization strategies (Kaiser & Warren, Chapter 16 of this volume; Warren & Rogers-Warren, 1985). In addition, there have been other major changes in the issues that preoccupy language interventionists. In 1974 they were concerned about teaching syntax and semantic functions, about the relationships of receptive and expressive abilities, about formal programs of language instruction, about infant perception abilities, and about stages of language acquisition. Currently, we are additionally preoccupied with pragmatic functions and contextual variables, generalization, natural environments and functional language, mother-infant transactions and prelinguistic communication, intentions, communicative competence, and topics of conversation.

The major shifts seem to be from language structure and formal language training to functional language and training language in the natural environment. Also, we have moved from preoccupying concerns with individual language users to transactional variables. Finally, we seem to have moved from a preoccupation with standard language issues to concern with individualized language variables affecting communication.

As we have shifted from our earlier preoccupations, however, we have not abandoned them but have simply shifted the emphasis to the impact of language on peoples' living environments. While this shift has had an important impact on research designs, data formats, and theoretical explanations, the impact on intervention strategies has been extraordinary.

The reasons for the environmental shift have been many. Included among these reasons are the findings of Hymes (1964, 1971), Slobin (1967), Gordon and Ervin-Tripp (1984), and many other sociolinguists, ethnographers, and psycholinguists. These scientists have concluded that formal rules of grammar simply do not explain all the performance features emitted by language users in various contexts and that a much broader knowledge of language competence must be accounted for. Also included among the reasons for the emphasis on environment are the observations of Stokes and Baer (1977) that formally taught language often does not generalize beyond the instructional setting and that recently acquired language often does not appear to serve a functional purpose for the learner. These issues are highly relevant to the substantive and theoretical shifts presented in this introduction.

## REFERENCES

Dore, J. (1986). The development of conversational competence. In R. L. Schiefelbusch (Ed.), *Language competence: Assessment and intervention* (pp. 3–60). San Diego: College-Hill Press.

Gordon, D., & Ervin-Tripp, S. (1984). The structure of children's requests. In R. L. Schiefelbusch & J. Pickar (Eds.), *The acquisition of communicative competence* (pp. 295–321). Austin, TX: PRO-ED.

Hymes, D. (1964). Formal discussion. In U. Bellugi & R. Brown (Eds.), *The acquisition of language*. Monograph Social Research Child Development *29* (1, Serial No. 92).

Hymes, D. (1971). Competence and performance in linguistic theory. In R. Huxley & E. Ingram (Eds.), *Language acquisition: Models and methods* (pp. 3–24). New York: Academic Press.

Schiefelbusch, R. L. (Ed.). (1980). *Nonspeech language and communication: Analysis and intervention*. Austin, TX: PRO-ED.

Schiefelbusch, R. L. (1986). *Language competence: Assessment and intervention*. San Diego: College-Hill Press.

Schiefelbusch, R. L., & Bricker, D. D. (1981). *Early language: Acquisition and intervention*. Austin, TX: PRO-ED

Schiefelbusch, R. L., & Pickar, J. (1984). *The acquisition of communicative competence*. Austin, TX: PRO-ED.

Schieffelin, B., & Eisenberg, A. (1984). Cultural variation in children's conversations. In R. L. Schiefelbusch & J. Pickar (Eds.), *The acquisition of communicative competence* (pp. 377–420). Austin, TX: PRO-ED

Slobin, D. (1967). *A field manual for the cross-cultural study of the acquisition of communicative competence*. Berkeley, CA: ASUC Bookstore.

Staats, A. W. (1974). Behaviorism and cognitive theory in study of language: A neopsycholinguistics. In R. L. Schiefelbusch & L. L. Lloyd (Eds.), *Language perspectives—Acquisition, retardation, and intervention* (pp. 615–646). Austin, TX: PRO-ED.

Stokes, T. F., & Baer, D. M. (1977). An implicit technology of generalization. *Journal of Applied Behavior Analysis, 10*, 349–367.

Warren, S., & Rogers-Warren, A. (1985). *Teaching functional language*. Austin, TX: PRO-ED.

SECTION I

# *Early Developmental Issues*

RICHARD L. SCHIEFELBUSCH, EDITOR

# 1

# *The Context of Language Development*

ARNOLD J. SAMEROFF AND
BARBARA HARRIS FIESE

Language has been seen as the most human of human characteristics. The ability to communicate complex ideas through an organized system of meanings supports not only everyday social interchanges but may play a major role in the cognitive development of each human individual. Despite the logical complexity of adult linguistic skills, "Language is learned, in the normal course of events, by children bright and dull, pampered or neglected, exposed to Tlingit or to English" (Gleitman & Wanner, 1982). In fact, one of the major figures in linguistic theory was led to the conclusion that language acquisition is one of the greatest intellectual feats a human is asked to perform (Bloomfield, 1933). Exactly how difficult this task is has become a source of debate. The universality of its appearance in humans has led to a view that it may emerge rather than be acquired. The linguistic "revolution" of the last few decades was based on the nativist view that human infants are born with the biological capacities to learn natural languages (Chomsky, 1965).

The purpose of this chapter is not to resolve whether language is learned or emerges, nor even to assume an interactionist position devoted to determining what proportion of language acquisition can be attributed to biological or environmental determinants. The purpose is rather to place language acquisition in a developmental context where performance is viewed as the outcome of a biological organism interacting with a human

---

Preparation of this chapter was supported in part by a MacArthur Foundation Fellowship while the senior author was a Fellow at the Center for Advanced Study in the Behavioral Sciences at the University of Illinois at Chicago.

social environment. In such a view there is no separation between child and context (Sameroff, 1983). Without the society of other humans there would be no language, and without the unique biological and cognitive characteristics of human beings there would be no language.

One of the more exciting research issues in recent times has been the debate over whether language acquisition is uniquely human. A series of attempts to teach language to other primates has met with varying degrees of success (Gardner & Gardner, 1980; Premack, 1971; Savage-Rumbaugh & Rumbaugh, 1980). Maratsos (1983) concluded that if language is defined as the ability to use signs to communicate meanings, then it seems clear that apes can learn language. On the other hand, if language is defined as containing the complex grammatical structure that characterizes human speech, then demonstrations of ape language have not been successful (Terrace, Pettito, Sanders, & Bever, 1979). Although the easiest conclusion from such data is that apes do not have the *biological* requisites for language acquisition, an equally compelling argument could be made that apes do not have the *social* requisites for language acquisition. In this view the social organization of meanings in ape cultures does not support the complexity of communication found in human cultures. For example, Savage-Rumbaugh, Rumbaugh, and Boysen (1980) observed that apes in language studies do not engage in the turn taking that is characteristic of the interindividual behavioral regulation of human language. Further evidence for this position would be found in an analysis of the evolution of human language in relation to the evolution of human society.

The study of biological evolution is made quite difficult by the spotty historical record. The study of behavioral evolution is many times more difficult, because it can only be inferred from the discovery of human artifacts. In the case of language, the only clear evidence would be from the existence of written records. This lower bound would place the clear existence of language at only 5,000 years ago. If language were thought to be inherent in human biology, then the upper bound would be over 2 million years ago with the evolution of Neanderthal man. Yet there is precious little archeological evidence for even simple cultures or technologies up until around 40,000 years ago. To a historically distant observer it appears that for the longest period of human existence there just wasn't that much to talk about. The need for the complexities of what we call language arose in the context of communicating over technological or social advances, such as how to chip a flint stone or plant some grain seed. Jaynes (1976) argues that before such advances can be identified in the archeological record, there is no reason to assume that humans had communication needs of sufficient complexity to require a language. Jaynes raises the question as to how, in the absence of language, early man communicated. His answer is very simple. Early man lived and communicated much like current apes do, with an abundance of visual and vocal signals that are very different from syntactically organized language.

The comparative and evolutionary evidence for the connection between being a human and having acquired language is still far from satisfactory. It is clear that humans raised in current societies acquire language. It is not clear whether this is a unique circumstance based on being human or a fortuitous one emerging from a combination of human social and biological evolution.

Although we have argued that the nature/nurture debate is not the most fruitful approach to understanding language acquisition, much of the field does not share this view (see Maratsos, 1983, or Wanner & Gleitman, 1982). Despite over 400 years of scholarly research, the nature/nurture issue remains central in discussing language development. Crudely, two perspectives predominate in the current literature. One perspective focuses on the formal linguistic aspects of language development. By this we mean an emphasis on the acquisition of grammatical structures. The linguistic approach presupposes a significant innate contribution to language development. The second major perspective is the communication view. By this we mean an emphasis on the communicative interchange characteristic of language development. The communication approach presupposes that early nonlinguistic social interactions are significant contributors to language development. These two views differ in the sources of their evidence and the role they assign to the learner.

## ORIGINS OF LANGUAGE UNIVERSALS

Universals are considered a central component of any theory of language development. Those who propose that innate characteristics make a significant contribution to language development often base their argument on the universal characteristics of language. All normal children learn language, therefore it is universal, therefore it must be innate. The ubiquitous development of noun and verb phrases across languages is proposed as evidence that the structure of language itself is innate. The arguments run from innate general tendencies such as tendencies to process and organize linguistic material in a given manner (Roeper, 1982) to innate structural characteristics such as unique characteristics of the brain or at least of the human organism that allow for language development. Universal rules are also proposed that are assumed to reflect the innate organizational features of language development (Roeper, 1982). In this view the systematic aspect of rule governed speech across languages is considered evidence for innate contributions to language development.

The characteristic of universality in itself need not presuppose that language is innate. There are also social universals. Those who emphasize the communicative features of language development also accept a set of universal characteristics. At least two people are considered necessary for language to develop. There must be both a sender and a receiver for communication to continue. This holds true across all languages and all levels of language development. Rules must be accepted by the speaker and listener in regard to turn taking, topic switches, and even grammatical structures such as familiar versus formal address systems. Typically, when one of these universal characteristics is violated, the nature of language and communication is altered.

Universality in itself is not an indication of unique innate characteristics. Shatz (1983) has pointed out that oath taking involves a system of turn taking but that this form of turn taking bears little communicative similarity to natural conversations, although linguistically the structure may be similar. Other social rituals and conversational characteristics are also universal, yet they are rarely explained as the result of innate operations.

Even if a unique innate contribution is required for language acquisition, it could occur at a number of different levels (Maratsos, 1983). Strong arguments for innateness include the unfolding of a genetic blueprint specific to language (Caplan & Chomsky, 1980). Weak arguments rely on smaller contributions by emphasizing an innate processing ability rather than the existence of a specific linguistic structure (Roeper, 1982). Similarly, social interaction in itself does not address the relative contributions of other systems such as cognitive and biological regulators. Reliance on single contributors even at the level of universals does not explain the course of language development or the context in which it occurs. Indeed, universality may be a reflection of the common ease by which certain features are acquired in different languages rather than a common set of linguistic patterns believed to be structurally innate (Slobin, 1982).

For our current purposes the context of language development may be broken into the assumed properties of the learner, the properties of language as a system, and the context in which the interaction between learner and language is regulated. In this context the systems of language and learner form a mature system of language use and production. The assumptions underlying each property as proposed by the linguistic and communication approaches are briefly reviewed below.

## Nature of the Learner

The properties of the language learner are assumed to be different according to each theoretical position. According to the linguistic approach, the goal of learners is to become competent grammarians. The learner must ultimately master the rules of generative grammar which are considered universal (Chomsky, 1968). The learners are motivated to attain the adult form of language representation. The end result of successful language learning is measured by the production of grammatically mature responses. Frequently, the fact that only humans develop mature forms of language is taken as evidence that there are innate contributors to the structural characteristics of language. This viewpoint is particularly evident in "learnability" theories that emphasize adult representation as a central principle to be explained (Wexler & Culicover, 1980). Language has been "learned" when it is equivalent to the adult forms of language.

An important part of this view is that learners (i.e., young children) are assumed to have a limited cognitive capacity. Because this limitation is viewed as a constraint on the system, a more powerful force must be assumed to be guiding the movement toward linguistic maturity. This force acts outside the system of normal cognitive development. The acquisition procedure itself is considered innate. A process of inductive reasoning is used to solve the task of language learning (Chomsky, 1975). Mistakes in production are taken as evidence that the learners are linguistically immature and have not yet mastered the rules of mature organisms. The structure for the rules is given in the underlying structure of the organism. However, the expression of the rules must wait for linguistic maturity.

Developmentally, little emphasis is put on contributions of linguistic acquisition mechanisms prior to the occurrence of at least single-word speech. The generation of rule-guided speech focusing on rules of combination and order is not evidenced until at least the level of two-word utterances. The system of rules includes how the individual word units are combined to form meaningful and grammatically acceptable phrases and sentences. It is only when words are produced by learners that the rules of acquisition can be applied.

The communication approach considers the child to be motivated by a need to be understood. The child's goal is to become a competent transmitter, which subsumes the more specific aspect of becoming a competent grammarian. The system relies on rules that are generated out of social interaction and the need to maintain contact and shared understanding. The structure of communication, then, is inherent in the system of early interaction. Language development is seen as a channel by which patterns of living are transmitted (Halliday, 1975). Rather than viewing language as a uniquely human achievement, phylogenetic differences are viewed in terms of the significant contribution of specific nonlinguistic skills such as imitation and tool use (Bates, 1979). The argument that only humans develop true language does not necessarily indicate a strong innate feature of language development. It is the development of certain nonlinguistic skills that is considered part of the process leading to universal human language achievement.

The limited capacity of the learner is not taken as evidence of innate structural contributions but is seen as a contributor to the behavior of the receiver. The way in which mothers talk to their young infants ("motherese") may be seen as an attempt by the mother to find ways to be "understood" or at least to maintain contact with her immature communication partner. Motherese may be seen as an indication of communication failure on the part of the speaker in order to be understood by an immature listener (Bates, Bretherton, Beeghly-Smith, & McNew, 1982). Even young preschool children will adapt their language behavior to immature listeners. Systematic efforts to adjust conversation are guided by the goal of understanding (Shatz & Gelman, 1973). The limited capacity of the learners is seen as a feature that regulates early interaction.

A goal of communication is considered to be sharing attention to some common occurrence. This may include a wide range of everyday events such as attention to the infant's smile, a colorful mobile, or the sound of a barking animal. Constraints operate on the level of shared attention and reference, with the more competent communicator providing a scaffold for the less mature communicator (Bruner, 1975). The mother then "fills in the gaps" to aid in the goal of her infant being able to understand. Early interaction prior to speech production is seen as a significant contributor to laying the foundation for later communication. The interaction acts as a way to fine-tune the system toward more mature forms of communication (Newport, Gleitman, & Gleitman, 1977). The infant's initial reaching behavior may develop into pointing for a desired toy. Nonverbal behaviors such as pointing and reaching are seen as significant precursors to linguistic requests. Communication becomes more ritualized resulting in an economy of the signal. The child is becoming a more effective communicator when he or she can use a shared symbol such as pointing or saying "want" rather than using arm waving as an all-around request behavior. The development of economy of the signal and shared symbols makes it easier for the listener to understand the speaker. Random gestures develop into synchronous gestural intentions that have a systematic effect on the listener (Bates, Camaioni, & Volterra, 1975).

In this view language is learned through a deductive reasoning process that maps nonlinguistic features onto linguistic structures. These early nonlinguistic interactions include requesting, demonstrating, and turn taking, which are seen as the foundation for similar properties of linguistic production. Even errors in production are seen as reflections of systematic reorganizations that occur in accord with developmental and cognitive changes (Bowerman, 1982). The active construction of rules is reflected in linguistically immature responses.

## Nature of Language

Both the linguistic and the communication approaches view the system of language as rule-governed. The level at which these rules operate and the type of system that they regulate are different. For the linguistic approach, the rules of grammar are seen as separate from the rules of meaning (Chomsky, 1968). The system is hierarchically organized based on generated rules of grammar. Rules must account for the systematic relationship between underlying base structures and observable surface structures. The rules themselves or the structures in which they operate may not be directly observable but must be induced in principle (Wexler, 1982). The rules must ultimately explain how only grammatical sentences are generated. Rules must conform to grammatical boundaries such as tense, combination order, and phrase agreement.

The communication approach views organization on the level of social interaction. Rules of turn taking, reversals, and topic comment are emphasized. The rules are generated from a perceived structural similarity between early social interaction and later linguistic development (Bruner, 1978). It is not only on the level of grammatical structures that rules operate, but also the illocutionary force or intention of the speaker (Searle, 1969). The intention behind the utterance is just as important as the grammatical structure. For example, one might say, "Is anyone else cold?" not looking for a weather report but actually intending for someone to close the window. Whether the speaker is understood in part determines the successful use of these rules.

While the radical behaviorist view that language development is caused by feedback in the form of reinforcement of correct utterances has been generally disproved, there is much more evidence that the system is regulated by feedback for truth (Maratsos, 1983). Parents correct young children according to the semantic accuracy of their statements much more than the grammatical uracy. The signs and the users are systematically related (Morris, 1946). Utterances are adjusted according to whether they are understood and according to the social dictates of the situation. Meaning plays an important role in distinguishing meaning as an object and meaning as an act. Meaning is more crucial in regulating the system than a match of grammatical forms. The unit of analysis is action and effect rather than individual words and phrases. The development of rule systems can be directly observed through reorganizational principles in studying production errors (Bowerman, 1982). A hierarchy is evident here in which the rules may rely on meaning and context of use (Blewitt, 1982).

## Context of Language Development

The ways in which information is received by the learner differ according to theoretical perspective. Those who emphasize the linguistic aspects of language development and consider innate contributions as significant consider the input to the learner as variable and chaotic. To minimize the effects of this chaos, the system of the learner must have some built-in constraints so that there is some order in an otherwise unpredictable situation. These constraints are considered structural characteristics in the organism that allow for the regulated development of grammatical forms. The environment is seen as providing too limited a base for such complex functions to develop (Bowerman, 1982).

Those who focus on the communicative aspects of language view input as systematically regulated rather than chaotic. The context provides meaningful support for the immature learner. The social environment minimizes the demands on the child by providing a structure to facilitate the learning process (Snow, 1977). Meaning is considered central, and there are several ways to solve the problem of being understood. The output is regulated by understanding rather than grammatical correctness.

When addressing the issue of the context of language development, the two major perspectives presented in this chapter rely heavily on their own theoretical assumptions concerning the nature of the learner and the nature of the system of language. A view that addresses the concerns of both perspectives but in a complementary fashion would interpret the linguistic environment as far from the chaos assumed by the linguistic perspective but would also argue for a contribution from the mental organization of the child.

The synthesis requires looking at both child and context in dynamic rather than static terms. If the language productions that the child hears are interpreted statically, they can easily appear to be chaotic and unorganized. However, when they are embedded in the flow of activity that characterizes human social interaction, they take on clear meanings. On the child's side, when behavior is examined for specific language acquisition mechanisms, they are difficult to identify. However, when the child's activity is viewed dynamically as a solution to a series of increasingly more complex cognitive tasks, then it is clear that the child develops specific skills to solve successively more complex problems. Although adult speech may contain far more linguistic information than the child is able to understand, the total context in which the speech is embedded is generally adapted to a level where the child is capable of understanding the communicative intent.

There is a mutual dynamic regulation of the child's capacities to understand and the experiences that are presented to be understood. A good example of how this relationship is conceptualized can be found in the discussions of the "zone of proximal development" by Vygotsky (1978) and his interpreters (Rogoff & Wertsch, 1984). This zone is defined as the difference between the developmental level of the child when independently engaged in problem solving and the level demonstrated when guided by adults or in collaboration with more capable peers. The concept of the zone implies a social pacing in the presentation of problems that children need to solve on the road to adulthood. The initiative remains with the child, but the direction of that initiative is channeled by the context.

The zone of proximal development concept has been most frequently used in analyzing the effects of educational efforts (Griffin & Cole, 1984), but it easily can be related to the task of language acquisition. Understanding the complexity of adult linguistic behavior is one of the problems for children to solve. In this view the presentation of language is embedded in a larger socialization scheme that needs to be identified. The source of this scheme is in the regulatory code for each society. Before examining such social regulatory functions, we need to examine the general issue of developmental regulation.

## A BIOLOGICAL MODEL OF DEVELOPMENT

At the outset we defined our task as placing language acquisition in a developmental context that transcended any debate over the relative contributions of nature and nurture. We have described two perspectives that search for either innate or experiential roots of language performance. To fully appreciate the need for an inclusive model, we need to examine how other developmental systems are organized in both the biological and behavioral domains.

All development seems to follow a similar biological model. In this biological model outcomes are never a function of either the individual taken alone or the experiential context taken alone. Outcomes are a product of the combination of an individual and his or her experience. To predict outcome, a singular focus on the characteristics of the individual—in this case, the child—or the context will frequently be misleading. What needs to be added is an analysis and assessment of the experiences available to the child and the capacities of the child to interpret these experiences.

A view of development that included both the child and the child's experiences was suggested by Sameroff and Chandler (1975). Within this "transactional model" the development of the child was seen as a product of the continuous dynamic interactions of the child and the experience provided by his or her family and social context. What was innovative in the transactional model was the equal emphasis placed on the effect of the child on the environment, so that the experiences provided by the environment were not independent of the child. The child by his or her previous behavior may have been a strong determinant of current experiences. For example, a complicated childbirth may have made an otherwise calm mother somewhat anxious. The mother's anxiety during the first months of the child's life may have caused her to be uncertain and inappropriate in her interactions with the child. In response to such inconsistency, the infant may have developed some irregularities in feeding and sleeping patterns that give the appearance of a difficult temperament. This difficult temperament decreased the pleasure that the mother obtained, so that she spent less time with the child. By interacting less with the child, and especially by speaking less, the mother may be diminishing the child's chances of developing the language skills necessary to pass preschool language tests.

In the preceding example the outcome was not determined by the complicated birth nor by the mother's consequent emotional response. If one needed to pick a cause it would be the mother's avoidance of the child, yet one can see that such a view would be a gross oversimplification of a complex developmental sequence. The important proximal cause of the language delay, avoidance of the child by the mother, can be multiply determined in a single child and determined by many different factors in different children. This conclusion is supported in Decarie's (1969) study of thalidomide children with severe limb deformation. She found a higher correlation between language performance and the degree to which parents interacted with their child than the degree of the handicap.

The transactional model is not a new model, it is merely a new emphasis on some very old traditions in developmental theory, especially theories of the dialectic in history and philosophy (Sameroff & Harris, 1979). A more cogent empirical referent is in biological research, where transactions are a recognized essential part of any developmental process. In the study of embryological development, for example, there are continuous transactions between the phenotype and the genotype (Ebert & Sussex, 1970; Waddington, 1957). A simple view of the action of genes is that they produce the parts that make up the organism. A brown eye gene may be thought to produce a brown eye. In reality there is a much more complex process of mutual determinism. The material in the fertilized egg cell will turn on or off specific genes in the chromosomes. The turned-on genes will initiate changes in the biochemicals in the cell. These changed biochemicals will then act back on the genetic material, turning on or off more genes in a continuous process usually producing an adult organism.

In certain circumstances, as in the case of eye color, there is an illusion of a linear relationship between a particular gene and a particular feature of the phenotype. In reality, however, there is never a linear determinism because of the complexity of biological processes. What then creates the illusion of causality? The answer is in the regulatory system that buffers development, what Waddington (1957) described as canalization. Within all the complex interactions between genotype and phenotype is a regulatory system that monitors developmental changes to assure that they stay within defined bounds. This regulatory system and the bounds are the result of an evolutionary process that occurred across myriad generations and now assures a particular outcome.

With eye color the regulatory system is hidden because it is so tightly buffered, that is, regulated. If one knows the structural genes, one can predict the outcome. However, there are some simple examples where the regulatory system is quite evident. In the case of identical twins, a single fertilized cell splits in two. Shouldn't the result be two half-sized children? The genetic regulatory system ensures that this is not the outcome. Compensations are made so that the resulting infants will all be of normal size. In the case of genetic dominance, the result for a homozygous individual is the same as for a heterozygous one. If there are two brown eye genes, the eyes are no browner than if there were only one. A regulation has occurred.

A more complex example is the result of the translocation in Down syndrome. In the meiotic process of forming a germ cell, there is a breakage in a chromosome that results in one of the germ cells having too much genetic material and the other having too little. In the cell with too much, the Trisomy 21 condition, regulations can occur that compensate for much of the anomalous genetic condition. A child is born that looks much like other human infants. In the case of the germ cell in which there is too little, regulation fails and the zygote is aborted. From another perspective regulation succeeded in the aborted cell and failed in the trisomy cell, but that issue will not be dealt with in this presentation.

## CULTURAL CODES AS REGULATORY SYSTEMS

In a moment we will begin to apply these notions of biological regulation to the problem of understanding psychological development, but first we must deal with the issue of discontinuity. If indeed there were no discontinuities in development, there would be no need to attend to context. The analysis of behavioral development would be restricted to the understanding and manipulation of gene action. The transactional model shows that such is not the case. The development of life, and particularly human life, is filled with transitions. In these transitions, the previous state of the child contributes to, but does not determine, the new state because many other factors may be involved. For example, if one were to make developmental predictions from newborn condition based on a model of continuity, one would argue that normal infants should have the best outcomes, infants with birth complications should have less positive outcomes, and children born with handicaps should have deviant outcomes. These predictions would be correct if one were restricting the definition of outcome to physical condition, especially in the case of handicapped infants. If a child is born blind, deaf, or with cerebral palsy, the child will continue to be blind, deaf, or motorically impaired. But if one is predicting psychological outcomes, the situation is quite different. Infants from any of these categories can end up quite normal or quite deviant in intelligence and mental health (Sameroff, 1975). There is a discontinuity between biological and psychological functioning. To understand biological development, one must understand the workings of the biological regulatory systems. To understand psychological development, one must understand the workings of another regulatory system, the psychological one.

Just as there is a biological system, the genetic code, that regulates the physical outcome of each individual, there is a behavioral system, the cultural code, that regulates the way human beings fit into society. This cultural code guides cognitive and social-emotional development so that individuals will be able to fill social roles defined by that society.

The genetic code has two properties that permit it to maintain its superordinate biological regulatory role: It is transmitted as an organized system through time from one individual to another, and it is not affected by the individual action of those who carry it. The cultural code has the same two properties: It also is transmitted through time as an organized system from one individual to another (Berger & Luckmann, 1966), and it is not affected by the individual action of those who carry it.

The importance of identifying the sources of regulation of human development is obvious if one is interested in manipulating that development, as in the case of child rearing or educational programs. The failures of such efforts can only be understood in terms of a failure to understand the regulatory system.

The cultural code can be broken down into sets of regulatory functions that operate across different magnitudes of time. The longest cycle is associated with the *macroregulations* that are a culture's "developmental agenda." The developmental agenda is a series of points in time when the environment is restructured to provide different experiences to the child. Age of weaning, toilet training, schooling, initiation rites, and marriage are coded differently in each culture but provide the basis for socialization in each culture. The validity of such agendas is not in their details but in the fact that the culture is successfully reproduced in generation after generation of offspring. These macroregulations are known to each member of the culture.

On a shorter time base are *miniregulations,* which refer to the caregiving activities of the child's family. Examples of such activities are feeding children when they awaken, changing diapers when they are wet, and keeping children warm. Both mini- and macroregulations are known to educated members of society and can be transmitted from member to member.

On the shortest time base are *microregulations,* which refer to the momentary interactions between child and caregiver that others have called "behavioral synchrony" or "attunement" (Field, 1979; Stern, 1977). Microregulations are a blend between the cultural and biological codes, because many of these activities appear naturally and even without awareness. These include the caregiver's smiling responses to an infant's smile or the putative matching of vocal and movement patterns between caregiver and child (Condon & Sander, 1974).

Although the cultural code can be conceptualized independent of the child, changes in the abilities of the child are major triggers for regulatory changes and in most likelihood were major contributors to the evolution of the code. In most cultures formal education begins between the ages of 6 and 8 (Rogoff, 1981), when most children have acquired the cognitive ability to learn from such formalized experiences. On the other hand, informal education can begin at many different ages depending on the culture's attributions to the child. For example, the Digo and Kikuyu are two East African cultures that have different beliefs about infant capacities (deVries & Sameroff, 1984). The Digo believe that infants can learn within a few months after birth and begin socialization at that time. The Kikuyu wait until the second year of life before they begin serious education.

## CHANGING SOCIAL REGULATIONS

The concept of a cultural code that regulates child development can be combined with the transactional model to provide a framework for understanding intervention efforts. The case of phenylketonuria (PKU) is a good example. A child is born with a biological deficit, an inability to metabolize phenylalanine. The biological deficit is thought to produce mental retardation. However, it is not the genetic problem that produces the deficit; rather, it is the deficit plus a diet that contains phenylalanine. The retardation is an interactional effect of the child and his or her experience. The normative experience in this case will produce mental retardation. However, if a different experience occurs, if a diet is provided that is phenylalanine-free, retardation would not be an outcome. What is necessary is a transaction—the child must affect the environment so that the different diet is provided. This is now possible through the evolution of the medical system. There is now a test that is given to most babies for the diagnosis of PKU. If the test results are positive, a transaction occurs in which the behavior of the environment is changed by the behavior of the child; the diet is changed. The outcome of this transactional system is that the child does not become mentally retarded.

A similar analysis can be applied to the relation between deafness and language delay. Deafness by itself does not produce language delay. If a child is born totally deaf and the only experience he or she gets is vocal language, then there will be a major retardation in the development of language. If, on the other hand, there is a transactional regulation, this result need not be the case. If the infant is tested at birth and the deafness recognized, then a different experience can be planned (e.g., the use of sign language). Deaf children who are trained in sign language need not become language delayed.

The caregiving environment in every culture has evolved to provide normative experiences for the normative child. Should a child be born that does not fit the normative pattern, then new regulations must be made to restore the child to the appropriate developmental path. The activation of these new regulations requires transactions where the environment is sensitive to critical individual differences in the children raised in that environment.

In the above examples society found a way to adapt the cultural code to deal with a broader range of child conditions to change the context of development. How are we to interpret developmental disabilities that persist over time? The initial response is usually to attribute the disabilities to biological conditions that prevent normal development. The above analysis of context effects suggests another explanation. If developmental disabilities persist over time, it is because the regulatory mechanisms are inadequate, not because the child is inadequate. The regulatory mechanisms at fault may be biological ones, but they also may be cultural ones. Until the regulation of each developmental achievement is understood, the source of the failure to reach that achievement cannot be understood.

Another example using Down syndrome may illustrate this point. Children with this disorder are delayed in development and hardly ever attain normal adult language functioning. Is this deficit in language performance part of the biological syndrome or a deficit in cultural regulation? Nonhandicapped infants go through a stage of word play in the first and second years of life that consists of much babbling and is considered an important precursor to later language behavior. It is also considered to be cute behavior and stimulates much adult-child vocal interaction. Blank (1975) observed that Down syndrome children go through this stage during the third through fifth years of life. During this period babbling is considered socially inappropriate and generally discouraged by parents of delayed children, because it is seen as a sign of deviance rather than a normal stage in language acquisition.

## OVERVIEW

The conclusions of this discussion are not simple. Developmental achievements are the complex product of a specific kind of individual in a specific kind of context. Human achievements are the product of a human child growing in a human context. The outcome cannot be determined by an examination of the characteristics of either the child or the context alone (Rogoff, 1982). What has been described for development in general must also be true for specific developmental achievements such as the acquisition of language. Whatever accomplishments or disabilities are found in this domain will be the result of a particular child growing in a particular context, never a characteristic of the child or the context alone. Understanding of that achievement will require a dynamic analysis of the child in context—of the mutual interplay of the developing abilities of the child and the developmental agenda that society fits to those abilities.

## REFERENCES

Bates, E. (1979). The emergence of symbols: Ontogeny and phylogeny. In W. A. Collins (Ed.), *Children's language and communication. Minnesota Symposia on Child Psychology* (Vol. 12, pp, 121–155). Hillsdale, NJ: Lawrence Erlbaum.

Bates, E., Bretherton, I., Beeghly-Smith, M., & McNew, S. (1982). Social bases of language development: A reassessment. In H. W. Reese & L. P. Lipsitt (Eds.), *Advances in child development and behavior* (Vol. 16). New York: Academic Press.

Bates, E., Camaioni, L. & Volterra, V. (1975). The acquisition of performatives prior to speech. *Merrill-Palmer Quarterly, 21,* 205–226.

Berger, P. L., & Luckmann, T. (1966). *The social construction of reality.* Garden City, NY: Doubleday.

Blank, M. (1975). *Perspectives on the acquisition of language*. Paper presented at the biennial meeting of the Society for Research in Child Development, Denver, April.

Blewitt, P. (1982). Word meaning acquisition in young children: A review of theory and research. In H. W. Reese (Ed.), *Advances in child development and behavior* (Vol. 17, pp. 139–195). New York: Academic Press.

Bloomfield, L. (1933). *Language*. New York: Holt.

Bowerman, M. (1982). Reorganizational processes in lexical and syntactic development. In E. Wanner & L. R. Gleitmann (Eds.), *Language acquisition: The state of the art* (pp. 319–346). Cambridge: Cambridge University Press.

Bruner, J. S. (1975). The ontogenesis of speech acts. *Journal of Child Language, 2,* 1–19.

Caplan, D. & Chomsky, N. (1980). Linguistic perspectives on language development. In D. Caplan (Ed.), *Biological studies of mental processes*. Cambridge, MA: MIT Press.

Chomsky, N. (1965). *Aspects of the theory of syntax*. Cambridge, MA: MIT Press.

Chomsky, N. (1968). *Language and mind*. New York: Harcourt Brace Jovanovich.

Chomsky, N. (1975). *Reflections on language*. New York: Random House.

Condon, W. S., & Sander, L. W. (1974). Synchrony demonstrated between movements of the neonate and adult speech. *Child Development*, *45*, 456–462.

Decarie, T. G. (1969). A study of the mental and emotional development of the thalidomide child. In B. M. Foss (Ed.), *Determinants of infant behavior* (Vol. 4). London: Methuen.

deVries, M. W., & Sameroff, A. J. (1984). Culture and temperament: Influences on temperament in three East African societies. *American Journal of Orthopsychiatry*, *54*, 83–96.

Ebert, J. D., & Sussex, I. M. (1970). *Interacting systems in development* (2nd ed.). New York: Holt, Rinehart and Winston.

Field, T. M. (1979). Interaction patterns of preterm and term infants. In T. M. Field (Ed.), *Infants born at risk: Behavior and development* (pp. 332–356) New York: SP Medical and Scientific Books.

Gardner, B. T., & Gardner, R. A. (1980). Two comparative psychologists look at language acquisition. In K. E. Nelson (Ed.), *Children's language* (Vol. 2). New York: Gardner Press.

Gleitmann, L. R., & Wanner, E. (1982). Language acquisition: The state of the state of the art. In E. Wanner & L. R. Gleitmann (Eds.), *Language acquisition: The state of the art* (pp. 3–48). Cambridge: Cambridge University Press.

Griffin, P., & Cole, M. (1984). Current activity for the future. In B. Rogoff & J. P. Wertsch (Eds.) *Children's learning in the "zone of proximal development." New directions for child development* (No. 23., pp. 45–63). San Francisco: Jossey-Bass.

Halliday, M. A. K. (1975). *Learning how to mean: Explorations in the development of language*. London: Arnold.

Jaynes, J. (1976). *The origin of consciousness in the breakdown of the bicameral mind*. Boston: Houghton Mifflin.

Maratsos, M. (1983). Some current issues in the study of acquisition of grammar. In J. H. Flavell & E. H. Markman (Eds.), *Cognitive development* (pp. 707–786). Vol. III of P. H. Mussen (Ed.), Handbook of child development. New York: John Wiley.

Morris, C. (1946). *Signs, language and behavior*. Englewood Cliffs, NJ: Prentice-Hall.

Newport, E. L., Gleitman, H., & Gleitman, L. R. (1977). Mother, I'd rather do it myself: Some effects and non-effects of maternal speech style. In C. E. Snow & C. A. Ferguson (Eds.), *Talking to children: Language input and acquisition*. Cambridge: Cambridge University Press.

Premack, D. (1971). Language in chimpanzee? *Science*, *172*, 802–822.

Roeper, T. (1982). The role of universals in the acquisition of gerunds. In E. Wanner & L. R. Gleitman (Eds), *Language acquisition: The state of the art* (pp. 267–287). Cambridge: Cambridge University Press.

Rogoff, B. (1981). Schooling and the development of cognitive skills. In H. C. Triandis & A. Heron (Eds.), *Handbook of cross-cultural psychology: Developmental psychology* (Vol. 4). Boston: Allyn & Bacon.

Rogoff, B. (1982). Integrating context and cognitive development. In M. E. Lamb & A. L. Brown (Eds.), *Advances in developmental psychology* (Vol. 2, pp. 125–168). Hillsdale, NJ: Lawrence Erlbaum.

Rogoff, B., & Wertsch, J. V. (1984). *Children's learning in the "zone of proximal development." New directions for child development* (No. 23). San Francisco: Jossey-Bass.

Sameroff, A. J. (1975). Early influences on development: Fact or fancy? *Merrill-Palmer Quarterly*, *21*, 267–294.

Sameroff, A. J. (1983). Developmental systems: Contexts and evolution. In W. Kessen (Ed.), *History, theories, and methods* (pp. 237–294). Vol. I of P. H. Mussen (Ed.), Handbook of child psychology. New York: John Wiley.

Sameroff, A. J., & Chandler, M. J. (1975). Reproductive risk and the continuum of caretaking casualty. In F. D. Horowitz, M. Hetherington, S. Scarr-Salapatek, & G. Siegel (Eds.), *Review of child development research* (Vol. 4). Chicago: University of Chicago Press.

Sameroff, A. J., & Harris, A. E. (1979). Dialectical approaches to early thought and language. In M. H. Bornstein & W. Kessen (Eds.), *Psychological development from infancy: Image to intention* (pp. 339–372). Hillsdale, NJ: Lawrence Erlbaum.

Savage-Rumbaugh, E. S., & Rumbaugh, D. (1980). Language analogue project I, phase II: Theory and tactics. In K. E. Nelson (Ed.), *Children's language* (Vol. 2). New York: Gardner Press.

Savage-Rumbaugh, E. S., Rumbaugh, D., & Boysen, S. (1980). Do apes use language? *American Scientist*, 68, 49–61.

Searle, J. R. (1969). *Speech acts*. Cambridge: Cambridge University Press.

Shatz, M. (1983). *Communication*. In J. H. Flavell & E. H. Markman (Eds.), *Cognitive development* (pp. 841–889). Vol. III of P. H. Mussen (Ed.), Handbook of child psychology. New York: John Wiley.

Shatz, M., & Gelman, R. (1973). The development of communication skills: Modifications in the speech of young children as a function of listener. *Monographs of the Society for Research in Child Development*, *38* (5, Serial No. 152).

Slobin, D. I. (1982). Universal and particular in the acquisition of language. In E. Wanner & L. R. Gleitman (Eds.), *Language acquisition: The state of the art* (pp. 128–170). Cambridge: Cambridge University Press.

Snow, C. E. (1977). Mother's speech research: From input to interaction. In C. E. Snow & C. A. Ferguson (Eds.), *Talking to children: Language input and acquisition*. Cambridge: Cambridge University Press.

Stern, D. (1977). *The first relationship: Infant and mother*. Cambridge, MA: Harvard University Press.

Terrace, H. S., Pettito, L. A., Sanders, R. J., & Bever, T. G. (1979). Can an ape create a sentence? *Science*, *206*, 891–900.

Vygotsky, L. S. (1978). *Mind in society: The development of higher psychological processes*. Cambridge, MA: Harvard University Press.

Waddington, C. H. (1957). *The strategy of the genes*. London: Allen & Unwin.

Wanner, E., & Gleitman, L. R. (Eds.). (1982). *Language acquisition: The state of the art*. Cambridge: Cambridge University Press.

Wexler, K. (1982). A principle theory for language acquisition. In E. K. Wexler & P. Culicover, *Formal principles of language acquisition* (pp. 228–315). Cambridge, MA: MIT Press.

Wexler, K., & Culicover, P. (1980). *Formal principles of language acquisition*. Cambridge, MA: MIT Press.

# SECTION II

# *Symbolization and Lexical Development*

STAN A. KUCZAJ II, EDITOR

# 2

# The Symbolic Nature of Words in Young Children

Stan A. Kuczaj II

Regardless of theoretical differences about the nature of language and its acquisition, all scholars concerned with these topics agree that language is a symbolic system, that is, a system in which elements of the system represent other things. Although there are many types of symbols and many difficulties inherent in the study of symbols (as discussed in Chapter 3), there can be no question that language involves symbols and their manipulation. We use the symbols of language to represent real, possible, or imaginary aspects of our universe. Although other types of symbols may be used to represent aspects of our experience, the symbols of language are unique in that they are conventional and arbitrary, yet shared by all normal members of any language community. Although other symbolic systems may be arbitrary and conventional (e.g., mathematics), the prevalence of the symbols of language in human cultures over other arbitrary conventional symbolic systems suggests that the symbolic system of language involves the most basic type of arbitrary conventional symbols.

This introductory chapter is concerned with the symbolic nature of words in young children. Words are certainly symbols—namely, sound patterns that speakers use to represent aspects of their experience, whether individual objects, classes of objects, or hypothetical ideas. The

The original research discussed in this chapter was presented at the Third International Congress for the Study of Child Language in Austin, Texas, July 8–13, 1984. I am grateful to my colleagues for their comments and suggestions about this work at that time.

acquisition of words and their meanings, although not well understood, has been the subject of considerable investigation (see Clark, 1983) in atypical as well as typical populations (as discussed by Leonard in Chapter 4). Rather than review this literature (readers who are interested in such reviews are referred to Kuczaj, 1982a, 1982b, and to a recent treatment by Clark, 1983), I shall consider an aspect of words as symbols in children that has long puzzled me. The ability to distinguish a symbol from that which it signifies would seem to be the most basic prerequisite for the emergence of symbolic activity. For example, the word *dog* and its referents are very different sorts of things. The word *dog* has certain phonetic properties, but lacks all of the properties of dogs—the word *dog* is not furry, does not bark or wag its tail, and is certainly not man's best friend. In fact, those of us who have attempted to study lexical-meaning acquisition have assumed that the meaning of a word is not an inherent part of the word and that children somehow come to attach the correct (or adult) meaning to words. The literature in this area is replete with examples of scholars assuming that, even for very young children, words are symbols that stand for something. Young children may err in what they believe a word represents, but most of us assume that they know (perhaps tacitly) that the word *dog* and the object *dog* are qualitatively different. One refers to the other, but they are not equivalent.

## NOMINAL REALISM

Over one-half century ago, Piaget (1929) suggested that young children do not recognize that words and the objects to which they refer are substantially different. To the contrary, Piaget assumed that young children believe that a word is either an integral part of or the same thing as the object to which it refers. Piaget referred to this misconception on the children's part as *nominal realism*. Other influential theorists of Piaget's era also assumed that young children fail to differentiate words and their referents (Vygotsky, 1962; Werner, 1940). More recently, studies support the notion of nominal realism. Osherson and Markman (1975), Papandropoulou and Sinclair (1974), and Scarlett and Press (1975) all reported data consistent with Piaget's claim that young children fail to distinguish words and referents. The results of this literature may be summarized as follows. First, although young children may agree that the name of an object could be changed, they also believe that changing the name changes properties of the referent object. For example, although a young child might agree that the word *dog* could be changed to *cat*, the child might argue that such a change would result in dogs meowing rather than barking. In the child's view, changing the word results in corresponding alterations in the properties of the referent objects. Second, young children frequently attribute properties of referents to words. For example, when asked about the word *rain*, a child might state that it is wet. Of course, the word *rain* is not wet, but instead refers to certain falling particles in the world that possess the property "wet." Finally, young children believe that the disappearance of a word's referents results in the disappearance of the word.

Nominal realism seems more likely to rear its ugly head in monolingual children than in bilingual children. Bilingual children seem to be more aware of the arbitrary conventional relation of words and referents than monolingual children (Ben-Ze'ev, 1977; Cummins, 1978; Feldman & Shen, 1971; Ianco-Worrall, 1972; Leopold, 1949; Slobin, 1978). In spite of observations that bilingual children do not always best monolingual children in studies of the word-referent relation (Pinker, 1979; Sandoval, 1976; both cited in Rosenblum & Pinker, 1983), the possibility that bilingual children grasp the distinction between words and referents at an earlier age than do their monolingual counterparts suggests that children's initial failure to discriminate words and referents and the later ability to do so is not a function of general cognitive abilities (unless one assumes different general cognitive abilities for bilingual children than for monolingual children). To the contrary, the data from bilingual children suggests that the ability to distinguish a word from its referents is a function of particular types of experience—those involving hearing the same object called by different names. This is something that bilingual children experience to a much greater extent than do monolingual children. The following describes an attempt to provide monolingual children with a miniature multilingual experience in order to assess the significance of such experience for children's ability to distinguish words and objects.

## TESTING FOR THE MULTILINGUAL ADVANTAGE

Eighty monolingual children ranging in age from 3-2 to 6-9 participated in our investigation. There were 20 children (10 males and 10 females) in each of four age groups (3-year-olds, 4-year-olds, 5-year-olds, and 6-year-olds). Each child was tested individually. Initially, children were shown an object (e.g., an airplane) and asked to name the object. They were then asked to pretend that all of the airplanes in the world had disappeared, to consider whether we could still have the word *airplane*, and to justify their response. Following this, children were asked to imagine that nobody in the world ever said the word *airplane*, to consider whether there would still be airplanes in the absence of the word airplane, and to justify their response. This procedure was repeated until each child had responded to questions about six words and their referents.

As shown in Figure 2.1, children of all ages were more likely to agree that objects could exist in the absence of words than to agree that words could exist in the absence of their referents. Nonetheless, both the frequency with which children agreed that words could exist in the absence of their conventional referents and the frequency with which children agreed that referents could exist in the absence of their corresponding words increased with age.

These data provided the basis from which we elected to assess the significance of our miniature multilingual experience. Based on their responses to the questions in the first testing session, the 80 children were divided into two groups—a control group and an experimental group. The two groups had an equal number of males and females, an equal number of children from each age group, and were composed such that the two

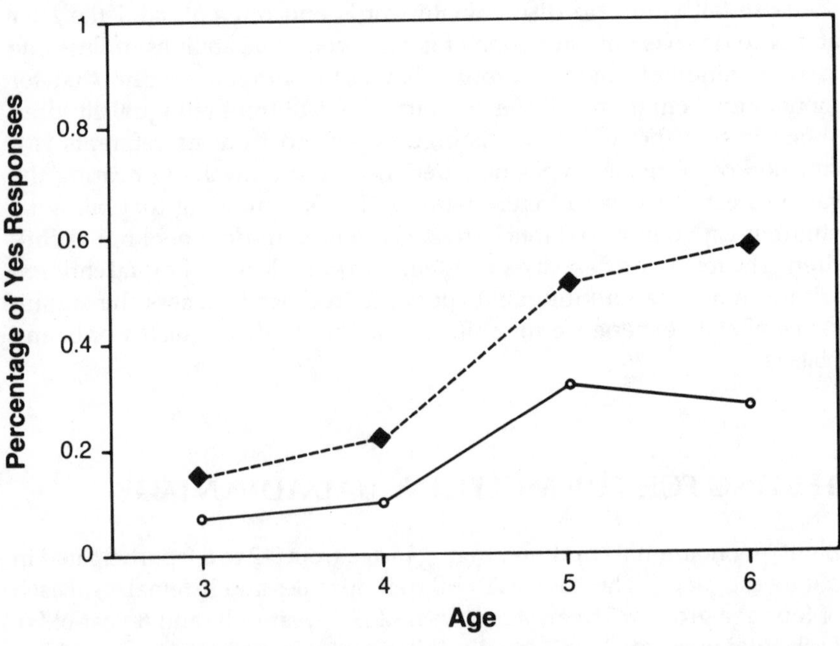


**Figure 2.1.** Percentage of "Yes" responses to questions about whether objects could still exist in the absence of their corresponding words (dashed line) and about whether words could still exist in the absence of their corresponding objects (solid line).

groups were matched as closely as possible in terms of their responses in the first testing session.

The children in the experimental group were introduced to three puppets and told that each puppet spoke a different language. The children were asked to learn the words that each puppet used to refer to a given referent so that they could talk to the puppets using the words that the puppets used. These children were then exposed to three objects (none of which had been used in the first testing session), heard each of the puppets call each object by a different nonsense name, and tried to learn these novel names.

All of the children were subsequently given a task identical to that used in the first testing session, the only difference being the objects that were used. Six objects that had not been used in the first testing session or in the puppet condition for the experimental group were used in the second testing session.

The results from the second testing session are shown in Figures 2.2 and 2.3. The absence of a significant difference between the experimental group and the control group demonstrates that experience with the puppets did not significantly improve the children's ability to recognize that words could still exist in the absence of their referents. However, in comparison to the control group, the experimental group did improve significantly in regard to their answers to questions concerning the possibility of referents continuing to exist in the absence of words. Thus, the miniature multilingual experience given to the children in the experimental group improved the children's ability to recognize that objects still exist even if the words typically associated with them have disappeared. However, the same experience did not influence the children's ability to understand that words might still exist if the objects typically associated with them had disappeared.

These results suggest that experience with objects being referred to by different names helps children to recognize the distinction between words and objects, although the children were more likely to recognize the independence of objects than the independence of words. These results accord well with the notion that bilingual children benefit from their experience with hearing the same object labeled with different terms. However, it is a bit surprising that the experience given to the children in the experimental group proved as effective as it did. After all, it was a very limited experience—three objects were each labeled with three different novel names. It seems unlikely that such limited experience could have altered children's understanding of the word-referent relation. Perhaps it simply awakened their ability to deal with the questions being posed to them.

Rosenblum and Pinker (1983) compared the performances of 12 monolingual children and 12 bilingual children on questions concerned

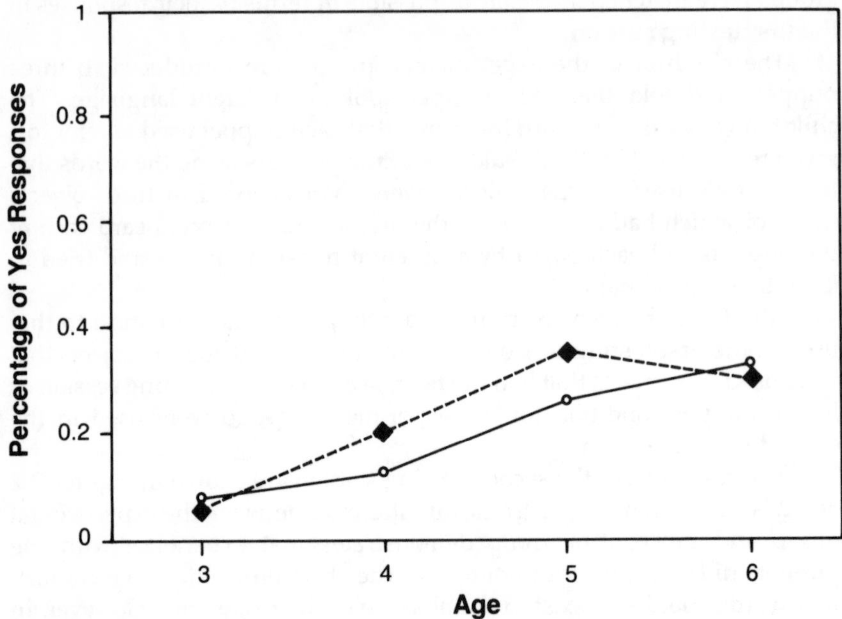


**Figure 2.2.** Percentage of "Yes" responses to questions about whether words could still exist in the absence of their corresponding objects. Dashed line denotes the experimental group. Solid line denotes the control group.

with the relation of words and their referents. Specifically, Rosenblum and Pinker asked the children if the names of certain objects could be changed and requested them to label objects with nonsense names or names for other objects. Contrary to previous research suggesting that bilingual children are precocious in regard to understanding the distinction between words and objects, Rosenblum and Pinker found comparable abilities in monolingual and bilingual children. In fact, neither group of children exhibited much evidence of nominal realism. Rosenblum and Pinker noted that it is incorrect to assume that bilingual children hear an object labeled by more than one name whereas monolingual children do not. Monolingual children do hear objects called by different names. There are synonyms as well as different ways of describing a given object. For example, a dog might be referred to as *Sparky*, *dog*, *poodle*, *pet*, *animal*, or *living thing*. Bilingual children are also exposed to this sort of information, but they also learn that a given object has a different name depending upon the language being used. Thus, monolingual and bilingual children learn that an object has different names depending on the salient properties to which one wishes to refer, but bilingual children also learn that

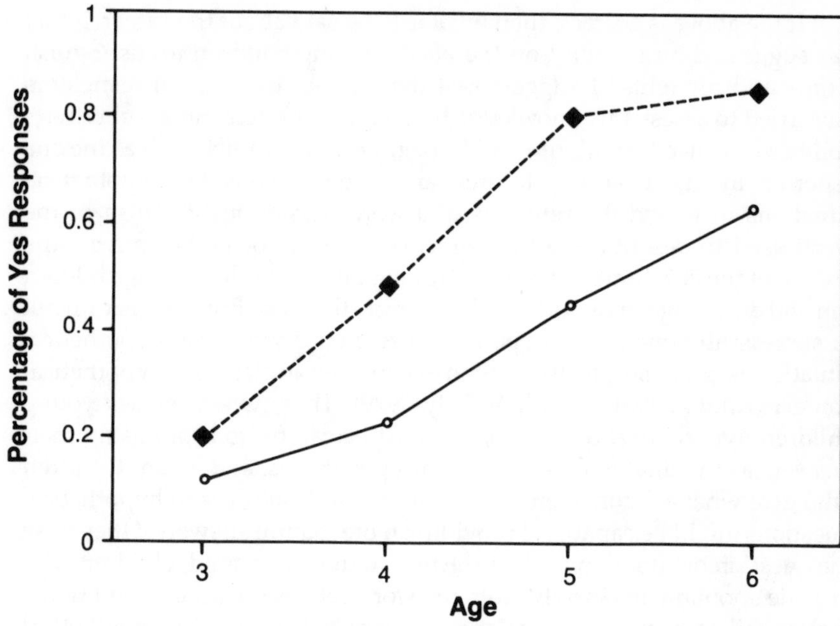


**Figure 2.3.** Percentage of "Yes" responses to questions about whether objects could still exist in the absence of their corresponding words. Dashed line denotes the experimental group. Solid line denotes the control group.

different discourse contexts may lead to different words being used to refer to a given object.

## A THEORY ABOUT WORDS AND THEIR REFERENTS

Rather than suppose that young children must learn to distinguish words and their referents, I should like to suggest that children recognize the difference between words and objects from the very beginning of the lexical-meaning acquisition process (see also Bates, 1979; MacNamara, 1982). In fact, given the nature of lexical-meaning acquisition, it is difficult to imagine that it could be otherwise. Children learn much about the world before they begin to acquire words. As they begin to ascertain the significance of words, they attempt to determine the appropriate meaning of each word. They do not believe that a word and an object are identical but know from the beginning that words are used to label objects.

If the above is correct, then what is to be said about the research that has suggested an inability on the part of young children to distinguish words and referents? I suggest that the manner in which investigators have tried to assess this knowledge has led us to underestimate children's abilities (see also Rosenblum and Pinker, 1983). In studies such as the one reported in this chapter, children are asked to consider hypothetical situations in which the referents of a word mysteriously vanish or the word used to describe a set of referents is mysteriously taken from the lexicon of the children's language. Although it is clear that young children can and do engage in hypothetical reference, they also find it more difficult to successfully engage in hypothetical reference when the hypothetical situation is proposed to them than when they initiate the hypothetical context (Kuczaj, 1981; Kuczaj & Daly, 1979). Thus, when we ask young children hypothetical questions, we must be careful to avoid using their answers as the final word on their concepts, values, and so on. Children who give what are considered to be "immature" answers to hypothetical questions might be capable of providing more mature answers if they pose the question or situation to themselves. On the other hand, children who provide spontaneous insights into the word-referent relation might nonetheless fail to provide correct answers if asked to answer hypothetical queries about the same topic.

The data obtained from a study in which I asked adults the same sorts of questions that we asked children in the study reported in this chapter support the notion that we might expect too much from children in such contexts. All of the adults queried recognized that referents would still exist even if the words usually used to refer to the referents had disappeared. However, approximately 40% of the adults' answers indicated that a word would not exist if its referents had disappeared. Adults, then, are much like children in the manner in which they view the relation of a word and its referents. Objects are more significant than words, and so are more likely to be viewed as being able to exist in the absence of words than are words likely to be viewed as being able to exist in the absence of objects. Objects are salient independent entities, whereas words are symbols used to refer to such entities. Markman (1976) has suggested that young children fail to differentiate words and referents because they focus on the empirical properties of referents rather than because they believe that words are part of the referent. Adults and children may recognize the independence of words and objects but more readily accept the continued existence of objects than the continued existence of words in hypothetical situations such as those used to assess nominal realism. This is due to the greater salience of objects as objects than words as objects. An object is a salient thing, while a word is salient only insofar as it signifies something else. Moreover, the knowledge that words are arbitrary conventional symbols may in fact lessen our ability to realize that words may exist in the absence of their referents. Having learned that a particular word is meaningful because of its relation to some aspect of our world, it seems to be more difficult to realize that words may continue to exist but with some different meaning if their referents disappear than it is to realize that objects continue to exist if the word disappears. Words are significant aspects of our lives, but not as significant as those aspects to which they refer. We learn that there are many ways to refer to entities such as dogs, depending on exactly what we elect to emphasize and the language to be spoken. Perhaps as a result of this, objects achieve a level of significance in our conceptual system that words do not.

Given all this, what may be said of the finding that the miniature multilingual experience helped children recognize that objects could exist in the absence of words? I suspect that such experience helped the children process the hypothetical queries directed toward them in regard to the word-referent relation. The contrived multilingual experience did not teach children the distinction between words and objects, this being something that children "know" from the beginning of the lexical-meaning acquisition process. Instead, the experience helped children employ the distinction when confronted with one of the hypothetical situations. Specifically, in order to truly consider the possibilities raised in the hypothetical questions, one must separate the conceptual representation of a word as word from the conceptual representation of its referents and independently act on each representation. Hearing the same object labeled with different names, particularly in a situation such as that of the miniature multilingual experience, may help children realize that conceptual representations and activities are involved in such questions.

## CONCLUDING REMARKS

Nominal realism, then, is an epiphenomenon. It is not a universal characteristic of early childhood. Some, but not all, children exhibit behavior consistent with the notion of nominal realism, the incidence of nominal realism depending on the particular task used (some tasks are easier than others) as well as on the nature of the sample (e.g., bilingual vs. monolingual children). Moreover, when children do seem to exhibit nominal realism, it is likely that they do not understand the question and respond in terms of their bias toward thinking and talking about objects rather than words. Although young children possess certain metalinguistic skills (e.g., Sinclair, Jarvella, & Levelt, 1978), they probably find using language to talk about language a relatively novel experience. Thus, they may reasonably assume that the conversation uses words to refer to objects, not realizing that words are being used to refer to words and to objects.

Although I have argued that children rarely if ever confuse words and objects (at least in the sense of equating the two or believing that the word is an inherent part of the object), the issue of how children come to use symbols is a very important, if unresolved, topic. In the next chapter, Richards and Richards examine the central concerns involved in the study of symbols and symbolization. While their chapter and this chapter deal with issues relevant to the development of the symbolic system of language, the chapter by Leonard (Chapter 4) is directly concerned with the acquisition of words and their meanings by young children. However, to fully understand lexical-meaning acquisition, we must understand the nature and development of other symbolic processes and the manner in which various types of symbols and symbolic processes interact throughout development. Thus, the chapters in this section are best viewed as interrelated parts rather than as isolated units.

## REFERENCES

Bates, E. (1979). The emergence of symbols: Ontogeny and phylogeny. In W. Collins (Ed.), *Children's language and communication*. Hillsdale, NJ: Lawrence Erlbaum.

Ben-Ze'ev, S. (1977). The influence of bilingualism on cognitive strategy and cognitive development. *Child Development, 48*, 1009–1018.

Clark, E. V. (1983). Meanings and concepts. In J. H. Flavell & E. M. Markman (Eds.), *Handbook of child psychology: Vol. 3. Cognitive development*. New York: John Wiley.

Cummins, J. (1978). Bilingualism and the development of metalinguistic awareness. *Journal of Cross-Cultural Psychology, 9*, 131–149.

Feldman, C., & Shen, M. (1971). Some language-related cognitive advantages of bilingual five-year-olds. *Journal of Genetic Psychology, 118*, 235–244.

Ianco-Worrall, A. (1972). Bilingualism and cognitive development. *Child Development, 43*, 1390–1400.

Kuczaj, S. (1981). Factors influencing children's hypothetical reference. *Journal of Child Language, 8*, 131–138.

Kuczaj, S. (1982a). *Language development: Syntax and semantics*. Hillsdale, NJ: Lawrence Erlbaum.

Kuczaj, S. (1982b). The acquisition of word meaning in the context of the development of the semantic system. In C. Brainerd & M. Presley (Eds.), *Progress in cognitive development research. Vol. 2. Verbal processes in children*. New York: Springer-Verlag.

Kuczaj, S., & Daly, M. (1979). The development of hypothetical reference in the speech of young children. *Journal of Child Language, 6*, 563–580.

Leopold, W. (1949). *Speech development of a bilingual child. Vol. 4. Diary from age two*. Evanston, IL: Northwestern University Press.

MacNamara, J. (1982). *Names for things*. Cambridge, MA: MIT Press.

Markman, E. (1976). Children's difficulty with word-referent differentiation. *Child Development, 47*, 742–749.

Osherson, D., & Markman, E. (1975). Language and the ability to evaluate contradictions and tautologies. *Cognition, 3*, 213–226.

Papandropoulou, I., & Sinclair, H. (1974). What is a word? *Human Development, 17*, 241–258.

Piaget, J. (1929). *The child's conception of the world*. London: Routledge and Kegan Paul.

Pinker, S. (1979). *Bilingual and monolingual children's awareness of words*. Unpublished bachelor's thesis, McGill University, Montreal.

Rosenblum, T., & Pinker, S. (1983). Word magic revisited: Monolingual and bilingual children's understanding of the word-referent relationship. *Child Development, 54*, 773–780.

Sandoval, J. (1976). *Aspects of cognitive development in the bilingual: An exploratory study of word-object separation*. Unpublished master's thesis, University of California at Los Angeles.

Scarlett, H., & Press, A. (1975). An experimental investigation of the phenomenon of word realism. *Merrill-Palmer Quarterly, 21*, 205–226.

Sinclair, A., Jarvella, R., & Levelt, W. (Eds.). (1978). *The child's conception of language*. New York: Springer-Verlag.

Slobin, D. (1978). A case study of early language awareness of a bilingual. In A. Sinclair, R. Jarvella, & W. Levelt (Eds.), *The child's conception of language*. New York: Springer-Verlag.

Vygotsky, L. (1962). *Thought and language*. Cambridge, MA: MIT Press.

Werner, H. (1940). *Comparative psychology of mental development*. New York: International Universities Press.

# 3

# *The Development of Language and Imagery as Symbolic Processes*

MEREDITH MARTIN RICHARDS
AND LARRY G. RICHARDS

Our ability to use symbols is often taken as the hallmark of our humanity. Man is a symbol-using animal, and in this way is distinct from all other known species. Philosophers (Cassirer, 1944; Langer, 1957) and humanistic psychologists (Kinget, 1975) have argued that the essential unique characteristic of the human species is our ability to use symbols. Although this assertion may be questioned in light of the experimental studies of language in primates and recent developments in computer simulation and artificial intelligence, the use of symbols is surely more elaborate, pervasive, and consistent among humans than among any other known species. It has been argued that man has a "need for symbolization" (Langer, 1957)—a need to find meaning and significance in the world. Our modes of perceiving and thinking about the world are symbolic; indeed, "symbolism is involved in one way or another in virtually all, if not all, human acts by the time adulthood is reached" (Bartley, 1958, p. 56).

Symbolization involves a symbol and its field of reference; a word has its meaning, a picture represents something. A third element is also required: a person or organism capable of generating or appreciating the symbolism. Many kinds of things can be symbols—marks on paper, bursts of sound, body movements, arrangements of matter in space—even patterns of neural activity in the brain and body of a person or animal, or electrical activity in the "brain" of a machine.

Symbols represent; they stand for, or mean, or convey information about objects and events to an appropriate recipient. Symbols serve two primary functions: They are the basis for thought and for communication. They allow us to talk to each other and to talk to ourselves.

Symbols are the tools we think with. They free us from the necessity for external stimulation to control our thoughts and actions (Gregory, 1970). We can behave without having to react to an external stimulus or situation. We can think about fish when none are present, and about skin diving when we are far from the sea.

Symbols are necessary for communication; they are the media through which it occurs. Effective communication requires shared symbols based on common experiences, contexts, or culture. The meanings of symbols are determined by the society and culture in which an individual is raised (Pollio, 1974). Nonetheless, most symbols are arbitrary. They are conventions individuals must learn from the society or group to which they belong. Even within a culture, individuals master different arbitrary symbols as they assume various careers or disciplines.

Symbols serve as internal representations of the external world. By manipulating symbols we can anticipate changes in the world, foresee the results of actions, and thus decide how or whether to act. Our facility with symbols allows us to adapt to the environment and to adapt the environment to us. Symbols are artifacts; indeed, as Simon (1981) notes, "symbol systems are almost the quintessential artifacts, for adaptivity to an environment is their whole *raison d'être*. They are goal-seeking, information processing systems, usually enlisted in the services of the larger systems in which they are incorporated" (p. 27).

## VARIETIES OF SYMBOLS

Alfred North Whitehead (1927) discussed the role of symbolism in human life and culture. He differentiated several levels of symbolism varying from primitive to complex. Most fundamental is the symbolism of perception. At a higher level, both language and mathematics are clearly symbolic. Complex symbolism is apparent in architecture, literature, religion, ritual, art, and ceremony.

Langer (1957) distinguished two types of symbolism. *Discursive symbolism* is represented by language. A language has a vocabulary and a syntax—a set of terms (words) and their definitions, and rules for combining the terms into larger units. The syntax imposes serial order on verbal expression. On the other hand, the products of the visual arts are examples of *presentational symbolism*. Drawings, paintings, and photographs all convey meaning to the human mind, yet they generally violate the principles of denotation that apply to languages. Presentational symbols are nondiscursive. In a picture all of the parts are presented simultaneously, and all enter into the meaning of the whole.

In *Languages of Art*, Nelson Goodman (1976) provides a more formal and precise treatment of many of the problems addressed by Langer (1957). He proposed a set of five formal criteria for a *notational system*. These criteria are logical and precise, and few symbol systems meet all of them. Symbol systems may be characterized by the degree to which they deviate from the strict criteria of notationality. The Western notation for musical scores satisfies all five of Goodman's criteria and thus is notational. But natural languages do not. Human languages allow ambiguities that are not permissible for a notational system. Painting and other visual arts are even less notational.

## SYMBOLS DISTINGUISHED FROM OTHER SIGNS

As noted above, a symbol is something that represents or stands for something else. But that definition can also apply to several other terms: signs, signals, symptoms, indices, and icons. These terms are all related, but there are important differences between them. *Sign* is the most general term; all of the others are types of signs. Pierce (1933) is usually credited with distinguishing three classes of signs: indices, icons, and symbols. *Indices* acquire meaning through de facto correlations existing in the natural environment. For example, a certain noise or nest indicates the presence of a particular type of animal. Indices have a causal connection to the object signified. *Symptoms* are a special case of indices; they indicate a change in state, usually an abnormality, in an object or organism. Thus, a change in body temperature is a symptom of disease. *Signals* are signs that control behavior. They may be either natural (e.g., sexual signals in primates) or artificial (e.g., traffic lights). *Icons* acquire their meaning from their similarity to the things they represent. Iconic signs embody shared features—as when we recognize an object in a picture because the representation shares features with the thing represented. *Symbols* acquire their meaning through conventional use and understanding: Language is symbolic in this sense. Symbols are designators, as opposed to operators. They are referential: "They tell *what* or *how* a thing is" (Kinget, 1975, p. 15). Symbols are part of the domain of meaning. They "are independent of the presence of sensory stimulation" and dependent on the person using them.

These distinctions are common in the philosophy literature, but psychologists do not generally adhere to them. In particular, several theorists whose work is described below make somewhat different distinctions.

## THE SYMBOLIC PROCESSES IN PSYCHOLOGY

What are symbols and symbolic processes from the psychological point of view? In his classic *Method and Theory of Experimental Psychology*, Osgood (1953) identifies problem solving and insight, thinking, and language behavior as symbolic processes. These symbolic processes had to be postulated to account for the many circumstances in which the observable responses of a subject (animal or human) could not be explained solely in terms of the current stimulus situation. Under such circumstances, the association between stimulus and response was said to be "mediated by a symbolic process" (p. 601). This approach represented behavioral psychology's attempt to deal with the fundamental problems of meaning and thought.

Twenty years later, Pollio's (1974) book *The Psychology of Symbolic Activity* also dealt primarily with language and thinking as symbolic processes, covering memory, concept learning, and problem solving from both the associative and information-processing perspectives. The two volumes edited by Weimer and Palermo (1974, 1982), *Cognition and the Symbolic Processes*, cover a much broader range of topics: awareness, meaning, comprehension, tacit knowledge, structural realism, perception, and neuropsychology.

Since 1954, a small group of researchers has attempted to program computers to display intelligent behavior in a large variety of tasks, including problem solving, theorem proving, game playing, inference, and design. According to Simon (1981), symbol use is the key to general intelligent action. A computer can be programmed to behave intelligently because it is capable of using and manipulating symbols. He argues that systems that exhibit "intelligence" will necessarily be symbol systems, and that physical symbol systems of adequate complexity and organization can be made to exhibit intelligent behavior (Newell, 1981; Newell & Simon, 1981). Simon (1981) and Newell (1981) strongly advocate computational theories of mental processes. More recent work by Kolers (1983) and Kolers and Smythe (1984) challenges the computational view of mind and argues that its adherents have too limited a concept of symbolism. The computational view focuses on consensual articulated symbols (such as those in natural language) and ignores other types of symbolism (as described by Langer, 1957, and Goodman, 1976).

Concern for the symbolic processes among psychologists has expanded greatly in recent years. Symbols are no longer simply constructs introduced into behaviorist theories to account for embarrassing phenomena, but rather represent areas of major theoretical and empirical concern.

## LANGUAGE AND IMAGERY AS SYMBOLIC PROCESSES

Although there are many symbolic domains, language and imagery represent the primary spheres of human symbolic activity. Words and images are used throughout our culture to communicate; visual and verbal concepts seem to occupy much of our thought. Writing and pictures are the two dominant ways to convey meaning over space and time. We will emphasize the symbolic properties of images and their role in thought as well as the relation of imagery to language. Our major focus will be on systematic theories of the development of language and imagery as symbolic processes.

### The Importance of Imagery

Arnheim (1969, 1979) asserts that all thinking is basically perceptual in nature. Thinking is in terms of images—not complete, detailed replicas of experience, but images that abstract its generic qualities. Images in thought reduce experience visually to a skeleton of essential dynamic features.

There is much literature establishing the facilitative effects of visual imagery in learning and memory, especially in paired associates learning, concept learning, free recall learning, and so forth (Paivio, 1972, 1978). This effect seems to increase, rather than decrease, with age in childhood (Reese, 1977). Here the visual image is used to facilitate recall of essentially verbal material. Of course, visual mnemonics (memory aids) have been used to enhance human memory since ancient times.

Bower (1972) and Paivio (1978) have developed dual coding theories for the representation of information in memory. Bower distinguishes two kinds of memory based on whether we remember in images or propositions. When remembering images, we call upon the appearance of the thing remembered and spatial information about it. Images are a way of "re-presenting to ourselves the appearances of past events we have witnessed" (Bower, 1972, p. 52).

Potter (1979) and Brewer (1974) propose an abstract level of meaning (i.e., ideas) underlying both language and imagery. They assume a deeper level of conceptual representation which captures the *idea* of an object. Words and images are merely access routes to concepts or ideas. This deeper level is characterized as amodal conceptual knowledge.

Berlyne (1965) has provided a cogent account of the role of symbols in human thought. To him, thinking is "any process that involves a chain . . . of symbolic responses" (p. 19). It can involve words, propositions, formulas, images, daydreams, and so forth. Directed thinking is focused on the solution of problems. Both words and images are important to directed thinking; they are examples of symbolism and may be components of transformational chains. Images may be transformations as well as states—an image is a means of thinking as well as something to think about. The spatial arrangements in the image can be used to make clear the relations between things. Berlyne speaks of an "informational isomorphism" between images and the objects or events they represent.

Harnad (1982) argues on logical and empirical grounds for a duality of mental function or a functional bifurcation of mental processing. *Bounded engrams* represent the results of categorical perception. There is more information in the world than is represented in our phenomenal experience. Furthermore, what we remember is a subset of what we perceive. Memory represents a reduction—a selective encoding—of experience. Indeed, what we achieve in memory is a "minimum set of invariants" which we can uniquely identify. These categories reflect "the invariant and recurrent" aspects of experience. We learn them by induction and are able to associate a unique arbitrary output (a name) with them.

However, a second kind of representational system must also exist. Both our immediate perceptual experience and our iconic imagery are rich and continuous. Neither reflects the kind of minimal representation appropriate for bounded engrams. Unbounded engrams are "analogs of our moment to moment experience"—that is, they are images. As such, each has an inherent uniqueness. However, taken as a set, there is a "great deal of overlap" and hence confusability. Unbounded engrams cannot be "reliably addressed"—they cannot be given names.

Symbols for bounded engrams can enter into propositions; unbounded engrams may appear in apposition. Harnad (1982) proposes that metaphor, which we usually think of as a linguistic phenomenon, is in fact mediated by unbounded engrams and involves processing of information in the nonverbal mode. Metaphor is effective because of the apposition of ideas or images rather than as a result of propositional expression. The unbounded system is also the domain of affect. Indeed, Harnad suggests that the emotional aspects of experience are irrelevant to most symbolic systems. Both of these ideas—metaphor as apposition and the emotional component of unbounded engrams—are important to understanding creative thinking.

## The Symbolic Nature of Images

Perception itself is symbolic (Bartley, 1958; Harnad, 1982; Whitehead, 1927); it is our internal representation of the external world. Perception involves sorting the world into meaningful categories of experience (Proffit & Halwes, 1982). We perceive objects, events, and features of the environment (Brunswick, 1950; Kohler, 1947). Imagery is very much like visual perception. It involves partitioning experience into the same kinds of categories, objects, events, and features. Neisser (1970) argues that it probably employs the same mechanisms as visual perception.

What are images like? For some people they are literally pictures in the mind's eye—visual representations of considerable detail and vividness. For others, images are vague, fleeting, uncontrolled segments of experience, and, for a few people, notions of mental images are treated as meaningless nonsense. However, both Bower (1972) and Neisser (1970) think that people who claim to have no mental imagery do not understand the question. In standard imagery tasks (e.g., count the number of windows in the back of your house, or how many turns are involved in traveling between two locations in a familiar town), most people consult an internal image, however faint or fleeting. That is not to say that images are reproductions; they usually are not. They are often constructions or reconstructions. They are influenced by our knowledge and expectations. They are often incomplete, lacking in all but the essential details. They may be elaborated or filled in as necessary to accomplish a task. Loftus (1979), in her work with eyewitness testimony, has concluded that eyewitnesses reconstruct, rather than reproduce, memory for the events witnessed. Information from other sources can alter the accuracy of the reconstruction, particularly for nonessential details of the event or scene.

Images are a special kind of representation. They are symbols that represent spatial or configural aspects of the world. By manipulating them, one can predict or assess changes in the world. Images are different from words or propositions. They provide different kinds of information to the thinker, and they are processed differently. Whereas words may be used to describe an object (to talk about the object), images may be used to "re-present" the object (to reconstruct its appearance) (Bower, 1972).

## DEVELOPMENT OF THE SYMBOLIC FUNCTION

Only a handful of developmental researchers and theorists have approached symbolic functioning as a domain of inquiry in itself, although many have studied it implicitly in research involving one or another particular symbol system (language, pictorial representation, imitation, etc.). In this chapter we deal with five systematic theories of the development of the symbolic function: those of Piaget, Bruner, Werner and Kaplan, Bates, and Gardner and his associates. Each of these theorists achieves a breadth of inquiry, recognizing symbolic development as a process that occurs in multiple modalities (bodily movement, visual perception and representation, sound and vocalization, etc.). The ontogenesis of symbols is seen as following constant laws across a variety of domains.

Our brief review of the major psychological and philosophical approaches to the nature of symbolic representation raises some important issues which any theory of the development of the symbolic function should address. The first issue deals with the mechanisms necessary for acquiring the meanings of symbols. Symbols may stand in different relations to the thing symbolized (Peirce, 1933), and different learning mechanisms are implied by these different types of relationship.

We acquire the meaning of iconic signs through abstraction. Since an icon bears a physical resemblance to the thing signified, its meaning is understood when the features in common with the referent are correctly apprehended. Although some icons lend themselves more readily to interpretation than others, recognition of pictorial representations is accomplished as early as 2 years of age (Hochberg & Brooks, 1962) and is universal in many respects (Kennedy, 1974). Children seem to be able to remember images very well; eidetic imagery is common among young children (Haber, 1969; Neisser, 1970).

Indices and symbols, on the other hand, require associative learning through contiguity and are indistinguishable in the early stages of learning. The word *train* is only one of a variety of sights and sounds that accompany the physical appearance of a moving train. To the young child the word is indistinguishable from the other associates that regularly occur in temporal contiguity with the object. The word, like other sights and sounds, serves an initial indexing function until its referential or "naming" function is understood. "The knowledge that indices and symbols are different is a very late development, and of no relevance to the acquisition of sign-referent relations by young infants" (Bates, 1979b, p. 51).

This suggests other important issues for developmental research: What are the early signs of the emergence of symbolization, when do they occur, and how does the child come to the metasymbolic awareness that arbitrary symbols are distinct from natural signs and indices? Werner and Kaplan (1963) speak of gaining psychological "distance" between the vehicle (symbol) and the referent, recognizing not only that these are distinct entities, but that one serves a general, referential function with respect to the other.

Imitation, gestures, and symbolic play are all important behavioral accompaniments to the process of learning language. How are these related to the onset and nurturing of the symbolic function; do they play a determining role, or is their correspondence during this period merely coincidental? One suspects, for instance, that the ability to substitute surrogate objects for familiar ones (e.g., a stick for a spoon or a gun) in play sequences implies recognition of the familiar object's constant and objective identity, surely a prerequisite to symbolic naming. Golomb (1979), finding that such substitutions are neither arbitrary nor egocentric (as Piaget believed them to be), argues for symbolic play as an early form of reversible thinking.

Another important type of play involves the manipulation of symbols for their own sake. Nursery rhymes, repetitive chants, songs, and rhythmic poems are examples. People have always derived pleasure from manipulating symbols apart from symbolization, from using symbols in a way that frees them from the necessity to represent. Children love to manipulate verbal, musical, gestural, and even pictorial symbols for the rhyme, meter, inflection, tension, pulse, contrast, and so forth, that they present in their material form as symbols, divorced from their representational content. Throughout history, cultures have developed such artifacts for children to learn. Their popularity may be due to the developmental function that is being served. These help the child gain psychological distance between symbols and their referents by objectifying the vehicle—the complementary process to objectifying the referent through symbolic play. Both forms of play help the child gain metasymbolic awareness.

Another issue for theories of symbolic development is the relative emphasis that is placed upon language as the medium of symbolization. There is overwhelming evidence that imagery, if not the "flesh and blood" of thought itself (as Arnheim, 1969, asserts), is at least one of the most powerful and productive forms of thinking available. The extent to which psychological accounts of the development of symbolization give forms of representation other than language a place in this process is a mark of their completeness.

## The Development of Symbolism in Piaget's Theory

Piaget attached great importance to symbolic activity in the growth of human intelligence. He referred to the "semiotic function" (Piaget, 1962) as the capacity to represent sensorimotor action through signifiers that are differentiated from their significates. The emphasis upon internalized actions ("operations") as the basic units of thought is central to Piaget's theory. Symbolic representation is essential to the gradual process of internalizing the action schemas that dominate the sensorimotor period.

Following Saussure, Piaget (1962) distinguished between two types of signifiers: the *signs* of language (which are learned, conventional, and communicable) and the *symbols* of deferred imitation, symbolic play, and mental imagery. Unlike linguistic signs, nonverbal symbols are uninstructed, idiosyncratic, loosely structured, and highly personal. For these reasons, Piaget considered such symbols to be far more revealing of stages in the development of logical thought and therefore of more interest to developmental psychology.

***Language vs. Imagery as Symbolic Modes.*** A common assumption in major contemporary theories of cognitive development is that visual imagery is prior to and necessary for the development of symbolic meaning, a first stage in the development of language as the mediator of thought. To theorists such as Werner and Kaplan (1963) and Bruner (Bruner, 1973; Bruner, Olver, & Greenfield, 1966), imagery is an ontogenetically early level of representation; it becomes less functional for the child as the more flexible and abstract linguistic modes of representation are acquired. These theorists hold that imagery is limited in its capacity for representing, processing, and schematizing information.

In sharp contrast, Piaget considered language to be the inferior form of semiotic functioning. Piaget argued that, as a "collective sign system," language necessarily consists of signs that generalize and classify experience, referring to properties of experience that are common to all individuals. Yet there are a great many forms of experience that language conveys badly. Piaget noted that, when listening or talking, individuals concretize the words by means of their own system of personal images. "For concepts strictly identical from one individual to the next, and strictly defined by a uniform vocabulary, there are countless corresponding personal images" (Piaget & Inhelder, 1971, p. 380). Nonverbal symbols are also indispensable for preserving past experience.

> It is clear . . . that if one wishes to evoke in thought some past perception, it is necessary to supplement the verbal sign systems with a system of imaginal symbols. The image, then, is a symbol in that it constitutes a semiotic instrument necessary in order to evoke and think about what has been perceived. (Piaget & Inhelder, 1971, p. 381)

***Role of Symbols in Operational Thinking.*** Gregory (1970) argued that the capacity for symbols releases humans from the tyranny of perception—from the dominance of the "here and now" in determining one's responses to a situation. Similarly, Piaget argued that symbolic thought releases the child from the "here and now" of immediate perception and direct action that characterizes sensorimotor intelligence.

The emergence of symbolic thought coincides with the onset of symbolic play and deferred imitation—two developments that mark the end of the sensorimotor stage of cognitive development. During the sensorimotor period, the child shows no capacity for imaginal representation. Expressing its emerging motor competencies, the infant performs physical actions upon objects, often in repetitive sequences (e.g., banging). In a later stage, the baby engages in "prelogical" actions upon objects (e.g., stacking cans or nesting cups). Both of these types of activity precede and seem to prepare the child for make-believe behavior, when objects are used routinely as symbols for others (Inhelder & Karmiloff-Smith, 1978). By the end of the sensorimotor period (about 1½ years), most children are engaging in the kind of imaginative play and deferred imitations that signal the onset of representational (semiotic) functioning. Thereupon the child begins the gradual development of the use of imagery as an instrument of thought.

Images, according to Piaget, consist of action schemata "played out" internally—sometimes with the assistance of overt gestures—in which the child imitates in thought the behaviors that would bring about a movement or transformation on an object. As such, images are an abstract representation of reality rather than a mere copy of it "in the mind's eye." Piaget explicitly contrasts his view ("Knowledge as Assimilation") with that of the early associationists, who considered perception to be a passive registration of the characteristics of the perceived world ("Knowledge as Copy") and the image to be a delayed evocation of such perceptions from memory.

***Piaget's Studies of the Image.*** Piaget and Inhelder (1971) reported extensive studies of imagery in their book, *Mental Imagery in the Child*. In these studies, Piaget deals with two types of imagery: *reproductive* (imagining experienced objects and events from "memory") and *anticipatory* (imagining objects and events in the absence of previous experience). Reproducing a stationary object from memory is the simplest form of imagery. Images of movements (change of position) or transformations (change of form) on the object are more involved. In kinetic and transformational imagery, the distinction between reproductive and anticipatory is largely technical: "In order to imagine a given movement or transformation, it is necessary to reconstitute them by the identical process by which unknown movements or transformations are represented. In other words, there is in most cases no essential difference between reproductive and anticipatory imagery" (Piaget & Inhelder, 1971, p. 354).

In his studies, Piaget had children view such events as a rod with differently colored ends falling end over end from a table, a wire strung through differently colored beads undergoing a 180-degree rotation about the horizontal axis, and many other examples of kinetic or transformational events. The child was asked to reconstruct, then subsequently to recognize (from pictures), the successive stages of change. For anticipatory imagery, Piaget asked children to imagine such things as the final pattern that would result from folding then cutting off one end of a piece of paper, or bending an arched wire into a straight line, and so forth. The child was then asked to construct or recognize the stages of change.

***Imagery in the Preoperational Child.*** Piaget observed that preoperational children often engage in gestural routines (e.g., rotating the hands while holding an imaginary wire, or folding in series the edges of an imaginary paper) as aids to anticipatory imagery. He concluded that such gestures reveal an intermediate stage in the internalization of the action schemas that constitute operational thinking; he took their existence as support for his definition of imagery as "internalized imitation."

Piaget also observed that the preoperational child can accurately reconstruct the beginning and end states of kinetic or transformational events (e.g., beads in original and reverse order) but frequently errs in reconstructing or recognizing the intermediate stages. From numerous instances, Piaget concluded that the preoperational child lacks kinetic and transformational anticipatory imagery. The images of the preoperational child are essentially static; the child ignores transformations in favor of configurations or states, with the result that the images of this level focus on the simplest elements available (i.e., the end states of movement and transformation).

The capacity for accurate anticipatory imagery does not emerge until well into the concrete operational stage, often as late as 10 or 11 years of age. One of the reasons is because accurate anticipatory imagery requires all of the logical operations of thought that emerge during this period: seriation, reversibility, decentration, and conservation.

Piaget observed fascinating examples of "pseudo-conservation" in the anticipatory imagery of the preoperational child. An example is conserving the shorter length of an arched wire in anticipating the length of a resulting straight wire. Another example is the reconstruction of stages in the horizontal displacement of one square in relation to another (the square on top is moved to the right of the square on the bottom). Many preoperational children try to conserve the overall boundary relations between the two squares by having the top square contract (so as not to project beyond the right edge of the lower one) or expand (so that its left edge stays in line with the lower one while its right edge extends beyond it). In other words, solutions to the problem center on ordinal properties of the extremities or boundaries rather than the metric property of length of the horizontal sides.

***Conclusions.*** Several compelling conclusions about the nature and function of imagery in the development of thought follow from Piaget's observations. First, the use of gestural aids in anticipatory imagery suggests that imagery is "internalized imitation" in which the imager symbolically represents the stages and consequences of imagined action schemas in thought. Second, the preoperational child's inability to reconstruct from memory all but the terminal stages of observed movement or transformations suggests that such images do not occur simply as a result of witnessing the event in question. The child has observed the intermediate stages through perception as surely as he or she has observed the end product. These images are not reproductions from memory, but imaginal anticipations deriving from intelligence. Third, the phenomenon of "pseudo-conservation" points to the active intervention of schemata that are appropriate to the level of cognitive development.

From observations such as these, Piaget concluded that the image, rather than being an accurate copy of perception, is a distortion and reconstruction of it. In this sense, he said, the image, like the word, is symbolic—it designates or signifies something, and its resemblance to the thing signified is determined by the intervention of intelligence.

## Bruner's Three Modes of Representation

To Jerome Bruner, cognitive growth progresses through three alternative forms of representation: enactive, iconic, and symbolic. Representation is defined as a system or set of rules "in terms of which one conserves one's encounters with events" (Bruner, 1973, p. 316). Enactive representation of an event is in terms of the actions it requires; iconic representation forms a picture or image of the event; and symbolic representation uses words or other symbols to refer to and think schematically about the event. Within each medium, representation is necessarily selective; we do not include all the information about something in its representation but select features that are determined by the medium and the purposes of the representation. Each medium of representation has its own constraints and characteristics.

***Enactive Representation.*** Enactive representation is constrained by the nature of action itself (i.e., it is sequential and irreversible). It is through the formation of habitual motor skills that the enactive mode becomes representative. Past events become inscribed into a persisting and transferable habit pattern. Such patterns become generative in the sense in which language is generative; that is, they allow us to substitute and recombine specific serial behaviors that fall within the general habit pattern.

The earliest form of representation in the child is enactive. Bruner's concern is to show how the child progresses from enactive to symbolic representation through the intermediate mode of imagery. At first, the infant does not separate a percept from an act. To restore an object lost from view, for example, the child will perform an act appropriate to it. Toward the end of the sensorimotor period, however, perception becomes autonomous from action, and the child has two independent systems of representation. Contributing to this separation is the formation of motor habits; these enable the child to abstract the action schema from the particular act of the moment and to form an action-free image of the spatial context or "layout" of the situation. Thus, habitual motor patterns become the basis for action-free imagery. Once the child has the capacity to represent the world in spatially organized, action-free perceptual schemata (images), the task is to translate between the two modes of representation, to coordinate how one behaves toward a thing with how it appears.

***Iconic Representation.*** Bruner treats iconic representation (images) as essentially static pictures "in the mind's eye." He states that pictures can be symbolic (as in a highly abstract circuit or wiring diagram), that they can be used to represent serial action (as in a flow chart), and that some logical problems (e.g., syllogisms) can be translated into images for solution (Bruner et al., 1966). Beyond that, however, Bruner gives little credit to the image as a medium for symbolic representation, for the representation of movement and transformation, or for problem solving. These functions of imagery are critically important to Piaget's analysis of semiotic functioning; the two theorists clearly differ in the importance they place on visual imagery and its role in symbolic thought and problem solving.

Bruner cites studies of conceptual sorting tasks in which children use the vivid, sensory aspects of objects, rather than more subtle patterns or functional uses of objects, as a basis for conceptual grouping. He concludes that imagery as a medium of representation concentrates upon the surface properties of the environment up to age 8 or 9. (High imagers are more likely to show inferior concept formation performance as a result of this tendency, although they will show superior ability to associate verbal labels with pictures.) Bruner refers to this property as *ostensiveness* of childhood imagery: The child matches something in his or her mind to something encountered in the environment by pointing to some particular sensory correspondence between the two. "It is only when he can go beyond this 'match by direct correspondence' that he comes to deal with such 'nonsensory' ideas as the relations between quantities, invariance across transformations, and substitutability within a conceptual category" (Bruner et al., 1966, p. 29).

***Symbolic Representation.*** To Bruner, the full characteristics of a symbolic system are not met through either enactive or iconic representation, but only through language. The following characteristics from Hockett's (1960) design features for a language are properties without which any symbolic activity would be "logically and empirically unthinkable" (Bruner et al., 1966, p. 47).

*categoriality*—Words cover classes of things, and these classes are rule-governed so that new members can be added. This includes morphology and syntax as well as semantics.

*hierarchy*—Any linguistic unit at one and the same time serves as a context for simpler units and/or finds its own context in a more complex linguistic unit.

*predication*—Subject-predicate relations, present in all languages, are an expression of the argument of a function: "x (subject) is a function of y (predicate)."

*causation*—Verb-object relations are a linguistic expression of cause and effect.

*modification*—An instance of the intersect of classes, for example, "a green apple," is an intersect of the class of all green things with the class of apples.

Bruner considers language to be the primary mode of productive thinking and problem solving. The ability to transform experience into new or altered forms through language (e.g., asking "What if . . .?" questions) permits experimental alteration of the environment without having to use trial and error or imagery. Finally, language alone permits the representation of things that are remote in time and space (displacement) to gain distance from a task by going beyond the immediate situation and dealing with its remote features. Bruner contrasts this characteristic with the domination of immediate perceptual features of situations (ostensiveness) that characterizes iconic representation.

From this discussion, the contrast between Piaget's views and those of Bruner is immediately evident. Piaget showed how imagery takes on anticipatory and manipulative functions that allow us both to experiment with alternative possibilities and to displace thinking from the constraints of immediate perception. Thus, Piaget has endowed the image with those characteristics of a symbolic system that Bruner takes to be necessary for productive thinking but ascribes only to language.

***Interaction Among Modes of Representation in Development.*** Bruner argues that cognitive growth is compelled by the disequilibrium that occurs when two systems of representation do not correspond. It is then that the child makes revisions in the way a problem is solved, resolving conflicts among enactive, iconic, and symbolic representations of the problem.

An experiment in volume conservation with the terms *fuller* and *emptier* (Bruner et al., 1966, chap. 8) illustrates the interaction and transition between the different modes of representation of the information in a task. Very young children will define the terms enactively—for example, *empty* is turn-overable after drinking and *full* is when you are about to spill. At the next stage (around age 5), *fuller* means the higher water level in the taller glass, and *emptier* means the lower water level in the shorter glass (regardless of volume of the glass). These children have fixed upon a single perceptual attribute to render their judgments. At the next stage there is a separation of the attributes used to deal with the two concepts. Now, *fuller* means the volume of filled space, and *empty* means the volume of empty space. However, with some displays (e.g., a tall narrow glass and a short fat glass, both half full), these two bases of judgment lead one to judge the same glass as both *fuller* and *emptier*. Many 7 to 9 year olds in fact give contradictory answers to these questions. Thus, the older child's iconic system of representation of the task is more complex. He or she is able to dissociate the situation into two variables (filled space and empty space) but is not yet able to relate the variables to a third (the volume of the container itself). "When the child can establish the relationship among all three terms—the amount of water, the amount of empty space, the volume of the container—he has a symbolic concept of proportion" (Bruner et al., 1966, p. 181). Thus, fitting previously separate perceptual cues into a structured relationship is achieved, according to Bruner, when the terms of the problem are recast into symbolic rather than iconic representation.

## Werner and Kaplan: Linear Representations, Mental Images, and the Beginnings of Language

In 1963, Heinz Werner and Bernard Kaplan published *Symbol Formation*, a major work in the ontogenesis of symbols. The book presented a psychological theory and a mass of original data pertaining to the nature and development of symbolic representation. Werner and Kaplan take the humanist position that symbolization allows humans to know, rather than merely react to, the world about them by providing them with the instrument of knowing—namely, language.

***Components of Symbolic Activity.*** Symbolic activity is conceptualized by Werner and Kaplan (1963) as consisting of four components: *addressor* (symbolizer), *addressee*, *vehicle* (the symbol), and *referent* (also called the *significate*). Symbolization occurs when the symbolizer uses the vehicle to represent or stand for the referent. Representation is the constitutive mark of a symbol; it distinguishes a symbol from a sign or signal, which merely anticipates rather than represents the referent. This corresponds to Peirce's (1933) distinction between a symbol and an index.

Representation, according to Werner and Kaplan (1963), implies an intentional act and some awareness, however vague, that vehicle and referent are not identical but are, in substance and in form, two totally different entities. Werner and Kaplan disallow imagery, dreams, and gestures from the category of true symbols on the grounds of intentionality. Although such forms may serve as symbolic vehicles for the addressee, they are simply a direct and unintentional expression of the referent from the point of view of the person producing them. Such vehicles directly "present" rather than "represent" the referent and lack the prerequisite "intention to represent" that characterizes a symbol. Werner and Kaplan call these forms *protosymbols*.

Protosymbols are extremely important in the genetic process of symbolization. Protosymbols are transformed into true symbols through the progressive differentiation of vehicle and referential meaning. In fact, symbolization develops progressively as a process of differentiation (distancing) between pairs of the four components of symbolic activity—addressor and addressee, addressor and referent, and vehicle and referent.

***Developmental Milestones in the Distancing Process.*** Werner and Kaplan (1963) surveyed an enormous body of literature (largely diary studies) for evidence of universal milestones in the process of distancing between the components of symbolic activity. One of the earliest of these is the onset of "indexical pointing" (pointing with the index finger to a referent object) around the age of 9 to 10 months. The antecedents to this behavior are reaching for, touching, and turning to the object, actions that fuse the child's motor activity with the object. The pointing gesture, however, signals the onset of motoric reference, a sign of distancing between the child as symbolizer and the object as referent. Similarly, early vocalizations (word sounds) are fused with action patterns, which together constitute an overall action schema with respect to the referent object. These separate at the point that children vocalize in the absence of the other constituent behaviors, differentiating themselves as vocalizers from the word as vehicle.

Another milestone is the onset of delayed imitation and gestural depiction (prototypical gestures made in the absence of their concrete referents). These signal an increasing distance between the gestures and the contents they depict; for the gestural depiction to take place requires an internal model or schema of the content. This reflects a considerable development in representational activity in which children learn to control their own bodies to form vehicles of representation. A similar development takes place in vocal depiction, in which words eventually become *decontextualized* from the concrete contents they represent (see Bates, next section).

***Empirical Studies of Linear Representation and Imagery.*** Werner and Kaplan (1963) believed that they could recapitulate important trends in the development of linguistic representation by studying more "primitive" representational forms in the adult. Their experiments deal with interpretive line drawings and hypnotically induced imagery in response to linguistic stimuli. Werner and Kaplan offer the following rationale in support of this paradigm. Speech symbols in the adult have already been structured into highly conventionalized and habitual forms, whereas nonphonic media have not. Thus, the latter provide a better picture of the beginnings of formation of symbolic vehicles. Further, nonverbal media are relatively closer to the experiences they represent, entailing minimal distance among symbolizer, symbol, and referent. Hence, they provide a paradigm of the genetically early stages of symbolization.

Werner and Kaplan (1963) had subjects draw simple configurations interpreting linguistic statements in four domains: naming (actually, descriptors such as "joyous," "dark," "longing," etc.), temporal variations of an event (e.g., "He is running," "He was running," "He will run"), agent-action-object statements (e.g., "He catches a fly"), and abstract thought relations (sentences with *and*, *but*, *if*, or *because* clauses). Hypnotically relaxed subjects also produced mental images of these linguistic materials. The resultant lines, squiggles, and verbal protocols were then compared to genetically early stages in the acquisition of language, as exemplified by the language of children and primitive cultures.

As an example of Werner and Kaplan's (1963) findings from their study of adults' line drawings, consider the agent-action-object relationship. Typically, there is no overt representation of the agent as distinct from the action, and no overt or independent representation of the object as distinct from agent and action. The representation of the action is typically object-specific—given a new object, the representation of action is altered accordingly. Werner and Kaplan conclude that the lack of differentiation and articulation among the components of an event, plus the frequent omission of one or more of these components, suggest operation at a more primitive level of symbolization, where the distance between symbolizer and vehicle is small. Linear representation of agent-action-object resembles the primitive forms of concrete-depictive languages and parallels early stages in the acquisition of syntax by children.

***A Note of Exception.*** Werner and Kaplan (1963) studied the simple line drawings of adults in a society dominated by verbal communication. Most of us ceased attempting line drawings of the experienced world after grade school. It is no surprise that Werner and Kaplan's subjects produced fairly primitive and unarticulated drawings, given their lack of development in this medium.

However, as Arnheim (1969) makes clear in his analysis of visual media, art and imagery are not limited to expressive rather than representational content. Accomplished artists understand well how to represent complex relationships among their subjects, and between the subjects and their settings, as well as temporality, causality, emotionality, and so forth, using the media of lines, paint, or sculpting material. These are instances of intentional representation by the artist. The same can be said of the actor or mime artist, who consciously manipulates gesture for the meaning it depicts. In relegating gestures, drawing, and imagery to the status of "primordial" representation, Werner and Kaplan (1963) have seriously neglected the symbolic possibilities of these media.

## Bates's Biological Model of the Ontogeny of Symbols

Elizabeth Bates (1979a, 1979b) is concerned with determining the nonverbal "prerequisites" of symbolic reference and communication and with placing the development of language in an evolutionary context within the biological sciences. Bates sees language as a system that evolved out of separate, nonlinguistic capacities, present to some degree in primates, that were recombined in the human species in a way that was largely task-determined. This evolutionary path to language is recapitulated in the human infant, who develops language through a combination of nonlinguistic skills (prerequisites), the outcome of which is constrained by the nature of these skills and the nature of the communication task.

From biology, Bates adopts the model of homology through shared origins: Both language and its prerequisites emerge from a common origin of underlying "software." As a consequence of this model, we would expect (a) that the developmental sequence between language and its prerequisites is optional rather than fixed and (b) that the effects of training are bidirectional, training in its prerequisites influencing language and vice versa. As a test of her model, Bates (1979b) conducted systematic observations of a sample of 25 American and Italian infants at regular intervals during the first 13 months of life.

***"Two Moments in the Dawn of Language."*** Communication in the first 9 months of infancy is largely a built-in reaction to an internal state. Given a goal and an adult within view, the infant will fuss and reach to obtain the goal but will not turn and look at, or vocalize or gesture to, the adult to obtain the goal.

Around 9 months of age, however, the infant begins to interrupt his or her goal-oriented behaviors to look toward the adult, eye contact sometimes shifting back and forth between the adult and the goal. This is the first controlled, intentional use of human agents as a means to a nonsocial goal—a behavior Bates terms the *protoimperative*. At about the same time, the infant begins to give or show objects (accompanied by vocalizing and gestures), with no discernible goal other than to obtain adult attention. This tendency to share attention toward an external referent Bates terms the *protodeclarative*. Bates concludes that the *idea* of intentional, conventional signaling requires some underlying development that does not occur before 9 months of age.

The age of onset and frequency of ritual signaling prior to language is positively correlated with the development of early reference. Communicative signals also occur in chimpanzees, but only as protoimperatives (i.e., in the service of an external goal) rather than as protodeclaratives. "The motivation of shared reference, developed in human children before language, may be one of the nonlinguistic factors that predispose our species toward the discovery and exercise of the naming function and toward the use of the speech channel (or some other channel) for information exchange" (Bates, 1979a, p. 143).

Bates sees the development of intentional control over previously unconventional, goal-oriented gestures and vocalizations as a manifestation of the human capacity for tool use. Both the protoimperative and the protodeclarative are examples of the use of social tools in relation to objects. From Bates' investigations and those of others (Harding & Golinkoff, 1977; Sugarman, 1973), it appears that this development is significantly correlated with the development of object-to-object (nonsocial) tool use at 9 to 10 months. Bates argues that the use of social and nonsocial tools can emerge in either sequence, indicating that both emerge as a result of the development of some common underlying capacity.

***Decontextualization and the Onset of Symbolic Communication.*** Bruner (Bruner et al., 1966) spoke of displacement and Werner and Kaplan (1963) spoke of distancing as hallmarks in the use of words as symbols. Both studies were referring to the dissociation and differentiation that occurs between a vehicle and its referent when the vehicle is truly used symbolically. Bates operationalizes this concept through her observations of *decontextualization* of both language production and comprehension.

The first "vocal gestures" and wordlike sounds of the infant typically accompany ritualized requests, playing, or showing sequences and emerge around 9 or 10 months. These often recognizable sounds are functionally equivalent to the other, nonvocal, gestures that are also part of those sequences. They exist as part of a procedure occurring in fixed contexts rather than as names for their referents. Comprehension of words is also largely dependent upon context during this period.

The slow process of decontextualization begins around 12 or 13 months, when the child begins to widen the contexts in which a particular sound is used and in which comprehension is exhibited. Decontextualization signals the onset of symbolic communication, "when we can infer that the child has *objectified* the vehicle-referent relationship to some extent, realizing that the symbol or vehicle can be substituted for its referent for certain purposes, while at the same time realizing that the symbol is not the same thing as its referent" (Bates, 1979a, p. 144). From that point on, new words enter the vocabulary at a fast pace; it is not necessary for each new word to undergo the process of decontextualization, as the child now has the idea of referential naming.

*Nonverbal Correlates of Symbolic Naming.* Piaget (1962) considered symbolic play to be one of three sources of the semiotic function in childhood. Bates's research shows that the emergence of symbolic and gestural schemes in play coincides both in time and in quality with the onset of decontextualized naming. The onset time for both behaviors is around 13 months. In addition, the repertoire of referents for symbolic play is almost identical to the referents in the child's vocabulary of symbolic names. From these data, Bates concludes that the new symbolic capacity is essentially modality free. "There is as yet nothing unique, special, or in any way privileged about naming in the vocal channel" (Bates, 1979a, p. 148).

Other nonsocial correlates of the onset of referential naming were found in measures of imitation, tool use in problem solving, and complex object-to-object manipulations in nonproblem-solving situations. Symbolic naming did not correlate with measures of either spatial relationships or object permanence.

*Conclusions.* Bates concludes with an evolutionary model in which certain components of the capacity for symbolic communication—namely, tool use and manipulative play, imitation, and the social motivation to share reference to objects—evolved separately in primates but reached the criterial levels necessary for symbolic functioning in humans. The timing of emergence of these prerequisite skills in humans permits them to combine into the requisite configuration necessary for the development of symbolic communication.

## Harvard Project Zero

One of the most prolific writers on symbolism has been Howard Gardner. He and his coworkers at Harvard Project Zero have been studying the acquisition of symbol systems and their productive use in children from 1 to 7 years of age. They have conducted both concurrent and longitudinal studies of symbol production in a variety of domains.

In early childhood children engage in undifferentiated symbolic activity. As they develop the conception of different media with different means and rules for symbol use, their behavior focuses on specific modes of symbolization at different times. For a variety of symbol domains, one fact is clear: The productive use of symbols is absent in 1-year-old children but is well developed in most children by age 7.

*The Harvard Project Zero Data Base.* Gardner (1982) reports on a pilot study of 12 middle class children. They varied in age from 2½ to 5 and included both sexes (numbers of each not cited). They were observed over several months in both their daily preschool activities and four controlled observation sessions. We are assured that all the "usual experimental procedures were followed" (1982, p. 117).

In the experimental sessions, children performed four tasks in each of four symbolic media, resulting in 16 conditions for each child. The symbol domains were language (story telling), symbolic play (acting out events with blocks), and two- and three-dimensional depiction (drawing and clay modeling). The tasks were spontaneous production, completion, assembly of a whole from parts, and copying. We are spared the details of the data analysis and results, and no numbers, graphs, or hypothesis tests are presented. Instead, some generalizations are given based on this study. We are told some children were verbalizers and others visualizers; some self-starters, others completers; some were person-centered, others object-centered; a variety of sex differences were noted; and, finally, children varied in their reliance on fixed themes in their performances. This is an impressive number of distinctions to base on a sample of 12 children of various ages. The correlations between the dichotomous classifications are not discussed. Nor does Gardner (1982) refer us to a primary reference for the details of this study and its quantitative results.

In later papers all these distinctions are boiled down to one between dramatists and patterners. Wolf and Gardner (1979) describe this difference in terms of the behavior of two children. However, they do not indicate what the distribution of these categories is in their sample of children.

In their major empirical effort, Gardner and his coworkers at Harvard Project Zero followed the development of symbolic skills for a range of symbol domains in 9 middle class children from the Boston area (3 males, 6 females). A cross validation sample of 70 other children performed "specimen tasks" in each domain. The 9 children were followed longitudinally over a 6-year period—from age 1 through age 7. They were regularly observed in free play and periodically given experimental tasks in each of the symbol domains.

*A Theory of Symbolism.* Gardner has developed a structural and behavioral description of the acquisition of symbol systems. This framework for the development of symbolic skills involves four distinctions. Seven types or *domains* of symbols were investigated: language, two- and three-dimensional representation, number, music, symbolic play, and bodily gesture. Patterns of development within each domain are characterized as "*streams* of symbolization." Performance on tasks within each domain led to ordinal scales for each stream and little apparent influence of the streams on one another.

However, there were some similarities across domains that led to the assumption of "*waves* of development"—cognitive processes assumed to underlie performance across symbolic domains (Gardner & Wolf, 1983). Wolf (1983) identifies three such waves which occurred at 2-year intervals in this sample of children.

The first wave is *event structuring*, which occurs when children start to identify actors and objects and sequences of activity involving them. Event structuring results from the child's core understanding of roles and sequence, which is nonsymbolic and is acquired as early as age 2. In the second wave, acquired by age 4, children learn to represent structures, shapes, and features of objects. This is called *topological mapping*. A third wave, identified as *digital mapping*, involves both counting (numerosity) and measuring (metric concepts). The concept of number and ordered relations is manifest in several symbol systems by age 5. Each of these three waves is said to be overgeneralized in that it affects symbolic activity in domains and ways that seem inappropriate to an adult observer. The concept of waves of symbolization is intended to account for the observed correlations of developments in different symbol systems (e.g., between productive language and play skills).

Finally, "*channels* of symbolization" describe the differential development of the skills within a domain and are largely the result of how the child's societal or cultural context molds his or her skills. Davis and Fucigna (1983) describe drawing and mapping as "two channels of graphic symbolization." When children come into school at age 5, they can make reasonable pictures, but they cannot make maps. They acquire these skills during elementary school. They learn that different rules (conventions) apply to map making than to drawing pictures. These include the use of aerial perspective, landmarks, minimal representation of objects, and attempts to capture spatial relationships accurately. According to these authors, none of their subjects could make distinctions between maps and pictures until age 7.

One important concern of Gardner and his coworkers is with the development of metasymbolism: the awareness and self-conscious modification of one's own symbolic activity (Phelps, 1983). Examples are interpreting, evaluating, and editing one's symbolic products. Metasymbolic activity involves reflection on the act of symbolizing. It apparently develops when children learn that symbols function in communication.

Gardner's work is descriptive, taxonomic, and apparently post hoc. It does not really represent a theory of symbolic behavior, but rather provides an *empirical framework* (Gardner uses this term) within which a theory might be developed. His account does not provide the ability to make predictions, but rather describes patterns observed in his data. He provides no compelling a priori rationale for selecting the seven particular symbol domains he chose to study, except that they somehow relate to Goodman's (1976) characterization of symbol systems. It is also unclear, independently of the data, how one differentiates streams from waves from channels.

These authors fail to discuss the role of formal instruction, societal expectations, and demand characteristics in their findings. Observing regularities in performance as a result of the natural unfolding of cognitive competence is one thing; but some of these regularities may be heavily influenced by what children are taught and when.

A final problem with this work concerns the type, amount, quality, and analysis of the data. Most of Gardner's reported findings are based on observations of fewer than 25 children scattered among different studies and conditions. Although he has a validation sample of 70 additional subjects, Gardner (1983, p. 4) states that their performance differs in significant ways from the primary (longitudinal) sample. We need to see the tasks, the data, and their analysis in detail to assess the adequacy of Gardner's findings and theory. We look forward to the publications that will provide these details.

***Frames of Mind.*** The recent thrust of Garcher's work is his theory of multiple intelligences outlined in *Frames of Mind* (1983). In this work, Gardner attempts to reformulate our ideas about intelligence to conform to his analysis of symbol systems. He proposes six complexes of abilities—linguistic, musical, logical-mathematical, spatial, bodily-kinesthetic, and personal—and identifies each as an "intelligence." Although Gardner claims to "introduce novel scientific concepts" (p. 70), all of these abilities have been discussed before in the mainstream psychological literature (Anastasi, 1961; Cronbach, 1970), although most authors identify them, more conservatively, as abilities, aptitudes, interests, or skills rather than intelligences.

Why these six clusters of abilities? Gardner "discovered" this set of intelligences by applying eight criteria. The signs of an intelligence are that (a) it be potentially isolatable by brain damage; (b) there exist special individuals in that domain (e.g., prodigies, idiot savants); (c) the domain have a core set of basic information-processing operations; (d) it have a distinctive developmental history in the life of the individual and a set of specifiable end states indicating expert performance; (e) it exhibit an evolutionary history; (f) there exists evidence for it from experimental psychology; (g) psychometric findings support it; and (h) it be encodable into a symbol system. As a set of criteria for significant clusters of abilities and skills, this list is actually quite good. Taken together these criteria could help ensure a meaningful theory whose concepts had construct validity. However, Gardner doesn't weight these criteria equally. He seems to base his concept of intelligences primarily on criteria h, a, and b—in that order. He makes least use of criteria f and g, virtually ignoring 100 years of research in quantitative and experimental psychology.

Certainly, of the three criteria Gardner emphasizes, the relation of symbol systems to "intelligences" is most important. Tests of intelligence assess knowledge of and ability to manipulate symbols (Tyler, 1963). However, the concept of intelligence in the psychological literature has focused on what Kolers and Smythe (1984) call "consensual, articulated symbols." It is important to establish how humans develop skills in a variety of symbolic domains. Goodman's analysis of types of symbol systems is a good place to start. But the psychological relevance of his distinctions must be established by experiment rather than assumed. Gardner has some interesting ideas and insights about the acquisition and use of symbol systems. It remains for others to test them and establish their theoretical utility and empirical validity.

***Observations*.** The attempt of Gardner and his colleagues to study the development of symbolization across a variety of cognitive and behavioral domains is an important step. We need research that applies the same methods to study the development of different symbol systems and then locates the findings within a unifying theoretical framework. However, we are concerned that Gardner's work does not meet the standards of replicability and public inference normally applied to psychological research: No hypotheses are tested, inferences are post hoc, and the theoretical framework emerges as a consequence of what appears to be informal and ad hoc observation. This is fine for exploratory research, but additional empirical studies must be done before this work contributes to our understanding of symbolic development.

## Conclusions

In our survey of major studies of the development of the symbolic processes, we noted similarities and differences among these approaches. However, little or no borrowing of ideas and information has occurred among theorists.

The critical issues set forth earlier for a theory of symbolic development have been incompletely addressed by these theories. Bates recognizes that signs come in different types, and that these may require different learning processes. Piaget, Werner and Kaplan, and Bruner discuss the role of imagery in symbolic development. Werner and Kaplan use pictorial symbolism as their main source of data, while Piaget argues that imagery is the basis for the logical operations of thinking. Bruner incorporates imagery in his theory only as an intermediate stage in the progression to symbolic (linguistic) thought. Gardner attempts to trace developmental trends in a variety of symbolic domains.

Bates and Piaget are the most successful at tracking the development of the symbolic capacity in infancy. They see symbolism following from more basic cognitive developments, including objectifying vehicles and referents and recognizing these as separate from oneself and from one another. These steps toward metasymbolic awareness can be observed through an analysis of play, imitation, vocalization, and problem solving in infancy.

These theorists have turned to linguistics, philosophy, biology, and anthropology for critical insights. Each theorist builds a conceptual framework in which to place their work, and one must accept their assumptions before accepting the implications of their findings. For example, Piaget assumes that imitation and problem solving represent reconstructive, symbolic imagery; Bates assumes that the requirements for the ontogenetic emergence of certain capacities are the same as for their emergence in the species; Werner and Kaplan assume that presentational symbols are primitive precursors to the discursive symbolism of language, and so forth.

There are important insights concerning symbolism to be taken from each of these authors. None of them provide a theoretically complete treatment of symbolism, but their major findings must be incorporated into such an account.

## ISSUES FOR A THEORY OF SYMBOLISM

Any adequate theory of symbolism will have implications for a large number of important issues in psychology. These include the course of brain development, symbol use in other species (animal and machine), individual differences in modes and styles of thinking, the importance of dreaming and daydreaming, and perhaps even the problems of creativity, discovery, and innovation. A well-developed theory of symbolism will also profoundly affect educational theory and practice. Three selected issues are briefly discussed below, as are possible educational implications of coupling a theory of symbolism with modern computer technology.

### The Course of Brain Development

From both clinical and laboratory evidence, it is clear that the two hemispheres of the brain develop a dramatic separation of function during childhood. In addition to contralateral control over the right and left sides of the body, the hemispheres develop specialized control over particular modes of perceiving and styles of thought.

In general, the left hemisphere controls the verbal processes. It is predominantly involved with analytic, logical thinking; its mode of operation is linear and sequential. The right hemisphere is primarily responsible for visual and spatial thinking. Its mode of operation is parallel and simultaneous; it is involved in holistic, relational modes of perceiving and thinking and is associated with more intuitive, artistic, and integrative mental processes.

The verbal hemisphere assumes a disproportionate significance in determining the mode of thought in our Western culture. Some developmental theorists paint a picture that suggests the ontogenetically natural sequence is from iconic, spatial modes of representation to verbal, linear ones. However, while there is abundant scientific evidence that the hemispheres specialize during childhood, there is absolutely no evidence that the left hemisphere becomes naturally dominant over the right in determining how information is processed and stored. There is, to our knowledge, no natural predisposition toward verbal, linear, analytic, and propositional thinking in the human species.

As children enter the Western educational system, they are bombarded with verbally coded information. They are instructed in reading, writing, and the language arts; most other subjects are also presented verbally. There is nothing ontogenetically inevitable about the preference for left-brain processing that develops in Western society. Rather, we would argue, preference is determined more by experience than by nature. As Ornstein (1972) has observed, this is largely a societal, rather than a neurological, outcome.

Indeed, Gregory (1970) believes the brain, as a biological entity functioning naturally, is essentially an analogue device. Its ability to deal with discrete symbols is an artificial result of the structure of the symbol system that is language. Discursive symbols and our ability to handle them (via a culturally imposed artificial mode of processing) have extended the brain's capabilities and altered its mode of functioning.

## Individual Differences in Modes of Thought

As adults, people differ in their abilities to visualize—in the facility with which they can see things "in the mind's eye." There are people who can visualize objects very well and others who cannot. E. B. Titchener was an eidetic imager who read his lectures from scripts that he visualized, whereas John B. Watson maintained that he had no visual imagery whatever (Sommer, 1978).

Sommer (1978) categorizes people according to whether their dominant mode of thought is verbal or visual. Verbalizers think in words or abstract symbols; thinking is very much like talking to oneself. Visualizers think in images, which may be rich, vivid, and detailed. These modes of thought influence how each type of thinker approaches problems and tasks. Verbalizers approach problems in systematic ways; they proceed linearly, step-by-step. The information being used and the sequence of steps followed are known to the verbalizer, who tends to be aware of his or her problem-solving activities. Visualizers approach problems using spatial images or metaphors; they then attempt to structure and modify their images to move toward a solution. The solution often comes as a surprise, as an insight. It is reached spontaneously and often appears full-blown. The visualizer is often unaware of the thought processes that led to the solution. Bruner (1960) has made a similar distinction in separating analytic and intuitive problem solvers.

## Creativity, Innovation, Discovery

Problem solving and creativity are the results of our ability to represent the environment and manipulate that representation independent of the actual world. We can think of abstract ideas, and reason about things we cannot see. Works of art and literature, on the one hand, and science and mathematics, on the other, are artifacts produced as a result of human mental processes. By developing complex symbol systems, we are able to transcend the sensory world and through reasoning to reach conclusions about things remote from our direct experience (Gregory, 1970). Science is possible only because symbols permit higher order abstractions to be described and manipulated conceptually.

Shepard (1978) has compiled a set of case histories of individuals responsible for "major creative work of the highest order." He cites many examples of scientific, engineering, and artistic innovations resulting from spatial, visual, intuitive thinking. Shepard examines the conditions under which major scientific or technological discoveries were made, including Kekule's development of his theory of molecular structure, J. D. Watson's formulation of the double helix model for DNA, and Einstein's thought processes leading to the special theory of relativity. These case histories reveal the stages of (a) visual representation of the problem, (b) experimenting or playing with the visual images, and (c) sudden, often unexpected, realization of the solution. Shepard views "scientific theories and inventions as externalized mental images" (p. 134).

Such accounts are so frequent in the history of science that Gordon Hewes (1978) concluded that "to an overwhelming extent, science has advanced by finding means to *visualize* relationships and events" (p. 17).

Many authors have advocated training in visualization as a means of improving productive thinking and creativity (Adams, 1974; Arnheim, 1969; McKim, 1972). Sommer (1978) asserts that virtually all researchers who have studied visualization believe that these abilities can be improved through training.

## EDUCATIONAL IMPLICATIONS

Our conceptions of the mental abilities of children are limited by the environments they have typically encountered in our society. Formal educational experiences have been limited for most children until they entered elementary school. "Sesame Street" represented the first nationwide experiment in preschool education. With its format for presenting basic learning material in a captivating manner, it has had a marked effect on children's cognitive skills and their knowledge base (Salomon, 1979). It is now possible to go beyond television and film presentation to a new set of interactive instructional tools. With modern computers we can provide learning environments that are active, individualized, reinforcing, motivating, multimodal, and under the control of the child.

By coupling the computer as a symbol-manipulating device with a theory of symbol acquisition and use, we can develop powerful educational tools. Two major areas in which computers can be of significant educational value are interactive computer graphics and word processing. The ability to effectively use word processing will depend on the child reaching a certain level of verbal skill and motor coordination. But interactive computer graphics may be used to provide visual experiences to children at any age, perhaps from the crib on.

There are obvious possibilities for the use of computer graphics in perceptual learning, pattern recognition, and concept acquisition. These are tasks in which we need to learn what to see or attend to, or how to perceive the relevant aspects of a scene or event. By providing structured experiences on a display screen, we can structure the perceptions of the learner. The combination of computer graphics and voice-simulated output might be used effectively in language acquisition. By selecting, structuring, and systematizing nonverbal experience in conjunction with verbal output, the computer could help the child break the symbolic codes of meaning and syntax. The computer could become a scientifically programmed language input device.

In *Mindstorms*, Seymour Papert (1980) describes how the computer can provide models for children to use in comprehending the world. Indeed, computer graphics can be used to create models to simulate all kinds of "worlds"; it allows people to create and manipulate visual symbols (pictures) in ways unachievable with any other medium. Computer graphics can give concrete realism to abstract ideas; it can be used to illustrate phenomena that do not exist or are difficult to achieve in our physical world.

Computer graphics may also be used to help develop skills in visualization, spatial intuitions, problem solving, and productive thinking. Since imagery seems to be an important adjunct to productive thinking, we need to devise ways to train and enhance skills of visualization. For those with little or no natural imagery, interactive computer graphics may be an important prosthetic and educational device.

Finally, the computer may contribute to more creative thinking in yet another way. Strategies for fostering creativity usually suggest developing other modes of representation than the verbal, thus providing multiple avenues for thinking—including those off the main sequence (Neisser, 1963) or those that tap the unbounded system (Harnad, 1982). But there is another aspect to freeing oneself from the verbal mode: It involves escaping the rules or constraints of denotative representations. Creativity requires the ability to suspend the normal rules of rational thought, to transcend "functional fixedness," to escape the constraints of reality. Computer games and simulations will prove to be valuable educational tools, because they allow us to play with symbols and representations.

## REFERENCES

Adams, J. L. (1974). *Conceptual blockbusting*. San Francisco: Freeman.

Anastasi, A. (1961). *Psychological testing* (2nd ed.). New York: Macmillan.

Arnheim, R. (1969). *Visual thinking*. Berkeley: University of California Press.

Arnheim, R. (1979). Visual thinking in overview. Foreword in C. F. Nodine & D. F. Fisher (Eds.), *Perception and pictorial representation*. New York: Praeger.

Bartley, S. H. (1958). *Principles of perception*. New York: Harper & Brothers.

Bates, E. (1979a). The emergence of symbols: Ontogeny and phylogeny. In W. A. Collins (Ed.), *Children's language and communication* (pp. 121–155). Hillsdale, NJ: Lawrence Erlbaum.

Bates, E., (1979b). *The emergence of symbols: Cognition and communication in infancy*. New York: Academic Press.

Berlyne, D. E. (1965). *Structure and direction in thinking*. New York: John Wiley.

Bower, G. H. (1972). Mental imagery and associative learning. In L. W. Gregg (Ed.), *Cognition in learning and memory* (pp. 51–88). New York: John Wiley

Brewer, W. F. (1974). The problem of meaning and the interrelations of the higher mental processes. In W. B. Weimer & D. S. Palermo (Eds.), *Cognition and the symbolic processes* (pp. 263–298). Hillsdale, NJ: Lawrence Erlbaum.

Bruner, J. S. (1960). *The process of education*. Cambridge, MA: Harvard University Press.

Bruner, J. S. (1973). *Beyond the information given*. New York: W. W. Norton.

Bruner, J. S., Olver, R. R., & Greenfield, P. M. (1966). *Studies in cognitive growth*. New York: John Wiley.

Brunswick, E. (1950). The conceptual framework of psychology. *International Encyclopedia of Unified Science, 1*(10), 1–102.

Cassirer, E. (1944). *An essay on man*. New Haven: Yale University Press.

Cronbach, L. J. (1970). *Essentials of psychological testing* (3rd ed.). New York: Harper & Row.

Davis, M., & Fucigna, C. (1983). *Mapping and drawing: Two channels of graphic symbolization*. Paper presented at the Biennial Meeting of the Society for Research in Child Development, April 1983, Detroit.

Gardner, H. (1982). *Art, mind, and brain*. New York: Basic Books.

Gardner, H. (1983). *Frames of mind*. New York: Basic Books.

Gardner, H. & Wolf, D. (1983). Waves and streams of symbolization: Notes on the development of symbolic capacities in young children. In D. Rogers & J. A. Sloboda (Eds.), *The Acquisition of symbolic skills* (pp. 19–42). New York: Plenum Press.

Golomb, C. (1979). Pretense play: A cognitive perspective. In N. R. Smith & M. B. Franklin (Eds.), *Symbolic functioning in childhood* (pp. 101–115). Hillsdale, NJ: Lawrence Erlbaum.

Goodman, N. (1976).*Languages of art: An approach to a theory of symbols* (2nd ed.). Indianapolis: Hackett.

Gregory, R. L. (1970). *The intelligent eye*. New York: McGraw-Hill.

Haber, R. N. (1969). Eidetic images. *Scientific American, 220*, 36–44.

Harding, C., & Golinkoff, R. (1977). *The origins of intentional vocalizations in prelinguistic infants*. Paper presented at the Biennial Meeting of the Society for Research in Child Development, March 1977, New Orleans.

Harnad, S. (1982). Metaphor and mental duality. In T. W. Simon & R. J. Scholes (Eds.), *Language, mind, and brain* (pp. 189–211). Hillsdale, NJ: Lawrence Erlbaum.

Hewes, G. W. (1978). Visual learning, thinking, and communication in human biosocial evolution. In B. W. Randhawa & W. E. Coffman (Eds.), *Visual learning, thinking, and communication*. (pp. 1–19). New York: Academic Press.

Hochberg, J. E., & Brooks, V. (1962). Pictorial recognition as an unlearned ability: A study of one child's performance. *American Journal of Psychology, 75*, 624–628.

Hockett, C. D. (1960). The origin of speech. *Scientific American, 203*(3), 88–96.

Inhelder, B., & Karmiloff-Smith, A. (1978). Thought and language. In B. Z. Presseisen, D. Goldstein, & M. H. Appel (Eds.), *Topics in cognitive development* (pp. 3–10). New York: Plenum Press.

Kennedy, J. M. (1974). *A psychology of picture perception*. San Francisco: Jossey-Bass.

Kinget, G. M. (1975). *On being human: A systematic view*. New York: Harcourt Brace Jovanovich.

Kohler, W. (1947). *Gestalt psychology*. New York: Liveright.

Kolers, P. A. (1983). Perception and representation. *Annual Review of Psychology, 34*, 129–166.

Kolers, P. A., & Smythe, W. E. (1984). Symbol manipulation: Alternatives to the computational view of mind. *Journal of Verbal Learning and Verbal Behavior, 23*, 289–314.

Langer, S. K. (1957). *Philosophy in a new key: A study in the symbolism of reason, rite, and art*. Cambridge, MA: Harvard University Press.

Loftus, E. (1979). *Eyewitness testimony*. Cambridge, MA: Harvard University Press.

McKim, R. H. (1972). *Experiences in visual thinking*. Monterey, CA: Freeman.

Neisser, U. (1963). The multiplicity of thought. *British Journal of Psychology, 54*, 1–14.

Neisser, U. (1970). Visual imagery as process and experience. In J. S. Antrobus (Ed.), *Cognition and affect* (pp. 159–178). Boston: Little, Brown.

Newell, A. (1981). Physical symbol systems. In D. A. Norman (Ed.), *Perspectives on cognitive science* (pp. 37–85). Norwood, NJ: Ablex.

Newell, A., & Simon, H. (1981). Computer science as empirical inquiry: Symbols and search. In J. Haugeland (Ed.), *Mind design: Philosophy, psychology, artificial intelligence* (pp. 35–66). Cambridge, MA: MIT Press.

Ornstein, R. E. (1972). *The psychology of consciousness*. San Francisco: Freeman.

Osgood, C. E. (1953). *Method and theory in experimental psychology*. New York: Oxford University Press.

Paivio, A. (1972). A theoretical analysis of the role of imagery in learning and memory. In P. W. Sheehan (Ed.), *The function and nature of imagery*. New York: Academic Press.

Paivio, A. (1978). On exploring visual knowledge. In B. S. Randhawa & W. E. Coffman (Eds.), *Visual learning, thinking, and communication* (pp. 113–131). New York: Academic Press.

Papert, S. (1980). *Mindstorms: Children, computers and powerful ideas*. New York: Basic Books.

Peirce, C. S. (1933). *The collected papers of Charles Sanders Peirce*. Cambridge, MA: Harvard University Press.

Phelps, E. (1983). *Meta-symbolic awareness in early symbolic development*. Paper presented at the Biennial Meeting of the Society for Research in Child Development, April 1983, Detroit.

Piaget, J. (1962). *Play, dreams and imitation in childhood*. New York: W. W. Norton.

Piaget, J., & Inhelder, B. (1971). *Mental imagery in the child*. New York: Basic Books.

Pollio, H. R. (1974). *The psychology of symbolic activity*. Reading, MA: Addison-Wesley.

Potter, M. C. (1979). Mundane symbolism: The relations among objects, names and ideas. In N. R. Smith & M. B. Franklin (Eds.), *Symbolic functioning in childhood* (pp. 41–65). Hillsdale, NJ: Lawrence Erlbaum.

Proffit, D. R., & Halwes, T. (1982). Categorical perception: A contractual approach. In W. B. Weimer & D. S. Palermo (Eds.), *Cognition and the symbolic processes* (Vol. 2, pp. 295–319). Hillsdale, NJ: Lawrence Erlbaum.

Reese, H. W. (1977). Imagery and associative memory. In R. V. Kail, Jr., & J. W. Hagen (Eds.), *Perspectives on the development of memory and cognition* (pp. 113–175). Hillsdale, NJ: Lawrence Erlbaum.

Salomon, G. (1979). *Interaction of media, cognition and learning*. San Francisco: Jossey-Bass.

Shepard, R. N. (1978). Externalization of mental images and the act of creation. In B. S. Randhawa & W. E. Coffman (Eds.), *Visual learning, thinking, and communication* (pp. 133–189). New York: Academic Press.

Simon, H. A. (1981). *The sciences of the artificial* (2nd ed.). Cambridge, MA: MIT Press.

Sommer, R. (1978). *The mind's eye: Imagery in everyday life*. New York: Dell.
Sugarman, S. A. (1973). *A description of communicative development in the prelanguage child*. Unpublished honors thesis, Hampshire College, Amherst, MA.
Tyler, L. A. (1963). *Tests and measurements*. Englewood Cliffs, NJ: Prentice-Hall.
Weimer, W. B., & Palermo, D. S. (Eds.). (1974, 1982). *Cognition and the symbolic processes, Vol. 1 and 2*. Hillsdale, NJ: Lawrence Erlbaum.
Werner, H., & Kaplan, B. (1963). *Symbol formation: An organismic developmental approach to the psychology of language and the expression of thought*. New York: John Wiley.
Whitehead, A. N. (1927). *Symbolism: Its meaning and effect*. New York: Macmillan.
Wolf, D. P. (1983). *The origins of distinct symbol domains: The waves of early symbolization—the example of event-structuring*. Paper presented at the Biennial Meeting of the Society for Research in Child Development, April 1983, Detroit.
Wolf, D. P., & Gardner, H. (1979). Style and sequence in early symbolic play. In N. R. Smith & M. B. Franklin (Eds.), *Symbolic functioning in childhood* (pp. 117–138). Hillsdale, NJ: Lawrence Erlbaum.

# 4

# *Lexical Development and Processing in Specific Language Impairment*

LAURENCE B. LEONARD

Specific language impairment is a set of conditions in children characterized by a significant deficit in linguistic functioning in the face of normal hearing, age-appropriate performance on nonverbal psychometric intelligence tests, an unremarkable medical and developmental history, and the absence of gross neurological dysfunction. Children with specific language impairment (hereafter, "language-impaired children") constitute one of the most extensively studied clinical groups in the pediatric population. One reason for this is that the cause of these children's language difficulties is far from clear, opening the door for a wide range of research, speculative as well as theory-driven, into the nature of these children's problems. This research has been concerned with processes such as auditory discrimination, sequencing, memory, symbolic representation, and the planning of hierarchical units. In addition, a great deal of investigative attention has focused on language-impaired children's ability to produce or comprehend various aspects of language (see reviews by Johnston, 1982; Leonard, 1982). As a result, we know much about these children's phonological characteristics, the semantic relations reflected in their early word combinations, the syntactic structures that pose the greatest difficulty for them, and, more recently, these children's understanding and use of the pragmatic aspects of language. One aspect of these children's linguistic functioning about which we know relatively little, however, is their ability to learn, retrieve, and produce words.

The relative neglect of language-impaired children's lexical acquisition and processing is somewhat understandable given the theoretical frameworks that were dominant when investigators turned their attention to the difficulties experienced by these children. However, this neglect is puzzling given that lexical limitations are often part of the collection of behaviors used to identify these children as language impaired in the first place. For example, one of the hallmarks of language impairment is the late emergence of words (Leonard, 1979). Older, verbal language–impaired children, too, are sometimes distinguished on the basis of lexical limitations. For example, one subgroup of language-impaired children is described as exhibiting "word-finding" problems (Schwartz & Solot, 1980).

The purposes of this chapter are to review the available evidence on language-impaired children's lexical difficulties and to determine how our study of these difficulties may contribute to a better understanding both of the condition of language impairment and of children's acquisition, use, and processing of words in general.

There are two major reasons for studying the lexical abilities of language-impaired children. One of these, of course, is a practical one. By determining the specific aspects of lexical acquisition and processing that give language-impaired children the greatest difficulty, we can design more appropriate assessment tools and more effective treatment procedures to assist these children. The other reason is that the study of these children's lexical abilities may contribute to the refinement of theories of lexical acquisition. Allowing for a degree of individual variation, normally developing children show evidence of particular lexical attainments at a particular chronological age, at a particular level of intellectual and motor development, and after having received a particular amount of linguistic exposure. As a result, it is difficult to sort out the factors that are criterial for these attainments from those that are coincidental. On the other hand, language-impaired children provide evidence of these lexical attainments at a different (later) chronological age and level of intellectual and motor development, and after having received a greater amount of linguistic exposure. Consideration of data from language-impaired children, then, may enable investigators to separate previously confounded factors. For example, through study of these children it may be possible to determine whether the words used by children at the single-word stage vary as a function of intelligence and world experience or whether they are the same for all children at this stage, thus reflecting, in all likelihood, the natural constraints on communicating with single words.

## PRESCHOOL-AGED LANGUAGE-IMPAIRED CHILDREN

Most of the early reports of preschool-aged language-impaired children's lexical abilities have been case studies. These studies documented a number of clinical impressions that practitioners had had about these children: (a) They acquire their first words later than normal children, (b) they often acquire subsequent words more slowly than their normal peers, and (c) these children commit lexical errors on occasion. For example, Bender (1940) observed a child who failed to produce words until after age 4-0. A child studied by Werner (1945) did not begin using words until after age 5-0. In one of the few studies dealing with more than a single child, Morley, Court, Miller, and Garside (1955) noted ages of first-word acquisition ranging from 1-6 to 5-0 in 15 language-impaired children. Nice (1925) reported one child's subsequent lexical development. This child had acquired only five words by age 2-0 but had not yet acquired 50 words by age 3-0. Weeks (1974) reported a child whose expressive vocabulary did not reach 50 words until age 2-4. In contrast, it appears that normally developing children reach the milestone of 50 words by approximately age 1-6 (Nelson, 1973).

Information such as the age of first-word emergence and the rate of subsequent lexical development has provided an indication that language-impaired children have lexical learning problems, but these metrics have offered little insight into the nature of such difficulties. Reports of these children's lexical errors might have held more promise in this regard. Instances of "unusual" word usage were seen in the speech of the children studied by Nice (1925), such as "fu" for *blow* and "cuggan" for *sister*, and by Stumpf (1901), such as "aja" as an expression of joy. However, these investigators attributed these lexical forms to production patterns that were continued from the babbling period through their adoption by adults when speaking to the child. Weeks (1975) also observed an unusual form, "geekine," which was used in sentence slots appropriate for content words. However, this form, too, had a plausible explanation; it seemed to mean "this kind" and was used in instances where the child did not seem to know the appropriate word. Finally, other "unusual" errors, such as "brooming" and "barefeeting" noted by Weeks (1975), resemble the principled verb errors reported in the literature on normal language development (Bowerman, 1974; Kuczaj, 1978).

## Early Lexical Characteristics: Some Experimental Findings

Given that language-impaired children acquire their first words at older ages than is ordinarily the case, it is important to consider whether their early words resemble those seen for younger normal children at a similar stage of lexical development. Leonard, Camarata, Rowan, and Chapman (1982) examined the lexical distributions reflected in the spontaneous speech of a group of 3-year-old language-impaired children and a group of younger normal children matched according to expressive vocabulary size. For both groups, vocabularies ranged from 25 to 75 words with a mean of approximately 40 words. Nelson's (1973) lexical classification scheme was employed. No differences between the two groups were observed. General nominals (names of objects, substances, animals such as *block, milk, kitty*) constituted the majority (approximately 55%) of lexical types of each group of children. Words referring to actions and words referring to properties each represented about 12% of the lexical types for each of the groups. For both groups, each of the remaining lexical types constituted less than 10% of the children's expressive vocabularies.

One of the drawbacks to the use of spontaneous speech samples is that it is often unclear whether the observed utterances are representative of the child's speech or reflect a bias attributable to the means used to obtain that particular sample. Leonard et al. (*Early lexical acquisition*, 1982) used this limitation of spontaneous speech samples as a rationale for employing a controlled methodology to study 3-year-old language-impaired children's acquisition of words referring to actions and objects. These investigators used a procedure wherein names of novel objects and (intransitive) actions in uninflected form were presented an equal number of times, along with their object or action referents, in sentence-final position. The children's acquisition of these words in comprehension and production was carefully monitored. By controlling for linguistic input, Leonard et al. attempted to eliminate three of the factors often proposed as contributing to the earlier appearance and greater abundance of object names than action names during early linguistic development: (a) the more frequent appearance of certain object names, (b) their greater salience from occupying particular stressed sentence positions, and (c) their greater transparency from having fewer inflected variants (Gentner, 1982). One factor left remaining is the presumed difference in the nature of the categories reflected in the two lexical types. For example, unlike object names, the meaning of action names includes relational information such as, in the case of the words studied by Leonard et al., the involvement of an agent. The normal and language-impaired children serving as subjects were matched according to expressive vocabulary size, and were operating at the same levels of development as the children studied by Leonard, Camarata, Rowan, and Chapman (1982). Of course, this comparison pits young normal children against a group of children with similar vocabulary sizes but considerably more world experience who are operating at a higher level of intellectual functioning. Nonetheless, for comprehension the two groups acquired the same number of words and, significantly, both learned over twice as many object names as action names. Similar results were seen for production. However, the language-impaired children produced a greater number of action names than did the normal children.

These results were surprising for two reasons. First, it was expected that a smaller object-action name gap would be seen for the older, language-impaired children because these children, with normal intelligence and more world experience, should have been better prepared to grasp the presumed greater complexity of action names. Second, earlier studies had suggested that the subsequent lexical development of language-impaired children was slow. Yet the children in this study acquired as many names in the same time period as the normally developing children. Measures obtained from these children one year later indicated that they still exhibited significant language-learning problems. At this point, however, the acquisition of syntax appeared to be their biggest obstacle.

***Lexical Extension.*** Some caution should be exercised in interpreting the preceding results as support for the view that once lexical development is underway language-impaired children can acquire words with little difficulty. This work examined children's acquisition of words with a single object as referent, and it has been well documented that young normal children apply newly learned words to novel exemplars, even in studies employing experimenter-designed materials (e.g., Nelson & Bonvillian, 1973). This distinction is important, for as Greenberg and Kuczaj (1982) have pointed out, single-object concepts require only that the child can recognize that various instances of an object are instances of the same object. An ability to extend a term to a novel exemplar, on the other hand, is conceptually more complex, because it requires a decision that a particular object is an instance of a particular class of objects. Unfortunately, no study to my knowledge has explored language-impaired children's ability to acquire new words and extend them to other appropriate but newly introduced referents. Until these children's ability to use words reflecting such object-class concepts is examined, conclusions concerning their lexical skills must be drawn cautiously.

Although studies have not yet focused on preschool-aged language-impaired children's lexical extensions to novel but appropriate exemplars, preliminary evidence of a different type suggests that these children may be able to extend words to a range of referents. Inappropriate word extensions were the focus of a study by Chapman, Leonard, Rowan, and Weiss (1983). Nine of the 3-year-old language-impaired children studied by Leonard et al. (*Early lexical acquisition*, 1982) were also the subjects in this investigation. Each child was observed for 11 sessions. Cases in which a word appeared to be extended in production to an inappropriate referent were noted and subsequently tested more systematically in both comprehension and production. The percentage of words showing inappropriate word extension ranged from 3 to 63 across the children. The mean (19%) does not differ appreciably from the percentages reported to date for younger normal children (Gruendel, 1977; Rescorla, 1980). For the majority of cases, the referent receiving the inappropriate label was both perceptually and functionally similar to referents for which the label was appropriate. Of the 20 words tested in detail, 7 proved to be cases of analogy, where the child gave evidence of producing and comprehending the appropriate label and had apparently used the originally observed term to express a similarity between referents of the two classes. Only one case of overextension in both production and comprehension was observed, and no cases were reported of overextension in production but with appropriate comprehension. The latter finding in particular is surprising, for language-impaired children have often been described as experiencing word retrieval problems, as noted below. However, 50 of the 20 inappropriate word extensions tested represented an apparent competition between an appropriate and inappropriate term in production. This usage may have reflected a transitional point when a child's inappropriate name for a referent was giving way to the correct name. However, it is also possible that such usage may have reflected intermittent difficulties in word retrieval. Inappropriate word extensions of this type have been reported in only a few normally developing children (e.g., Gruendel, 1977).

***Comprehension-Production Relationships.*** Language-impaired children have been observed to differ in the extent to which their problems may include a deficit in comprehension ability or represent a problem limited primarily to production ability (e.g., Menyuk, 1978a). In many circles, these differences have led to the establishment of clinical categories representing primary areas of disturbance. For example, Benton (1978) has distinguished "expressive" language disorder from "receptive-expressive" language disorder. A careful inspection of the literature indicates that language-impaired children almost always exhibit production limitations, but that their comprehension abilities may range from those appropriate for their chronological age to those approaching the level of deficiency seen for their abilities in production. However, these descriptions have been based on results from rather global language measures, and therefore the relationship between lexical comprehension and production in these children has not been clear.

Some evidence of the lexical comprehension-production relationships among language-impaired children is available from Leonard et al. (*Early lexical acquisition*, 1982). These investigators studied only language-impaired children who showed some degree of comprehension deficit (at least 6 months below age level) on a global language measure. As noted above, these 3-year-old language-impaired children possessed expressive vocabularies of approximately 40 words on average. Due to the risks involved in assuming comparability of correct response probability on the comprehension and production tasks, Leonard et al. computed the percentage of experimental words the children produced out of the total that they comprehended. The language-impaired children were then compared to the younger normal children on this measure. No differences were seen; both groups produced approximately 30% of the words that they showed evidence of comprehending. Thus, although language-impaired children with age-level comprehension skills were excluded from this study, the same comprehension-production gaps often reported in the normal child were seen in these children as well. On a qualifying note, Leonard et al. observed several cases, for both the normal and language-impaired children, where an experimental word was produced but seemingly not comprehended. This type of finding has also been reported by several investigators of normally developing children's lexical development (e.g., Nelson & Bonvillian, 1978) and constitutes a phenomenon in great need of closer scrutiny.

## SCHOOL-AGED LANGUAGE-IMPAIRED CHILDREN

Reports of the lexical limitations of children with specific language impairment come from a variety of sources in the literature. One major reason for this is that children who continue to exhibit language-learning problems by school age are often given the psychoeducational label *learning disabled*. Of course, not all learning disabled children, even those experiencing difficulties with reading, give evidence of oral language deficits. For this reason, the literature included here is concerned only with children who were identified as having problems with oral language along with any specific educational deficits they may have exhibited.

The lexical limitation most frequently identified in the literature on school-age language-impaired children is a "word-finding" problem, that is, a problem generating the particular word called for in a situation (Kerschensteiner & Huber, 1975; Rapin & Wilson, 1978; Weiner, 1974). These difficulties have been variously described as "lexical look-up" problems (Menyuk, 1975b, 1978) or problems involving "delayed speed of word retrieval" (Schwartz & Solot, 1980). According to the clinical literature, the chief symptoms of word-finding difficulties are unusually long pauses in speech, frequent circumlocution, and/or frequent use of nonspecific words such as *that* or *it*.

The term *word-finding problem* has often been used to suggest that the child's difficulty with generating the appropriate word is due to a deficit in retrieval. That is, the word is present in memory, but the child uses an inefficient or inappropriate means of accessing it. However, clinical reports have not always provided evidence that the words were known by the children. A first step in providing this type of control has been through the use of formal naming tasks.

## Experimentation with Picture-Naming Tasks

The most frequently used naming task has been the confrontation naming task, in which pictures of objects are presented that the child is asked to name. Typically, language-impaired children commit a greater number of errors on this task than do normally developing children of the same age, even when they can identify the correct picture on a comprehension task (e.g., Rubin & Liberman, in press; Wiig, Semel, & Nystrom, 1982). Of course, because these children have language-learning limitations, the fact that they fail to name the depicted objects as accurately as their more linguistically advanced peers may simply mean that these children do not yet know the names of the objects well enough to retrieve them for production. A more telling measure is the speed with which the child produces the appropriate name. To ensure that the words are known by the children, response latencies are typically computed only for those pictures that are named correctly.

Probably the first study that examined naming latencies in language-impaired children was conducted by Anderson (1965). Language-impaired children (mean age 8-1) and chronological age–matched normal children named line drawings of common objects. Naming times were significantly slower for the language-impaired children. More recently, Wiig, Semel, and Nystrom (1982) compared the naming times of language-impaired children (mean age 8-1) and chronological age–matched normal children on tasks of pictured object naming and color and/or form (e.g., red triangle, blue square) naming. The language-impaired children showed slower naming times. It should be noted that the investigators' measure of naming time, the total time required to name all of the stimuli in each task, included latencies for incorrect responses.

Unfortunately, slow naming times even for correctly named pictures do not ensure that the children's poorer performance was attributable to retrieval problems. Storage-elaboration limitations may have played a role. Here, the degree to which a word is known is a relevant factor. Words that are better known are characterized as having stronger associations in semantic memory (e.g., Anderson, 1976) or, alternatively, more distinct representations in memory (e.g., Landauer, 1975) than less well-known words. In either case, retrieval would be more rapid for the better known words. Given that language-impaired children perform below the level of peers on tests of linguistic (including lexical) functioning, it would be safe to conclude that the same names may have fewer distinct representations in memory (or less associative strength) for the language-impaired children than for the normal children. Some evidence provided by Rubin and Liberman (in press) lends support to this view. These investigators analyzed the naming errors of language-impaired children ranging in age from 4-3 to 12-7 and identified a number of instances where the child only approximated the correct form of the word (e.g., "helidakter" for *helicopter*, "preztl" for *pretzel*).

Leonard, Nippold, Kail, and Hale (1983) attempted to disentangle storage from retrieval factors in language-impaired children's naming by using pictured objects whose names varied considerably in their frequency of occurrence. Normally developing children name objects with frequently occurring names more rapidly than objects with less frequently occurring names (e.g., Milianti & Cullinan, 1974). The explanations for this finding are precisely those given above, as frequency of occurrence is taken as an indirect estimate of the degree to which an individual knows a word. The paradigm used by Leonard et al. was sensitive to those retrieval factors related to frequency of occurrence. That is, if language-impaired children used frequency to direct retrieval in a manner akin to that of normal children, but did so more slowly, then the slope of the function relating naming time to frequency would be greater (i.e., steeper) for these children.

Younger (mean age 8-3) and older (mean age 11-10) language-impaired children served as subjects. These children's naming performance was compared to that of normally developing children matched according to chronological age and younger normally developing children matched with the language-impaired children according to composite language age derived from standardized language test results. The language-impaired children named the pictures less rapidly than their agemates, but more rapidly than the language controls. For all groups, naming times were significantly related to frequency of occurrence. Significantly, no differences were seen among the groups in the slope of the function relating frequency to naming time. Leonard et al. (1983) concluded that both storage and retrieval limitations may have accounted for the language-impaired children's performance, but if retrieval problems played a role, they must have affected those components of naming time uninfluenced by frequency of occurrence.

Ceci (1983) employed a different type of paradigm to examine the naming behavior of language-impaired children. He proposed a two-process model of semantic processing. According to Ceci, automatic processing occurs in cases where the presentation of a stimulus automatically activates the corresponding pathways containing its representation in memory. Presumably, this type of processing takes place without intention or awareness. Purposive processing, on the other hand, is a strategic form of processing which requires a conscious and deliberate plan to retrieve a word. Ceci suspected that language-impaired children's problems may be more related to the latter.

Ten-year-old language-impaired children, age-matched normal children, and 4-year-old normal children participated in the study. To ensure that all children could recognize the pictorial stimuli and could correctly name the pictures, each child was given considerable practice naming the pictures prior to the experiment proper. During the experiment, all picture presentations were preceded by a prime phrase. The condition designed to promote automatic processing and that designed to promote purposive processing were distinguished by the ratio of semantically related primes and pictures (e.g., "Here's an animal"—HORSE) to unrelated primes and pictures (e.g., "Here's a fruit"—HORSE). In the automatic processing condition, unrelated primes and pictures outnumbered related pairs and pictures four to one. The reverse ratio was used in the purposive processing condition. Neutral pairs (e.g., "Here's something you know"—HORSE) were also included in each condition to serve as a baseline by which one could judge the relative costs and benefits of the related and unrelated pair manipulations.

The results proved quite revealing. In the automatic processing condition, all three groups of children showed a moderate decrease in naming time, relative to neutral pairs, for related pairs and no increase in naming time for unrelated pairs. Identical results were seen for the language-impaired children and normal 4-year-olds in the purposive processing condition. However, in this condition the normal 10-year-olds showed a larger decrease in naming time for related pairs and a moderate to large increase in naming time for unrelated pairs. Ceci (1983) concluded from these findings that only the normally developing 10-year-olds actually engaged in active processing of the stimuli when the conditions indicated that this would be a useful approach to the task. Such processing resulted in even faster naming times for most items. However, on those occasions where the picture was other than that anticipated (unrelated pairs), naming time suffered. Ceci proposed that language-impaired children, like younger normal children, fail to engage in this type of purposive processing. Thus, these children seem to be exhibiting a strategic deficit.

## Experimenting with Recall Tasks

Kail, Hale, Leonard, and Nippold (1984) employed recall tasks to study the contribution of storage-elaboration and retrieval limitations in language-impaired children. One source of evidence was a comparison between performance on free and cued recall. Randomized lists of words from four different categories were presented to the children for recall. On free recall trials, the children recalled the words in any order. On cued recall trials, the category names (e.g., *animals*) were presented during the period for recall, and the children were asked to recall all words presented from that category. Kail et al. reasoned that if language-impaired children simply have less extensive lexical knowledge than normal children (i.e., a storage-elaboration limitation), they should recall fewer words in both free and cued recall. On the other hand, if language-impaired children's difficulties reside with the retrieval of adequately stored words, then differences between the two groups of children should be greater in free recall than in cued recall, because the category cues should facilitate the language-impaired children's otherwise inefficient word retrieval.

Repeated free recall served as the second source of evidence in this study. After the children had completed a free recall trial, they were asked to recall the words in the list again. This procedure was repeated twice, resulting in three recall attempts following one presentation of the word list. Kail et al. (1984) used a mathematical model to derive parameters of storage, retrieval, and forgetting to account for the patterns of performance that were possible on the three recall attempts. Several versions of the model were then fit to the data to determine which was the most consistent with the children's recall patterns.

Language-impaired children (mean age 10-0), age-matched normal children, and language-matched normal children served as subjects. Regarding free and cued recall, the language-impaired children recalled fewer words in each condition than the age controls and the same number as the language controls. For all three groups, cued recall was better than free recall. The difference between cued and free recall was no greater in the language-impaired children than in the other two subject groups. Regarding repeated free recall, the model that best fit the data for the language-impaired children and their age controls was one that assumed that the two groups differed in both storage and retrieval, but not forgetting. For the language-impaired children and their language controls, the best-fitting model was one in which retrieval and forgetting were similar in the two groups, but language-impaired children were more likely to store a word. Thus, both the free versus cued recall and repeated free recall analyses in the Kail et al. (1984) study found evidence for storage-elaboration limitations in the language-impaired children relative to normally developing children of the same age. However, only the repeated free recall task yielded data suggesting the possibility of an additional retrieval deficit in these children. This finding suggests that language-impaired children may experience retrieval problems, but only in cases where retrieval must be guided by constraints other than semantic categories and, given the findings of Leonard et al. (1983), frequency of occurrence.

Language-impaired children's word recall in larger, more natural linguistic contexts was examined by Leonard, Kail, and Hale (1984). The task employed was an adaptation of one used by Perfetti and Goldman

(1976). The children listened to stories containing brief pauses during which probe words were presented. Upon hearing each probe word, the children attempted to recall the word that had immediately followed the probe word in the story. The number of words intervening between the target word and the prompt to recall the word exceeds children's memory span for unrelated words. Therefore, successful performance on this task requires the child to make use of linguistic constituents in the form of clauses or sentences as units of analysis in short-term memory in order to recover the required word. The stories were constructed to examine the effects of two variables: (a) the distance, in number of words, between the target word and the recall prompt and (b) the type of clause, main or subordinate, in which the target word appeared. The types of words serving as targets were the same across all conditions. However, the probe or prompting words varied. For main clauses they were nouns or pronouns, and for subordinate clauses they were adverbials (e.g., *when*).

Language-impaired children age 8-0 to 13-0 served as subjects along with age-matched and language-matched normal children. The language-impaired children recalled fewer words than the age controls. However, the profiles of performance were identical in the two groups. Both groups showed higher recall scores when fewer words separated the target word from the probe word than when a greater number of words intervened, and both groups recalled a greater number of words from main clauses than from subordinate clauses. The performance of the language controls was similar to that of the language-impaired children in number of words recalled and in profile.

The stories used in this study were designed to be comprehensible to the language-impaired children. Indeed, a comprehension test dealing with material in the stories was administered following the task. The results indicated these children demonstrated adequate understanding. Thus, the poorer recall performance of these children relative to age controls was probably due to factors more closely related to recall.

The recall task employed in this study does not permit a differentiation of word retrieval and lexical storage-elaboration factors. For example, words may have been poorly recalled because the representations of these words in memory had few, or weak, associations. However, poor recall could also have occurred if the child had difficulty using the probe words to guide retrieval. Although the specific sources of the language-impaired children's poorer recall are not clear, the identical profiles seen in the language-impaired children and their age controls are significant. Although not performing at age level, the language-impaired children could use clauses as units of analysis in short-term memory and were no more influenced by the syntactic characteristics of the clause (subordinate vs. main) than were the children who were free of language-learning problems.

## CONCLUSIONS

There are a great many unanswered questions concerning language-impaired children's lexical development and processing. However, it is also clear that if the evidence available to date holds up under closer scrutiny, it will offer a number of suggestions for assessment and remediation with these children.

### Suggestions for Preschool-Aged Language-Impaired Children

With regard to younger language-impaired children, it does not appear that special clinical attention must be directed toward particular lexical categories rather than others. That is, judging from the lexical distributions reflected in language-impaired children's spontaneous speech, and their ability to learn action names as well as object names in experimental tasks, these children do not seem to be having specific problems with any particular lexical category.

In fact, the experimental task findings also suggest that the long-standing practice of teaching a number of object names to language-impaired children may be consistent with these children's lexical learning strengths, at least in comparison to their learning of words referring to actions. This characteristic of language-impaired children is similar to that seen in normal children. Yet these same findings suggest caution in using normal-child language findings as the sole basis for lexical training programs for children with specific language impairment. As a case in point, language-impaired children seem less averse to attempting action words than do normal children at the same general level of language development.

Research is clearly needed on language-impaired children's ability to extend words to new exemplars. We simply do not know whether these children show the same facility as young normal children in applying a newly learned word to novel yet appropriate instances of a concept. Such information would be of great value in determining a criterion of presumed mastery when teaching language-impaired children new words.

However, there is at least preliminary evidence that these children are capable of extending terms. This evidence comes in the form of these children's statements of analogy and occasional overextensions. It should be noted that in each of these cases, the child gives the impression of producing an inappropriate word extension. Thus, it is clear that comprehension testing should be conducted along with production testing when assessing the lexical abilities of language-impaired children. For instances in which the child produces a word to draw an analogy between two referents, treatment would not be indicated, and this type of response might even be encouraged. For cases of overextension in comprehension as well as production, intervention is probably in order. For example, a contrast approach might be applied where the clinician teaches the child the appropriate name for a referent to which another word had been extended and at the same time attempts to maintain the child's use of the extended term as the name for referents for which it is still appropriate.

Cases have also been noted in the literature where both inappropriate and appropriate terms are applied to a referent. Here, too, future research is needed. If such cases represent a transitional point where an inappropriate term is giving way to the appropriate name in the child's lexicon, training for such words should be given low priority. However, if these occurrences reflect genuine cases of confusion on the part of the child, the clinician may need to assist the child in learning the criterial attributes and boundaries of the concepts involved.

Results from experimental studies involving exposure of novel words indicate that young language-impaired children can learn to produce as well as comprehend new words without intervention focusing directly on production skills. In these studies, the children were free to imitate the experimenter and/or produce the words spontaneously. However, unlike many commonly used clinical approaches, production attempts were not solicited until posttesting. The word-exposure procedure had a greater impact on the children's comprehension than on their production. However, the same was true for the normal children serving as the comparison group, and in neither case was the ratio of comprehended words to words produced greater than that typically reported for this stage of development in normal children. Thus, this procedure should not be regarded as placing too great an emphasis on comprehension and may serve as a satisfactory approach to lexical training with language-impaired children.

## Suggestions for School-Aged Language-Impaired Children

A number of the studies of school-aged language-impaired children were concerned with uncovering the role of storage-elaboration and retrieval factors in word-finding problems. The evidence of storage-elaboration limitations in these children is undeniable. However, this is not simply a statement that these children, with documented language-learning problems, have acquired fewer words than normal children of the same age. Rather, once words have been acquired, in the sense that they are comprehended and produced routinely, their representations in memory seem less elaborate than is the case for children with normal language.

These findings indicate the importance of determining the degree to which a word is known by a child. A language-impaired child's appropriate production of a word does not seem to constitute a sufficiently stringent criterion for assuming adequate lexical knowledge. More detailed assessment is in order.

The interpretation that words are less elaborate in the semantic memory of language-impaired children suggests certain types of lexical training activities that may be appropriate. These activities would have as their aim the strengthening of the child's representations of the words in memory. This might be accomplished by providing the child with a richer base of information about each word such as the primary and secondary functions of the referent (e.g., the fastening and decorative functions of *cufflinks*), a range of nonidentical exemplars for each word (e.g., army, football, and hockey *helmets*), and referents from similar categories for purposes of comparison and contrast (e.g., similarities and differences among snakes and lizards).

To date the evidence of word retrieval limitations in language-impaired children is not as extensive as it is for limitations in storage-elaboration. However, two studies provide some evidence for such limitations. First, in repeated free recall tasks, language-impaired children were less likely than normal children to successfully retrieve a word, even when it had been stored initially. Second, purposive processing, where one spontaneously engages in a conscious and deliberate plan to retrieve a word, seems weak in these children. Data from cued recall tasks suggest that when directed by others, language-impaired children may be able to engage in such strategic behavior. For children showing retrieval limitations, then, training that emphasizes the spontaneous use of retrieval cues seems most appropriate. For example, the child might be taught to use superordinate category names (e.g., *furniture*), the initial consonants of words (e.g., [s]), or carrier phrases describing the object's function (e.g., "When I watch TV I sit on the ______") to retrieve names he or she is having difficulty accessing.

Finally, it appears that language-impaired children have some ability to use linguistic constituents such as clauses and sentences as units of analysis in memory in order to recover a required word. Thus, although it will be necessary to use a restricted level of syntactic structure in this material, given the known difficulties these children have in the comprehension of syntax, these findings nonetheless suggest that activities designed to aid the child's use of retrieval strategies can make use of natural language and need not be restricted to word lists.

## Theoretical Implications

The necessary distinction between words and concepts has long been recognized. Among the reasons for this are that words are linguistic in nature and hence may pertain only to those concepts that are relevant to communicate, and that even communicable concepts may be partitioned into words in different ways in different languages. In spite of this distinction, most theories of lexical development do not provide a clear separation of semantic memory from real-world knowledge (Nelson, 1978).

This constitutes one reason why study of the lexical development of language-impaired children is important. By virtue of their older ages and age-appropriate performance on nonverbal intelligence tests, these children show a discrepancy between their semantic development and their real-world knowledge. The overall similarities seen in the lexical development and processing of young normal children and older children with specific language impairment, then, suggest that the lack of distinction between semantic and real-world knowledge may not be a limitation of current theories. Further, the findings at this point suggest that previous proposals that young children's representations of words do not include episodic information as central components are probably correct. If such information were included, then language-impaired children, who have had much greater opportunity to learn the defining characteristics of words, would show lexical behavior quite different from that of younger normal children.

At the same time, the similarities in the lexical characteristics of language-impaired and young normal children suggest that even when children have had considerable world experience and demonstrate an ability to perceive and understand the events around them, the type of information they convey through words is still closely related to their vocabulary sizes. This clearly suggests that lexical acquisition and usage are separable from nonlinguistic aspects of development. However, it does not provide us with a precise indication of the source of language-impaired children's lexical constraints. Possibly, there may be a ceiling on the number of words these children can acquire in a period of time, and the ones they acquire are those that are most communicative. The similarities among language-impaired and young normal children would thus be explained on the basis that the latter group of children, too, select the words that are most communicative in the early going. A second possible source of constraints is that the words used by language-impaired, and young normal, children are those in which the word-to-concept mappings are the easiest to solve.

The second possibility is more likely. Although some of the words first acquired by both groups of children are highly functional and likely acquired early for just this reason, the lexical distributions of these children suggest a major role played by the mapping problem. Object names have a particularly transparent semantic mapping to the perceptual-conceptual word, and such words dominate the early lexicons of these children. However, although infants and toddlers demonstrate an ability to perceive the relations involved in actions, there are fewer psychological constraints on how these relations are parceled into lexical categories. Thus, children are less able to guess the meanings of action names solely on the basis of world knowledge (Gentner, 1982). The same might also be said for nouns applying to abstract notions (e.g., *job*), and, of course, such words are not seen at all in the early lexicons of younger normal or language-impaired children.

If we assume that the words used by school-aged language-impaired children were acquired at a later age (and at a more advanced level of experience and nonverbal intelligence) than the same words used by normal children, then another conclusion concerning the separation of lexical acquisition and nonlinguistic development is possible. Evidently, regardless of a child's world knowledge, the elaborateness of a word's representation in memory develops gradually. This finding, too, suggests the significant role that word-to-concept mapping plays in children's lexical development.

## REFERENCES


Anderson, J. D. (1965). Initiatory delay in congenital aphasoid conditions. *Cerebral Palsy Journal, 26,* 9–12.

Anderson, J. R. (1976). *Language, memory, and thought.* Hillsdale, NJ: Lawrence Erlbaum.

Bender, J. (1940). A case of delayed speech. *Journal of Speech Disorders, 5,* 363.

Benton, A. (1978). The cognitive functioning of children with developmental aphasia. In M. Wyke (Ed.), *Developmental dysphasia* (pp. 43–62). London: Academic Press.

Bowerman, M. (1974). Learning the structure of causative verbs: A study of the relationship of cognitive, semantic, and syntactic development. *Papers and Reports on Child Language Development, 8,* 142–178.

Ceci, S. (1983). Automatic and purposive semantic processing characteristics of normal and language/learning–disabled children. *Developmental Psychology, 19,* 427–439.

Chapman, K., Leonard, L., Rowan, L., & Weiss, A. (1983). Inappropriate word extensions in the speech of young language–disordered children. *Journal of Speech and Hearing Disorders, 48,* 55–62.

Gentner, D. (1982). Why nouns are learned before verbs: Linguistic relativity versus natural partitioning. In S. Kuczaj (Ed.), *Language development: Vol. 2. Language, thought, and culture* (pp. 301–332). Hillsdale, NJ: Lawrence Erlbaum.

Greenberg, J., & Kuczaj, S. (1982). Towards a theory of substantive word–meaning acquisition. In S. Kuczaj (Ed.), *Language development: Vol. 1. Syntax and semantics* (pp. 275–311). Hillsdale, NJ: Lawrence Erlbaum.

Gruendel, J. (1977). Referential extension in early language development. *Child Development, 48,* 1567–1576.

Johnston, J. (1982). The language disordered child. In N. Lass, J. Northern, D. Yoder, & L. McReynolds (Eds.), *Speech, language and hearing* (Vol. 2, pp. 780–801). Philadelphia: W. B. Saunders.

Kail, R., Hale, C., Leonard, L., & Nippold, M. (1984). Lexical storage and retrieval in language–impaired children. *Applied Psycholinguistics, 5*, 37–49.

Kerschensteiner, M., & Huber, W. (1975). Grammatical impairment in developmental aphasia. *Cortex, 11*, 264–282.

Kuczaj, S. (1978). Why do children fail to overgeneralize the progressive inflection? *Journal of Child Language, 5*, 167–171.

Landauer, T. (1975). Memory without organization: Properties of a model with random storage and undirected retrieval. *Cognitive Psychology, 7*, 495–531.

Leonard, L. (1979). Language impairment in children. *Merrill-Palmer Quarterly, 25*, 205–232.

Leonard, L. (1982). The nature of specific language impairment. In S. Rosenberg (Ed.), *Handbook of applied psycholinguistics* (pp. 295–327). Hillsdale, NJ: Lawrence Erlbaum.

Leonard, L., Camarata, S., Rowan, L., & Chapman, K. (1982). The communicative functions of lexical usage by language impaired children. *Applied Psycholinguistics, 3*, 109–125.

Leonard, L., Kail, R., & Hale, C. (1984). *Word recall in discourse by children with specific language impairment*. Paper presented to the International Congress for the Study of Child Language, July 9–13, Austin, TX.

Leonard, L., Nippold, M, Kail, R., & Hale, C. (1983). Picture naming in language–impaired children. *Journal of Speech and Hearing Research, 26*, 609–615.

Leonard, L., Schwartz, R., Chapman, K., Rowan, L., Prelock: P., Terrell, B., Weiss, A., & Messick, C. (1982). Early lexical acquisition in children with specific language impairment. *Journal of Speech and Hearing Research, 25*, 554–564.

Menyuk, P. (1975a). The language–impaired child: Linguistic or cognitive impairment? In D. Aaronson & R. Rieber (Eds.), *Developmental psycholinguistics and communication disorders* (pp. 59–69). New York: New York Academy of Sciences.

Menyuk, P. (1975b). Children with language problems: What's the problem? In D. Dato (Ed.), *Georgetown University Roundtable on Languages and Linguistics* (pp. 129–144). Washington, DC: Georgetown University Press.

Menyuk, P. (1978). Linguistic problems in children with developmental dysphasia. In M. Wyke (Ed.), *Developmental dysphasia* (pp. 135–158). London: Academic Press.

Milianti, F., & Cullinan, W. (1974). Effects of age and word frequency on object recognition and naming in children. *Journal of Speech and Hearing Research, 17*, 373–385.

Morley, M., Court, D., Miller, H., & Garside, R. (1955). Delayed speech and developmental aphasia. *British Medical Journal, 2*, 463–467.

Nelson, K. (1973). Structure and strategy in learning to talk. *Monograph of the Society for Research in Child Development, 38*, Serial No. 149.

Nelson, K. (1978). Semantic development and the development of semantic memory. In K. E. Nelson (Ed.), *Children's language* (Vol. 1, pp. 39–80). New York: Gardner Press.

Nelson, K. E., & Bonvillian, J. (1973). Concepts and words in the 18-month-old: Acquiring concept names under controlled conditions. *Cognition, 2*, 435–450.

Nelson, K. E., & Bonvillian, J. (1978). Early language development: Conceptual growth and related processes between 2 and 4½ years of age. In K. E. Nelson (Ed.), *Children's language* (Vol. 1, pp. 467–556). New York: Gardner Press.

Nice, M. (1925). A child who would not talk. *Pedagogical Seminary, 32*, 105–144.

Perfetti, C., & Goldman, S. (1976). Discourse memory and reading comprehension skill. *Journal of Verbal Learning and Verbal Behavior, 14*, 33–42.

Rapin, I, & Wilson, B. (1978). Children with developmental language disability: Neurological aspects and assessment. In M. Wyke (Ed.), *Developmental dysphasia* (pp. 13–41). London: Academic Press.

Rescorla, R. (1980). Overextension in early language development. *Journal of Child Language, 7*, 321–335.

Rubin, H., & Liberman, I. (1983). Exploring the oral and written language errors made by language disabled children. *Annals of Dyslexia, 33*, 110–120.

Schwartz, E., & Solot, C. (1980). Response patterns characteristic of verbal expressive disorders. *Language, Speech, and Hearing Services in Schools, 11*, 139–144.

Stumpf, C. (1901). Eigenartige sprachliche entwicklung eines kendes. *Zeitschrifft für Paedogogische und Psychologie, 6*, 420–447.

Weeks, T. (1974). *The slow speech development of a bright child*. Lexington, MA: Heath.

Weeks, T. (1975). The use of nonverbal communication by a slow speech developer. *Word, 27*, 460–472.

Weiner, P. (1974). A language-delayed child at adolescence. *Journal of Speech and Hearing Disorders, 39*, 202–212.

Werner, L. (1945). Treatment of a child with delayed speech. *Journal of Speech Disorders, 10*, 329–334.

Wiig, E., Semel, E., & Nystrom, L. (1982). Comparison of rapid naming abilities in language–learning–disabled and academically achieving eight-year-olds. *Language, Speech and Hearing Services in Schools, 13*, 11–23.

SECTION III

# *Language and Cognitive Development*

RICHARD F. CROMER, EDITOR

# 5

# *Differentiating Language and Cognition*

RICHARD F. CROMER

What effects does language have on thought? This question has interested philosophers and psychologists for many years. However, it is not a question of merely academic interest. Many people are concerned that the language we speak may affect our thoughts in subtle ways. Does sexist terminology and use, for example, lead people to believe implicitly that male domination in a number of areas is a natural state of affairs? Will a conscious effort to change language lead to a change in the way we think about the world? Conversely, should we ask instead whether the thoughts we have affect aspects of our language structure and language use? To continue the example, does sexist language merely mirror the commonly held assumptions in our culture, regardless of how they arose? To use another example, did the conscious suppression of the distinction between polite and familiar forms in French and in Russian at the times of revolutions in their respective countries affect people's thinking, or were these language forms reflections of preexisting categories that could not be changed merely by changing language patterns?

The language-thought question has more recently been broadened in various ways. One no longer considers thoughts in isolation; in addition, the effects of causation are no longer viewed in an all-or-none fashion, but are seen as partial and bi-directional. These two changes now make it more common to pose the question, "What is the relation between language and cognition?" One of the paths to future progress requires the differentiation of the two terms *language* and *cognition*. This is, of course, not the only way to proceed on this interesting issue. Atkinson (1982), who is highly critical of the state of child language development theory, appears to suggest that the only true advances in attempts to relate linguistic and cognitive development will occur when adequate formal descriptions of both systems are written which will allow their properties to be systematically related. As he puts it, in terms of linguistic descriptions, "the rules we formulate should have identifiable properties for which we can search in non-linguistic cognitive domains" (p. 203).

Linguists have indeed made important contributions in writing formal descriptions of linguistic structure, but psychologists have not been notably successful in writing formal descriptions of cognitive structures to which they can apply. Atkinson is pessimistic about the ability of psychologists and psycholinguists to arrive at meaningful conclusions concerning the relation between cognition and language until advances are made in the formal descriptions of linguistic and nonlinguistic cognitive functioning. There are, however, problems even in this enterprise. For example, there is no reason to expect that the same formalism would be appropriate to both fields. Furthermore, Atkinson fails to consider advances made possible by considering alternative approaches to the language-cognition relation. (See Bloom, 1984, for criticisms of Atkinson's approach as being limited.) Although it would mark a significant advance to be able to provide formal descriptions of the linguistic and nonlinguistic cognitive representations, a great deal can be learned of the relation between the two domains by the study of impaired functioning. Unlike Atkinson, I believe that plausible reasons can be advanced for postulating particular effects (or lack of them) of one domain on the other even in the absence of fully specified formal descriptions.

In this chapter I argue that a good deal about the relation between language and cognition can be learned by the study of language disorders and language deficiencies evidenced by various language disordered groups and individuals. The terms *cognition* and *language* are defined and differentiated. Studies of language functioning in the mentally retarded are then reviewed, both to demonstrate the need for such differentiation and to illustrate problems in the semantic component and possibly the morphological component of language in mentally retarded individuals.

## DIFFERENTIATING COGNITION

The *Oxford English Dictionary* (1933) defines cognition as "the action or faculty of knowing; . . . a product of such an action." This definition is interesting because it incorporates two important aspects that have not always been clearly separated by psychologists. First, there is the action of knowing, or what we might more commonly refer to as the mental processing of information. Second, there are the products of that faculty—the cognitions or concepts themselves. The former has been the primary concern of cognitive psychologists, especially those who take an information processing approach to cognition, while the latter has been the interest of philosophers and anthropologists and those psychologists who are more interested in the products of the thought processes. These two aspects of cognition also have implications for the type of research undertaken. Process-oriented researchers and theorists, for example, study human cognitive processing mechanisms in general and are often interested in cases where particular functions are impaired. Product-oriented researchers are interested in the cognitions themselves and often study cross-cultural differences in the content of thought or individual differences in attainment among members of the same culture. The actual content of the thoughts, of course, may reflect underlying processes. In the Piagetian framework, for example, the contents of thought are used to infer underlying cognitive structures and operations that vary at different stages of psychological development. These structures and operations are postulated on the basis of evidence other than the specific thought contents, and that is why Piagetians place great emphasis on *how* children at various stages reach their conclusions.

One important distinction, then, that can be made within *cognition* is between cognitive processes, on the one hand, and the concepts or "cognitions" to which these processes give rise on the other. Cognitive processes refer to the underlying faculties and representational operations that make thought possible. These include psychological faculties (e.g., memory and attention), the mechanisms that underlie these faculties (basic perceptual mechanisms, storage capacities, retrieval mechanisms, and other higher level abilities such as auditory sequencing and hierarchical planning ability), and basic psychological operations that can account for the manipulation of thought contents (e.g., those found in Piagetian theory). An examination of basic underlying cognitive processes is found in Chapter 7 of this book ("Cognitive Processes in Written Language Dysfunction") by Margaret Snowling and Dolores Perin, in which reading and spelling abilities are carefully analyzed and impairments in the processes underlying these abilities are explored by ingenious experimental techniques.

By contrast, the concepts or "cognitions" are the specific thoughts that are made possible by the basic underlying cognitive processes. In the consideration of the effects of language on thought, for example, it has been claimed that the language people speak either determines the concepts that they have or else strongly predisposes them to think in particular ways (e.g., see Carroll, 1956, for B. L. Whorf's selected papers). There are, however, a number of problems in the early research bearing on this issue. One of these is central to the argument being made here: Most of that early research examined the effect of the *lexicon* on particular categories or concepts. For example, it was claimed that the color vocabulary of particular languages affected the perception of (or at least the memory for) specific colors. But Whorf's argument for linguistic determinism was based not on the vocabulary differences of various languages but on differences in their basic structures. As Roger Brown (1977) put it, "Whorf had relatively little to say, in his work as a whole, about lexical differences. For the most part, he was concerned with semantic differences expressed in the grammars of languages, rather than in their lexicons. . . . But they have never been tested. Not because they are untestable, but because no psychologist has yet been sufficiently ingenious" (p. 187). In fact, since Brown wrote that, Alfred Bloom (1981) and Brown's own student, Terry Kit-fong Au (1983), have taken up the challenge and studied the possible effects of Chinese language structure on the understanding of counterfactual propositions. Bloom claims to have found evidence that when higher-level thought categories are considered, especially those based on grammatical structure rather than on lexical items, one does observe effects of language on thought. Au, however, criticizes aspects of Bloom's experiments. Her own experiments on Chinese speakers lead her to dispute his claims. In her chapter "Language and Cognition" in this volume, Au reviews the evidence for the claim that language determines thought and finds it for the most part wanting. Nevertheless, the important point here is that it is necessary to clarify what is meant by *language*; it may be that the effects of syntax differ from the effects of the lexicon. The term *language*, as well as the term *cognition*, is in need of differentiation.

## DIFFERENTIATING LANGUAGE

Language can be broadly defined as a body of words and methods of combining them. It is worthwhile to note that language and communication are not synonymous; a good deal of communication can be achieved by means other than language. Grammar, as defined by the *Oxford English Dictionary* (1933), is "that department of the study of language which deals with its inflectional forms or their equivalents and with the rules for employing these correctly; usually treating also of the phonetic system of the language and its representation in writing." The precise definition of the grammar differs from one language scientist to another and is greatly dependent on particular theoretical viewpoints. In the nineteenth century, grammar was morphologically based. In the first part of this century, the change in emphasis from historical to structural linguistics meant that grammar became primarily concerned with providing structural descriptions of sentences. Chomsky (1965), in turn, criticized traditional or structuralist grammars on the grounds that they did not go beyond mere classification of particular examples and were, therefore, deficient, since they did not express many of the basic regularities of the language. Chomsky argued that adequate grammars must be formulated in terms of rules that would describe the competence of the speaker/hearer. Most psycholinguists today would agree that the grammar must be formulated as a set of rules or principles rather than as a list of basic language forms.

Many people mistakenly believe that grammar is concerned only with syntax or, at most, with syntax and inflectional morphology. A broad definition of grammar, however, would include a number of basic subsystems. For the purpose of clarifying underlying cognitive processes and their relation to language, as well as for elucidating the problems observed in various language disordered groups, it is currently useful to subdivide the study of language into the language subsystems of syntax, morphology, semantics, phonology, and the not strictly linguistic category of pragmatics.

Syntax and morphology have often been treated together as the structure of language. Syntax refers to the way words are put together to form phrases, clauses, and sentences. Morphology, in its broad, general sense, is the study of the structure of words. The morpheme has often been defined semantically as the minimal unit of meaning (but see Aronoff, 1983, for criticisms of this). Some morphemes are bound and others are free. Bound morphemes are those that must be attached to other morphemes. Free morphemes are minimal meaning units that can stand on their own. Thus, for example, the past tense morpheme *-ed* is a bound morpheme that must be attached to some free morpheme. (See Fromkin & Rodman, 1974, for an introductory discussion of morphology.) Of particular interest to psycholinguists has been the class of morphemes called "inflectional morphemes." Inflections are the changes made in the forms of words that express their relations to other words in the sentence. Past tense *-ed* and plural *-s* are examples of inflectional morphemes. The use of inflectional morphemes was once thought to be determined by the syntactic rules of the language. Therefore, in many applied language studies, syntax and inflectional morphology have not been differentiated. It will be seen that the relation between syntax and morphology is not so straightforward as had been assumed. Furthermore, a careful consideration of the particular properties of language in some language disordered groups may require increased differentiation of the syntactic and morphological components.

Semantics is the study of the way meaning is encoded in language. This includes the words themselves (the lexicon) and the relations of those words to the concepts they exemplify and to one another. Phonology is the study of the speaker's knowledge about the sound system of the language. The rules of phonology are part of the speaker's grammar.

Pragmatics is concerned with the way language is used. Strictly speaking, it is not a subsystem of language at all but the way language is employed to achieve particular effects. Pragmatics includes studies of the ways sentences function in communication, how new information is related to known information, and the way features of the context interact with grammatical structure to determine particular meanings. Pragmatic considerations, by definition, cut across all aspects of language. Pragmatics determines the acceptable use of linguistic devices such as anaphora and ellipsis, particular structures (e.g., relative clauses) and forms (e.g., the use of polite and familiar forms where these are encoded in particular languages), and even the choice of lexical items.

A consideration of language in terms of its subsystems in various language handicapped groups can help to illustrate these subsystems. The language of mentally retarded individuals may be an especially valuable source of information on this topic. Therefore, what is known about linguistic functioning in the mentally retarded will be reviewed in some detail. By examining language in a more differentiated way, it may prove possible not only to learn more about language functioning in mental retardation but also to clarify the complex relation between language and cognition generally.

## LANGUAGE IN THE MENTALLY RETARDED

In the first edition of this volume (*Language Perspectives—Acquisition, Retardation, and Intervention*, Schiefelbusch & Lloyd, 1974), various studies of the language of mentally retarded individuals were reviewed in terms of delay, substandard but normal language, and in some cases the possibility of language differences (Cromer, 1974). In the following review, a similar format is followed. The purpose, however, differs in that the findings are interpreted in terms of the information they provide about the relation between aspects of cognition and language. In addition, those studies reviewed in the earlier edition are briefly mentioned, while only the more recent studies are treated in greater detail.

### Studies Showing Language Delay

One of the most commonly reported characteristics of mental retardation is that many developmental processes, while the same as in normal children, proceed at a slower rate and thus evidence delay in appearance.

Most of the studies of retardate language show this pattern. Karlin and Strazzulla's (1952) early study of 50 retarded children with IQs of 15 to 70 who were living at home revealed delayed linguistic development. They reported that the mean age of the first occurrence of babbling, single-word utterances, and sentences was increasingly delayed with lower IQ.

In the well-known study of Lenneberg, Nichols, and Rosenberger (1964), 61 Down syndrome children living at home performed like younger normal children on imitation tests. Furthermore, it was the passing of particular motor milestones that best predicted language development rather than the particular IQ level. More recently, Pennington, Puck, and Robinson (1980) found corroborating evidence of the predictive value of delay in passing motor and language milestones on later language development. They studied the language and cognitive development of eleven 47-chromosome, XXX girls who at the time of the report were between 6 and 14 years of age. These girls had been studied from birth as part of a longitudinal study of 51 children with sex chromosome variations. IQ data (WISC or WISC-R) were available for 9 of the 11 girls. Three girls had normal IQs, but the remaining 6 were mildly retarded with IQs ranging from 70 to 90 (median of 78). It was found that those girls who showed serious language and learning problems at the time of the study were those who had been significantly delayed in first walking or talking. As Pennington et al. put it, a milestone delay for either first walking or first talking identified the 7 girls with serious later problems and produced no false positives or false negatives. The 4 girls who had shown no delay in either motor or speech milestones were the 4 who were relatively unaffected by language or learning problems at the time of the current study. It is interesting to note from the table printed in Pennington et al. that the 7 girls with milestone delays and current language and learning problems comprised the 5 with the lowest IQ scores (70, 73, 76, 80, and 86) and the 2 for whom no IQ data were reported (they "were not given the WISC because one was too young and the other too language impaired"). Thus, there is more recent support for the Lenneberg et al. findings on Down syndrome children based on children with mild retardation of a very different etiology.

A study by Coggins and Morrison (1981) also supports particular aspects of the Lenneberg et al. (1964) findings. Coggins and Morrison studied the spontaneous imitations produced by four Down syndrome children during six individual half-hour sessions over a 4-week period. These children were all in the Stage 1 period of language acquisition as defined by evidencing a mean utterance length of between 1.00 and 2.00 morphemes. Their chronological ages ranged from 3-10 to 6-3. Like normal children, the Down syndrome children showed selectivity in their imitations. Coggins and Morrison assert that the slower rate of development in Down syndrome children will result in linguistic structures that will not differ greatly from those of normal children, since they are similar to normal language learners in the way they selectively imitate model utterances.

The review in the first edition of this book noted a number of studies that examined directly the linguistic structures used by retarded individuals and that gave evidence of normal but developmentally delayed language. A study by Graham and Graham (1971) of nine retarded children of mixed diagnoses showed correlations in the .90s between mental age and percentage of sentences using various numbers of transformations. Average sentence length increased steadily with mental age as did the use of more generalized transformations. Lackner (1968) wrote transformational grammars of the utterances of five retarded children suffering from congenital or early acquired encephalopathy. Sentence length was found to increase with mental age and was the same as for normal children at that age. Phrase structure rules developed regularly and became more differentiated at each increasing mental age, and none of the structures used was incompatible with normal adult usage. Similarly, in tests of imitation and comprehension, the number and types of transformations that were understood and used increased with mental age. Lackner concluded that the language of normal and retarded children was not qualitatively different; both groups followed similar developmental trends. Lovell and Dixon (1967) administered a version of the Fraser, Bellugi, and Brown (1963) test of imitation, comprehension, and production to 80 educationally subnormal children (mean IQ in the 60s) who were 6 and 7 years of age. They performed in the way younger normal children do, with imitation in advance of comprehension, which was in turn in advance of production for all 10 grammatical types tested. In fact, the 6-year-old subnormal children performed almost exactly like the 3-year-old normal children, while the 7-year-old subnormal children performed like the 4-year-old normals. These findings, then, are evidence of developmental delay.

## Studies Showing Mental Age Lag

Studies that show developmental delay in retarded children are not surprising nor are they thought to be difficult to interpret. By contrast, however, there have been a number of studies that show not only delay, but a delay that is greater than that which would have been predicted on the basis of mental age. This has been referred to as mental age lag (see, e.g., Spitz, 1982). Findings that indicate a mental age lag are open to a number of interpretations. Such observations in the domain of language may give some interesting clues as to differentiations needed in considering language and thought.

***Some Findings.*** In an early review, Spreen (1965) reported a number of studies that led him to conclude that retarded individuals show a small lag, as compared to mental age matched normals, on such language measures as sentence length and sentence complexity. For vocabulary size, however, retarded individuals were superior to mental age matched normals. Bartel, Bryen, and Keehn (1973) found that retardates were inferior to mental age matched normals in the use of grammatical categories, but they did not find the superiority in vocabulary; no differences were found in the use of lexical items by the two groups.

Naremore and Dever (1975) compared the language of educable mentally retarded children with mental age matched controls. In all, 30 children from each group were investigated. The groups comprised 6 children from each of the mental age levels 6, 7, 8, 9, and 10 years. The IQ range for the normal children was 100 to 110; that for the retarded children was 74 to 84. The retarded children had a chronological age range of 8 to 12 years. Two 5-minute speech samples were obtained from each child, who was given leading questions concerning programs watched on TV, school and holiday activities, and so on. Based on a syntactic analysis of the obtained utterances, Naremore and Dever report that the normal children were beginning to employ a range of syntactic devices of which the retarded children were taking less advantage. They report that the syntactic variables that discriminated the two groups were subject and predicate elaboration and the use of relative and subordinate clauses. In other words, for the same mental age, the retarded children were making less use of these forms.

McLeavey, Toomey, and Dempsey (1982) used an elicited imitation task to compare the language abilities of retarded and nonretarded children. The retarded group comprised 10 children whose mean IQ was 57 and who had a mean mental age (MA) of 5 years. Their mean chronological age (CA) was 8-7. No information is reported concerning etiology. These children were compared to two normal control groups. One group was matched for mental age (called the High-MA group), and they had a mean IQ of 114 and a mean CA of 4-5. The other group (the Low-MA group) had a mean mental age of 3-1. The mean IQ of this group was 106, and their mean CA was 2-11. The imitation task consisted of 70 sentences covering 18 syntactic structures. Subjects were instructed to repeat the sentences as presented. The results showed the mentally retarded subjects to be far behind their nonretarded mental age counterparts. They differed significantly on imitation of relative clauses, the conjunction *so*, prepositions, the auxiliary *have*, and *have got*. More strikingly, the performance of the retarded group was highly similar to the nonretarded low-MA group. That is, when the retarded children were compared to the normal children who were 2 years behind them in mental age, no significant differences were found on any sentence type.

Furthermore, the correlation of difficulty over the 18 sentence types was very high (.87). The results show, then, that mildly retarded children whose mean mental age was 5 years performed the imitation task at a level far below the nonretarded children of a similar mental age and in fact performed it similarly to nonretarded children whose mean mental age was only 3-1. Error analyses revealed that the retarded children used strategies for coping with difficult sentences that were highly similar to those used by the nonretarded group of a younger mental age.

Semmel, Barritt, and Bennett (1970) had used a Cloze task (where the child has to provide a missing word) to study the grammatical abilities of educable mentally retarded children of mean IQ 70. A tone was presented in the place of the missing word, and the child had to provide a word in order to "make good sense." On this task, the retarded children performed significantly worse than both the chronological age and the mental age matched controls. However, the retarded and the normal children showed similar trends on the same grammatical classes. That is, all groups found noun slots the easiest to fill and verb slots the hardest. It is of interest to note that the errors made by the retarded children were mainly of a type categorized as *nongrammatical and nonmeaningful*. They did not make significantly more errors of the class *nongrammatical, meaningful*, which might have been expected if the test were tapping only strictly grammatical ability. Furthermore, as Semmel et al. pointed out, the retarded children do possess grammatical competence in the encoding of grammatical sentences (i.e., as evidenced in their own spontaneous speech). They therefore concluded that such children have weak grammatical *decoding* habits. That is, Semmel et al. saw the poor performance of the retarded children on the experimental task as being due to differential efficiency between encoding and decoding skills. It is possible to argue, however, that the task is tapping other, nonsyntactic aspects of language, an idea that is developed below.

Lieber and Spitz (1976) studied the ability of retarded children to infer meanings from syntactic clues that were coupled with nonsense words. The background for their study was Brown's (1957) observation of the semantic implications of parts of speech. Brown had noticed that particular form classes have implications in child language: Verbs usually name observable actions, and nouns usually refer to concrete objects. He found experimentally that children could use grammatical class information encoded on nonsense words to determine whether those words named actions or objects. Lieber and Spitz were interested in whether retarded children would show the same ability as normal children to make such inferences. They tested 30 institutionalized retarded adolescents whose mean IQ was 57. The mean mental age of this group was 9 years, and the mean chronological age was 17. A group of 136 normal children ranging from 5 to 12 years of age was also tested. These children were divided into

4 groups with mean chronological ages of approximately 6, 8, 10, and 11½. The task was based on Brown's technique. For example, the child would view a picture in which an action (e.g., hands engaged in a kneading activity: a verb) was being carried out on a quantity of objects (e.g., tiny red shapes: mass noun), which were shown heaped into and spilling out of another object (e.g., a container: count noun). A nonsense word (e.g., *latt*) was used by the examiner to describe the picture in a way conforming to a verb, a mass noun, or a count noun. The child's task was to point to pictures of other exemplars of that word. For example, for a verb, the child was told, "Do you know what it means to latt? In this picture you can see latting. Now point to another picture of latting." For the mass noun, the verbalization was "Have you ever seen any latt? In this picture you can see some latt. Now point to another picture of latt." And for the count noun, it was "Do you know what a latt is? In this picture you can see a latt. Point to another picture of a latt." The results showed that only on count nouns did the retarded subjects perform at a level of accuracy expected at their mental age (9 years) as gauged by the normal group's responses. On the nonsense words presented as verbs, the retardates performed like the normal 8-year-olds, or about a year below their MA level; and on those words presented as mass nouns, their performance fell below that of any of the age groups of the normal children. Lieber and Spitz hypothesize that the performance of the retarded subjects reflects a basic deficiency in generalization ability. In addition, they noted a response bias in the retarded subjects toward choosing the count noun pictures on each set.

Studies using Berko's (1958) test of morphology have often shown performance by retarded individuals to be below that expected on the basis of their mental age. These studies were discussed in the 1974 review and will be only briefly mentioned here.

Newfield and Schlanger (1968) compared normal and subnormal children on the acquisition of morphological rules. They found that both groups learn morphology in a comparable manner, as evidenced by the fact that the order of acquisition was the same for the two groups. For the retarded children, the learning pace was slower, but the differences from normals was quantitative, not qualitative. One important aspect of their findings was that for both groups performance was better when morphological inflections had to be applied to real words rather than to nonsense words. That is, for example, children found it easier to supply the plural *glasses* for the singular *glass*, than to supply *tasses* for the nonsense word *tass*. They noted, however, that the retarded children were less able to generalize from the familiar words to the new (nonsense) words than were the normal children. Dever and Gardner (1970) independently obtained the same results, but they noted that the retarded children could and did produce the morphemes correctly in their spontaneous conversation. This suggested that their lack of generalization on the experimental task might have been due either to lack of knowledge of what was expected of them in the test situation or to unknown factors inherent in the use of nonsense words as test items.

The Berko (1958) test of morphology had also been used by Lovell and Bradbury (1967) to study 160 educationally subnormal children of mean IQ 70. These 14- and 15-year-olds performed more poorly than Berko's normal children at age 6. Lovell and Bradbury speculated that the subnormal children suffer from a reduced ability to generate the morphological endings of new words; they would, therefore, have to learn more of the specific inflections on particular words than normal children, who would more readily apply generalized rules to new words. In a later experiment on 18 educationally subnormal children, however, Bradbury and Lunzer (1972) obtained identical results for both the subnormal and normal children on a task that required the learning of nonsense particles marking plural, past, and possessive when attached to nonsense words. However, the subnormal children were less successful than the normal children when a transfer task to 30 new items presented only once was employed. Bradbury and Lunzer speculated that the poor performance on this new task might be attributable to something in the nature of the one trial method employed, or perhaps to the possibility that subnormal children, when faced with a new task, are less ready to search through and to use strategies available to them.

***Interpretations of the Mental Age Lag.*** It is clear that a number of studies have shown some sort of developmental lag in the language of various groups of mentally retarded individuals. Some aspects of their language, rather than being appropriate to their mental age, appear to lag behind what would be expected on the basis of comparisons to mental age matched controls. It is important to consider carefully what these findings might mean, since they may contain some important implications for the relation between language and cognition.

One possibility is that mental age does not reflect a meaningful dimension on which to equate performance when language is under consideration. Children are typically matched on mental ages derived from test performance, which measures a variety of skills. It is possible, for example, that language represents an autonomous faculty of the mind (cf. Fodor, 1983), and in part its development may proceed independently of other cognitive faculties. Whether one accepts the position of linguistic autonomy or not, the skills and processes tapped by most tests on which mental ages have been calculated nevertheless are not those most appropriate for linguistic competence. It might be more meaningful to match groups on some language-specific measure such as mean length of utterance (MLU), as is commonly done when comparing normal children of various ages on linguistic tasks. Miller and Chapman (1984) report that recent investigations on normal 3- to 6-year-old children (Paul, Chapman, & Wanska, 1980) revealed that MLU was a better predictor of complex sentence acquisition than was age or nonverbally measured cognition. They found that age or cognition accounted for additional variance instead on the semantic content—an issue that is raised in the next section. Developing language structures have been found to be related to measures of auditory short-term memory (Curtiss, Fromkin, & Yamada, 1978). Mental ages based solely on measurements of such memory may also be more meaningful than mental ages typically reported that represent a composite of various processes. When mental ages are based on linguistically appropriate measures, it may be that no developmental lag will be observed in the syntactic component of language.

However, even if the observed mental age lag on language is "real" and is not an artifact, problems of interpreting it remain. One controversy has been concerned with whether observed lags represent real deficits in cognitive functioning or whether there are motivational factors that depress test performance (see, e.g., Zigler & Balla, 1982). If part of the explanation for poor performance and poor learning in retarded individuals lies in deficient motivation, then that same low motivation might have had an effect during earlier language acquisition. (See, e.g., Moerk, 1976, for motivational variables in language acquisition.) However, as an explanation for mental age lag, this position is illogical, as Spitz (1983) points out; the same motivational deficiency that is thought to depress IQ (and thus mental age) can hardly be logically invoked again to explain performance on experimental tasks where retarded individuals perform even lower than their mental age level. A different interpretation of mental age lag focuses instead on whether retarded individuals are merely developmentally delayed or whether they are different in the sense that they have particular cognitive defects. Arguments pro and con are found in Zigler and Balla (1982). A mental age lag that could not be attributed to motivational or other test-taking factors would support the position that retarded individuals are cognitively different from normal individuals in specifiable ways. For linguistic tasks, one way to view such possible differences requires the differentiation of language into its subsystems. In order to see what can be learned from the language studies showing mental age lag, it is first necessary to examine the studies reported above more closely to see which aspects of language are in fact defective.

***Mental Age Lag Findings: A Closer Look.*** It will be recalled that some studies purported to show that mentally retarded individuals evidenced poorer syntactic abilities than their mental age matched controls. The Naremore and Dever (1975) study found that the retarded children made less use of subject and predicate elaboration and of relative and subordinate clauses than did normal children of the same mental age. Such a finding, while interesting, is not without its problems for understanding the language of retarded children. The data consisted of utterances made during two 5-minute periods in which spontaneous language was drawn out by the examiner through the use of leading questions. The problem with this procedure, which samples only a very small proportion of the child's speech, is that one cannot be confident that the language obtained really represents the child's competence. Furthermore, given the way the data were reported by Naremore and Dever, it is impossible to tell whether the language of the retarded group was totally lacking in any instances of these linguistic forms. Even if that were so for one particular form or another, one cannot know whether the children were *incapable* of using that form or if they merely failed to use it during those two 5-minute sessions. In addition, no analysis is shown of individuals, so it is impossible to know whether some forms were used by some children but not by others.

In the McLeavey, Toomey, and Dempsey (1982) study, the findings were based on a task involving elicited imitation. The retarded children performed below mental age level on imitation of a number of forms, but we have no way of knowing whether those forms are missing in the spontaneous speech of the children. Thus, the studies on syntax are not fully convincing in making the claim that retarded children are further behind in their development than would be predicted by mental age. This is especially so when one recalls that Lackner's (1968) study, which sampled spontaneous speech of five retarded children three times a day over an 8-week period, revealed a regular order of appearance of sentence types as mental age increased.[1]

In the Cloze task used by Semmel, Barritt, and Bennett (1970), the retarded subjects performed significantly below their mental age matched controls. But it will be recalled that Semmel et al. noted that these children in their spontaneous speech possessed grammatical competence for forms on which they performed poorly on the experimental task. This led them to conclude that the retarded children had weak decoding abilities but that their encoding abilities were adequate. Performance on the Cloze task, however, requires more than grammatical facility. To perform appropriately, one must also possess adequate semantic competence. Meaning plays an important part.

In the Lieber and Spitz (1976) study, children had to infer word class meanings from nonsense words marked either by inflectional affixes (*-ing*, as in "latting") or by other meaning-carrying units (e.g., *some* and *a* as in

---

[1] Although Lackner reported that sentence length increased with mental age and that this length was the same as for normal children of the same mental age, he did not report mental age comparisons for the developing syntax.

"some latt" vs. "a latt"). The child's responses can be affected by at least two nonspecifically morphological variables: (a) the understanding of particular meanings and (b) the ability to draw inferences about new instances used briefly during the experimental task. Lieber and Spitz reported, however, that of the three forms tested, the retarded children performed at a mental age appropriate level on count nouns; they performed below their mental age level on the verbs and mass nouns. This would seem to indicate that it is not the ability to make semantic inferences per se that was impaired but particular semantic inferences required by some of the tasks.

Paris, Mahoney, and Buckhalt (1974) had earlier demonstrated inferential ability on linguistic tasks by retarded individuals. Forty educable mentally retarded children of IQ 52 to 88 and whose chronological ages ranged from 7-5 to 13-5 were presented sentences that they were to try to remember. Passages such as the following were presented:

John is chasing the dog.

The dog is in the school yard.

The dog is white.

The first two sentences act as premises from which the inference can be drawn that John is in the school yard. In the recognition task that followed, various sentences were presented. The children were asked, "Did you hear this same exact sentence before?" Recognition sentences contained both true inferences ("John is in the school yard"), false inferences ("John is outside the school yard"), and both true and false premises ("John is chasing the dog"; "The dog is chasing John") to control for memory effects. A constructive approach to semantic memory would predict that subjects would confuse true inference sentences with actually presented acquisition sentences. The results showed that the average error rate on the true inferences was 50.0%, which was significantly greater than the error rates on the other three types (true premises: 18.8%, false premises: 20.6%, and false inferences: 28.8%). Paris et al. concluded that the retarded children in their experiment were clearly capable of spontaneous semantic integration and that educable mentally retarded children are capable of abstracting semantic relationships in a manner qualitatively similar to nonretarded children and adults. Their study lends support to the interpretation that the failure of retarded children in the Lieber and Spitz (1976) study can be attributed not to the inability to make semantic inferences but to particular semantic aspects of portions of the task.

In the studies mentioned so far, there is little firm evidence that syntactic aspects of language are especially deficient in mentally retarded individuals. By contrast, the results can be interpreted as showing a possible semantic deficit. The implications of this will become apparent when the effects of conceptual knowledge on specific subsystems of language are considered.

***Deficits in Conceptual Ability.*** The studies that most consistently have found a mental age lag in retarded children are those that have examined inflectional morphology using the tests devised by Berko (1958). Newfield and Schlanger (1968) found that while both normal and subnormal subjects appeared to learn morphology in a comparable manner, the retarded children were less able to generalize from familiar words to new (nonsense) words. Dever and Gardner (1970) obtained similar results. Lovell and Bradbury (1967) speculated on a reduced ability in the retardates to generate the morphological endings of new words. Bradbury and Lunzer (1972) also noted a generalization problem—at least to the new items that were tested on one trial only. They also speculated that retarded children are less able to make use of the available strategies that they do have.

Explanations based on lowered efficiency in generalization ability are not totally convincing, however. There is evidence, for example, that even severely retarded children are capable of generalization (O'Connor & Hermelin, 1963), and the children tested in the morphology experiments were only mildly retarded. Furthermore, Dever and Gardner (1970), who obtained similar results in their morphology experiments, noted that the children they studied did in fact generalize in their spontaneous speech. They felt that the explanation, therefore, must lie either in a lack of knowledge of what was expected in the test situation or in unknown factors associated with the use of nonsense words as the crucial stimuli.

Another possibility is that the deficit lies in conceptual ability, which would have effects on specific subsystems of language. It may be significant that the studies on language that have found a greater deficit than would have been predicted on the basis of mental age have been studies of inflectional morphology. Rosenberg (1982), in reviewing these studies, notes that Brown (1973) had found that both grammatical and semantic complexity predicted the order of acquisition of inflectional morphemes. Rosenberg points out that the use of these inflectional morphemes requires the mastery of both linguistic structures and the semantic phenomena they modulate. As mentioned earlier in this chapter, many child language researchers have treated syntax and inflectional morphology together as constituting the structure of language. Since there seems to be some differential disability in performance on these two aspects of structure, however, it may be increasingly useful to treat these as two separate subsystems of language. Aronoff (1983) has recently provided an excellent summary of recent linguistic work in morphology. As he points out, it is difficult to separate out morphology from the syntactic, semantic, and phonological components of the grammar. Morphology in fact consists in large part of the interaction of these other three subsystems of the grammar. A deficit in conceptual ability may have important effects on the semantic component of the grammar, as will be seen in the next section. Therefore, it may be that limited conceptual ability in mentally retarded individuals also has an important effect on those aspects of morphology that are especially tied to the semantic subsystem. These would certainly include those morphological entities that Berko's (1958) test examines—the encoding of past time, possession, plurality, and the like. If this is so, then some new predictions become possible. Aronoff specifies some parts of word formation morphology that, like inflectional morphology, verge on semantics. For example, the attachment of the suffix *-ism* to nouns is used to form new nouns that denote a system of beliefs, as in "Platonism," "vegetarianism," "socialism," and so forth. The attachment of the suffix *-able* results in derived adjectives that are passive and potential—something is "readable" if it can be read; it is "repeatable" if it can be repeated, and so on (Aronoff, 1983). If part of the explanation for some aspects of deficient language in retarded individuals lies in the effect of a limited conceptual system on semantics and morphology, then one might expect to find deficits in the generalized use of these word formation suffixes as well.

It may be useful to summarize the argument to this point. Studies of the language of mentally retarded individuals show either a delay in acquisition or, in some cases, a delay that is even more pronounced than would be expected on the basis of mental age. Questions were then raised concerning the appropriateness to language of most measures of mental age. Even if this mental age lag is accepted as real, then those studies that show such a lag in syntax are nevertheless subject to some doubt. This is because these studies were based on tasks that did not necessarily show that retarded children lacked particular structures, but merely that they either did not use those structures in short, spontaneous interviews to the extent that normal children did (Naremore & Dever, 1975) or that they did not imitate such structures to the extent that their mental age matched controls did (McLeavey et al., 1982). In the study using the Cloze task (Semmel et al., 1970), the experimenters noted that the retarded children did possess grammatical competence in their own spontaneous speech. Furthermore, it was pointed out that the task could be tapping other nonsyntactic abilities. By contrast, those studies that have given evidence of a mental age lag are those concerned with the morphological subsystem of language. This has led to the claim that the reason the morphological component may be especially affected is that it is closely tied to the semantic subsystem of language. The basic claim that will be made is that the semantic subcomponent in the language of retarded children reflects their conceptual deficits. Let us examine this claim more closely.

***Conceptual and Linguistic Knowledge.*** It is first necessary that a distinction be made between concepts and semantics. Many psychologists have mistakenly viewed conceptual knowledge (i.e., thoughts and concepts) as synonymous with semantic knowledge. This confusion makes it impossible to study the relationship between the two in development. It should, therefore, be emphasized that *semantics* is a linguistic term that refers not to meaning but to meaning-in-language. Semantic knowledge is not identical to thoughts and concepts but is instead the knowledge of what aspects of meaning receive linguistic marking in a particular language and how that encoding is carried out. Rice (1983; see also Rice & Kemper, 1984), in an excellent account of the cognition/language relationship and its implications for models of language disorders, makes the distinction between linguistic knowledge and nonlinguistic knowledge especially clear.

There is experimental evidence of the distinctness of the two domains. Potter (1979), for example, argued that abstract information is part of one's conceptual system rather than part of one's verbal system; this contrasts with views that identify abstract knowledge with the verbal system. She reported experimental evidence from Potter and Faulconer (1975), who used drawings and words that had been equated by a masking procedure to take the same amount of time to be seen correctly. Tasks included naming these drawings and words as well as categorizing them into superordinate categories such as *food* and *furniture*. Consistent with the findings in other experiments, it took subjects longer to name drawings than to name words—in this experiment, 260 msec. longer. But it took the same subjects 50 msec. *less* to *categorize* the drawings than to categorize the words. Potter interprets these results as supporting the position that associations between an item (e.g., *shoe*) and an abstract category (e.g., *clothing*) are part of an amodal conceptual system, not part of the verbal system as other theories have proposed.

Given the distinction between conceptual and linguistic knowledge, it is possible to trace the influence of one on the other. This is essentially what Carey (1978) has done in her experimental study of word acquisition in 14 normal children who were 3 and 4 years old. She introduced a rare word, *chromium*, for olive-colored objects in natural situations in their nursery school. By noting the labels the children had originally used for this color (usually "green" or "brown"), Carey was able to study the way the children changed both their color concepts (conceptual knowledge) and their terminology (semantic knowledge).

Being clear about this distinction also makes it possible to understand the effects of limited conceptual ability—for example, in retarded individuals—on language. I have argued elsewhere (Cromer, 1981) that limited conceptual knowledge may affect language acquisition—not by directly influencing the structure, but by affecting the semantic component of language. Miller and Chapman (1984) reach a similar conclusion. The study by Paul et al. (1980) had revealed that MLU was a better predictor of complex sentence acquisition than was age or nonverbally measured cognition. But age or cognition accounted for additional variance in the *semantic* content. Miller and Chapman interpreted this as suggesting that cognition is more closely tied to semantic aspects of development than to syntax. Rosenberg's (1982) argument, noted earlier, extends this to the morphological component; insofar as morphology depends on conceptual knowledge, deficits in that knowledge will affect the morphological subsystem of language as well as the semantic component itself.

The view that the morphological deficits observed in retarded children can be explained in terms of conceptual deficits that affect the semantic component of the grammar is not without its problems, however. It is not always the case that there is a one-to-one correspondence between morphological affixes and particular meanings. That is, inflections do not encode specific meanings, even though psychologists often assume that they do so. For example, past tense forms such as *-ed* are often mistakenly said to refer to past time. However, it is understood among linguists that, as Jespersen (1965) had pointed out, one must keep the two concepts of time and tense strictly apart. There is no single linguistic form for referring to a particular time, nor is any particular time necessarily referred to by a particular linguistic form. The present tense can refer to the future, as in "The boat *leaves* tomorrow" and to past time as in "He *says* 'yes,' then he didn't go, so I went alone." Past tense forms can refer to present time in conditional sentences such as "I wish I *had* money enough," and even to the future in sentences like "It's time you *closed* the window and *went* to bed." The analysis of precisely what it is that cognitive principles and conceptual knowledge contribute to the acquisition and use of the linguistic subsystem of morphology needs to be more detailed than most present studies have allowed for. Our currently naive formulations in this area will have to give way to more sophisticated accounts of the relation between the subsystems of language and the meanings they encode.

There is a further problem in interpreting the mental age lag in inflectional morphology as being due solely to the conceptual meanings that those inflections encode. As has been seen, there is little evidence that the syntactic component similarly suffers a mental age lag in retarded individuals. But it can be argued that particular syntactic operations encode or affect meaning. If the conceptual limitations of retarded individuals lead to a deficit in morphology, surely those limitations should affect particular aspects of syntactic acquisition as well. There are, then, problems for the interpretation of the mental age lags that are observed in the language of the mentally retarded as being solely due to conceptual deficits. However, there are aspects of language in some mentally retarded individuals that give more direct evidence of the influence of conceptual knowledge on language and that thus shed light on the relation between "thought" and "language."

## Cocktail-Party Syndrome in Mentally Retarded Children

Some children with internal hydrocephaly have been reported by clinicians to talk excessively, but their language, if they are mentally retarded, is often lacking in content. Taylor (1959) described these children in their preschool years as shining in their verbal fluency: "Most of them have an impressive vocabulary of 'big' words. . . . Some have a tendency to talk like grown-ups" (p. 219). Hadenius, Hagberg, Hyttnäs-Bensch, and Sjögren (1962) examined 23 of the 85 survivors from an original 180 untreated children who had a natural history of infantile hydrocephalus. Only cases in which an abnormally rapid increase of head circumference had taken place during the first year of life had been included in the original sample. They reported a syndrome in 6 of the 23 in which mental retardation was observed along with "a peculiar contrast between a good ability to learn words and talk, and not knowing what they are talking about" (p. 118). They went on to describe these children as loving to chatter, but thinking illogically, and coined the term *cocktail-party syndrome* for the condition. Ingram and Naughton (1962) described 16 cerebral palsy patients with arrested hydrocephalus, 9 of whom fit this description. The parents had often commented on the disparity between what the child could do and what he or she could say. Ingram and Naughton noted that these 9 had been described as "chatterboxes," "excessively talkative," or as "bletherers"; the term *chatterbox syndrome* has now also come to be used to describe these hyperverbal children.

Fleming (1968) formally studied 11 children with internal hydrocephaly aged 4-0 to 8-1. Their IQs ranged from 73 to 110, with a median of 94. The productive speech of these children, collected from a task of describing 10 pictures from the *Children's Apperception Test* (Bellak & Bellak, 1974), was compared to that of 11 normal controls who had been matched on chronological age, IQ, sex, race, socioeconomic status, and school grade placement. Fleming found no significant differences between the groups on measures of total number of responses, total number of words, and average length of response. She did report, however, that some hydrocephalic subjects gave the impression of verbosity because of the "personal and socially aggressive nature of their spontaneous conversation" (p. 81). It should be noted, however, that Fleming's group consisted of children primarily of normal or near normal intelligence, as she herself pointed out, whereas most hydrocephalic children who show the chatterbox syndrome have especially low intelligence, as will be seen below.

Furthermore, my own experience with such children shows that a picture description task of the type used by Fleming fails to elicit the hyperverbal behavior typical of these children.

Fraser, Agnew, and Grieve (1975), however, also failed to find differences in productive language measures when retarded hydrocephalic individuals were examined. They compared 5 adult hydrocephalics of mixed etiologies whose WAIS full-scale IQs were between 51 and 59 (mean = 53) with 5 high-grade mentally handicapped controls who were of the same chronological ages, of approximately similar institutional experience, and who were matched approximately on IQ (range: 47 to 72; mean = 55). Two assessments of language abilities were made. One was based on a partially structured conversational interview, and the other was the *Illinois Test of Psycholinguistic Abilities* (ITPA) (Kirk, McCarthy, & Kirk, 1969). Results of the conversational analysis were described as remarkably similar for the two groups—but this analysis consisted only of counts such as number of utterances, number of morphemes, mean length of utterance, and the numbers of inappropriate responses, false starts, overlaps, and the like. However, results on the ITPA revealed two statistically significant superiorities in the hydrocephalic subjects over the controls. These were on the Grammatical Closure subtest (the ability to make use of redundancies of oral language in handling syntax) and the Auditory Closure subtest (the ability to fill in deleted phonemes in auditory presentation).

***Intelligence Level.*** Tew (1979) studied 49 children who were taken from 59 survivors of 145 originally unselected cases of spina bifida cystica born in South Wales between 1964 and 1966. The language of these children was evaluated while they were undergoing assessment in an informal setting. They were classified as showing the cocktail-party syndrome if they met four of the following five criteria: (a) a perseveration of response (either echoing the examiner or repeating earlier self-made statements), (b) excessive use of social phrases, (c) overfamiliarity in manner not normally expected in a 5-year-old child, (d) introducing personal experience into the conversation in irrelevant and inappropriate contexts, and (e) fluent and normally well-articulated speech. Unfortunately, measurements of these criteria are not specified, and the assessment appears to have been made on rather impressionistic grounds, which may contaminate the results. Tew reported that 20 of the 49 children (40.8%) were judged by these criteria to show the cocktail-party syndrome. These children were then compared to the remaining 29 spina bifida, noncocktail-party syndrome children as well as to a group of normal controls with a Wechsler full-scale IQ mean of 106 who were matched for sex, place in family, social class, and area of residence. Tew reports that the cocktail-party syndrome was diagnostically indicative of low intelligence. The interesting differences are between the two subgroups of spina bifida children. Those children classified as evidencing the cocktail-party syndrome scored between 26 and 32 IQ points lower than the other spina bifida children on all three measures of IQ (verbal, performance, and full scale). The mean verbal IQ of the cocktail-party syndrome group was 65. This compares with a mean of 92 in the remaining spina bifida children. Full-scale IQ scores in these two groups were 55 and 88. On the *Reynell Developmental Language Scales* (Reynell, 1977), both the noncocktail-party spina bifida children and the normal controls scored at about the 5- to 5½-year-old level on both expressive and comprehension tests. By contrast, the mean expressive language age of the cocktail-party syndrome children was 3-1, and their mean verbal comprehension age was 3-8. It may seem odd that cocktail-party syndrome children score so poorly on the language tests, especially on the expressive language measures, given that such children are defined in terms of what appears to be their good expressive language. One problem is that such tests do not distinguish between the structural aspects of language and its ability to express meaning.

***Inappropriate and Bizarre Language Use.*** Swisher and Pinsker (1971) studied 11 children with Spina bifida cystica and a history of hydrocephalus who had been followed by the Spina Bifida Clinic of the New York University Medical Center. Children were included only if they were considered by clinicians to be hyperverbal. At the time of the study the children ranged in age from 3-2 to 7-10. They were compared to a control group, matched for age, that consisted of subjects who had been born with one or more extremities absent. This allowed for matching on the additional bases of history of a congenital physical handicap and history of exposure to hospitalization. The average IQ of the hydrocephalic children was 88 (range: 65 to 106) as obtained from hospital records and based on a variety of tests including the Stanford-Binet, WISC, or Merrill-Palmer. Each child was tape-recorded in a conversational setting with the investigator. Results were based on various measures of quantity of output, and descriptive categories were used for quality. Swisher and Pinsker found that, unlike some of the earlier studies reported above, there was a quantitative basis for the clinical impression that these children were hyperverbal: They used significantly more words and vocal response units and initiated more speeches than the control group. A high negative correlation (–0.73) between word output and type-token ratio suggested that the more talkative hydrocephalic children were more repetitive in language use. This relationship was not found in the control group. Utterances were classified for their quality into three descriptive categories: appropriate, inappropriate, and bizarre. Eight of the 11 hydrocephalic children used some language that was either inappropriate or bizarre, but only 2 of the control subjects did so. In fact, of these 8 hydrocephalic children, 6 showed both inappropriate and bizarre language in their samples, while none of the controls had entries in both of these categories.

Swisher and Pinsker (1971) note that none of the 3 oldest hydrocephalic children used any language that was categorized as either inappropriate or bizarre. A number of possibilities are entertained to explain the more appropriate verbal output and the decrease in unusual quality of language with increasing age in the hydrocephalic group. But a closer examination of their data shows that an alternative interpretation to age is possible. These 3 oldest children were also the 3 hydrocephalic children with the highest IQs; indeed, all 3 are in the normal range—98, 103, and 106. By contrast, those children with either inappropriate or bizarre language (usually both) had IQs ranging from 65 to 86. It would be possible to argue that low conceptual ability is what makes otherwise fluent-appearing language contain bizarre or inappropriate elements. Swisher and Pinsker note that the syntactical aspects of language of this group were better than comprehension and expression of the meaning of the words.

Earlier, the poor performance of retarded children was noted especially on inflectional morphology, where they evidenced developmental delays beyond what would be expected on the basis of mental age. It is, therefore, somewhat surprising to find the claim in Swisher and Pinsker (1971) that hydrocephalic children "are able to stretch the rules of English morphology to the extent of forming nonsense words for use in simple contexts" (pp. 746–747) as efficiently as controls of a higher mean IQ—a claim said to be based on findings by Parsons (1968). I can find no evidence of this in the paper by Parsons. In his study, he compared 30 children with hydrocephalus, aged 5 to 7½, to 18 normal controls on the Berko task of extending morphological rules to nonsense words in simple contexts. The controls were a cross-section of the normal child population who were under treatment for physical ailments; the groups were matched overall for age and intelligence. It should be noted that there was no evidence of any attempt to test *hyperverbal* hydrocephalic children. Rather, based on the fact that hydrocephalic children have often evidenced vocabulary subscale scores superior to their general psychometric status, Parsons merely predicted that hydrocephalic children would be more efficient at the Berko morphology test than the normal controls. He reports that in fact no difference was found between the two groups. Actual performance scores are not reported in the published paper.

***Measurement of Syntactic Abilities.*** Spain (1974) studied 145 spina bifida children who were 3 years of age. These children were tested on two scales from the *Griffiths Mental Development Scales* (Griffiths, 1951) and with the *Reynell Developmental Language Scales* (Reynell, 1969). She reports that on the subtest that measures language structure, the children had a grasp of syntax that was normal for their age. This was true even for children with poor performance ability on the mental scale. In fact, Spain notes that hyperverbalism or the cocktail-party syndrome was more likely to be found in children with poor performance ability. Such children tended to produce a characteristic pattern of scores on the verbal subtests, a pattern described as showing below average scores on the content subtest and on tests of verbal comprehension, but with average scores for syntax development. In fact, Spain reports that "of all the tests used, both verbal and non-verbal, only on the test of syntax development did this group produce scores comparable to those of the children within the average range of ability" (p. 776).

Anderson and Spain (1977) report follow-up studies of these children at age 6. The Structure (syntax) subtest of the Reynell Expressive Scale showed that within the group as a whole, use of syntax was quite normal for the age of the child, even in those children with low performance IQs. In addition, the studies at age 6 used other measures of syntax such as sentence length and the use of conjunctions. In general, the findings show that "spina bifida children are more likely to use complex syntax than normal children matched for ability, although they do not always use it appropriately" (p. 126). In their findings, Anderson and Spain report that about 40% of the spina bifida children at age 6 show the hyperverbal syndrome, although only about half of that number exhibit it to a significant degree. Such hyperverbal children were typically female and were poor intellectually, with considerably higher verbal than performance skills. They further report that analysis of the children's spontaneous speech showed that the hyperverbal group "differed remarkably" from a group of normal children matched on the *Wechsler Preschool and Primary Scale of Intelligence* (WPPSI) (Wechsler, 1967) for verbal ability. "They used quite complex syntax, but often inaccurately, and produced more bizarre utterances, with a tendency to change subject midflow, to give more false starts to sentences and more incomplete sentences. They produced a much higher rate of clichés, or adult-type phrases, although they rarely gave the impression of understanding their meaning" (pp. 129–130). Anderson and Spain present a short protocol extracted from the recorded speech of one child of IQ 55. It shows that the child uses some quite complex sentences and has an extensive vocabulary. But, as Anderson and Spain summarize, "The child declaims rather than converses, tends to drift from one topic to another only loosely related and clearly does not really understand what he is saying" (p. 130).

It seems clear that within the subnormal population, there exists at least one subgroup—hydrocephalic children—some of whom evidence the peculiar feature of possessing quite complex language in spite of moderate or severe subnormality. As this short review of various studies of these children indicates, the content of their language does not match its structural characteristics. In the extreme form of this hyperverbal behavior, cocktail-party or chatterbox syndrome, fluent speech is coupled with poor understanding. Such children present in clearest form the effects of cognition on language—or, more precisely, the effects of a limited conceptual system on particular subsystems of language. The findings from some studies suggest that, while the syntax (and phonology) remain relatively unimpaired, the semantic subsystem is greatly affected. I have also speculated that particular aspects of the morphological system may be affected by limited conceptual ability as well, and it will be seen that those same limitations also affect the pragmatic component.

## Other Examples of Semantic Deficits in Retarded Children

Most of the studies of the language of retarded children have used either standard tests or, when spontaneous language has been analyzed, usually a system of counting items such as the number of words or the length of utterances (Lackner's 1968 study being an important exception). By contrast, probably the most sophisticated analyses of subnormal language have begun to appear in the work of Curtiss and her colleagues. These researchers are concerned with the relationship between language and cognition in development and have presented clear evidence that limited conceptual abilities have specific effects on the semantic and pragmatic components of the grammar but not on the syntax. Curtiss (1981) has summarized two of the cases studied by her group. Here it will be useful to note some particular observations taken from the more detailed descriptions.

Curtiss and Yamada (1981) report their study of Antony, who they observed and tested extensively from the time he was 6½ years of age until he was 7. A psychological evaluation when Antony was 5-2 reports a Leiter IQ of 50 and a mental age of 2-9. Curtiss and Yamada tested Antony on a variety of nonlanguage cognitive tasks including various forms of conservation, classification, localization of topographical stimuli, drawing, copying, nesting of objects, spontaneous play, hierarchical construction, logical sequencing, auditory memory span, the *Benton Visual Retention Test* (Benton, 1965), *Knox's Cube Test* (Stone & Wright, 1980), figure-ground perception tests, tests of embedded figures, and the *Mooney Faces Test* (Mooney, 1957). On most of these tests, Antony scored either below all norms or below the 2-year-old level. On only one test—auditory (verbal) short-term memory—did he show normal (i.e., age-level) capacity.

Antony's language was examined through the use of a specially designed battery—the Curtiss Yamada Comprehensive Language Evaluation (CYCLE) in both its receptive and spontaneous speech forms. Curtiss and Yamada (1981) report that Antony performed poorly on the comprehension tests due to such factors as attentional deficits that made it difficult for him to consider all of the choices. Nevertheless, his best performances were on tests of syntactic structure: active-voice word order, subject relativization, *Wh-* subject questioning, and *Wh-* object questioning (receiving a perfect score on the last two). By contrast, Antony's worst performances were on tests of lexical semantics or lexically coded linguistic information: *before* and *after*; the tense and aspect forms *will*, *gonna*, and *finish*; disjunction; and the locative prepositions *in*, *on*, *under*, *over*, *next to*, *in back*, and *in front*. His best performance on any of these was only at the 2-year-old level. Furthermore, Antony did poorly on tests of inflectional morphology, scoring at the 3-year-old level on *-ing* and below the 2-year-old level on past tense. His comprehension in informal conversation showed that while he could respond appropriately to different kinds of questions (*yes/no* questions and *Wh-* questions), he could not respond correctly to *Why* or *How* questions (i.e., to the content). Antony could not respond to hypotheticals—for example, to "What would you do if you were at home and you wanted some ice cream?" he responded in a way implying he didn't have an ice cream—and he showed limited interpretations of other items. For example, *of* appears to have been understood only in its possessive (genitive) meaning. Curtiss and Yamada (1981) note the following exchange:

> E: Draw a picture of Vivian. (pointing to blank paper)
> A: No. It's not Vivian's, it's mine.
> E: Draw a picture of Mrs. W.
> A: No. It's not Mrs. W's. (p. 73)

He also seems unaware of the indefinite use of *you*:

> E: You sew with that. (referring to a spool)
> A: No, I don't sew with that. (p. 73)

In his spontaneous speech, Antony evidenced no noticeable phonological impairment. Of his syntax and morphology, Curtiss and Yamada (1981) note that he used 61 of the 68 different elements and structures of the grammar that they analyzed, including infinitival and sentential complements, relative clauses, and other subordinate clauses. In addition, he used a variety of morphological features that appeared consistent and well formed. Nevertheless, a number of his grammatical forms evidenced inappropriate use. Curtiss and Yamada summarize Antony's performance by noting, "His ability to use a wide range of syntactic devices . . . to encode his limited and confused thoughts, illustrates the discrepancy between Antony's grammatical knowledge and his conceptual/cognitive knowledge" (p. 75). They further point out that there were certain errors he never made.

> He did not place verb markers on nouns or vice-versa, did not use clausal connectors within VP's or NP's, nor use affixes as prefixes or vice-versa. His errors consisted exclusively of omissions and semantically inappropriate use. Antony appeared to have extracted purely syntactic and morphological constraints without the semantics which they normally encode. (p. 77)

It is instructive to apply this view to some of the findings cited earlier on inflectional morphology in retarded children generally. It was noted that their performance on Berko-type tests was poor—below the level of what would be expected on the basis of their mental age. But it was also noted by various researchers that the spontaneous language of these same children contained generalized use of inflections. In comprehension tests, interest is focused directly on the meaning and, in particular, the abstract meaning that the particular inflection encodes. Thus, to be able to add the plural inflection to one nonsense item called a "tass" when two are then shown to produce the form "tasses" may require a different level of semantic ability than producing the word "glasses" when first one glass and then two are shown. Curtiss and Yamada (1981) remark that they were struck by the poor grasp Antony had on the semantics that many of the grammatical forms he used were meant to encode. This is again evidence of the disparity between conceptual content and grammatical form.

Curtiss and Yamada (1981) also give evidence of the dissociation between conceptual ability and language demonstrated by Antony's lexical uses. They cite, for example, his use of pronouns. He rarely made any errors on pronoun case categories (only 2 errors in 347 pronoun uses), correctly marking subject and object forms of his pronouns. But they report that he made frequent errors with gender and number. Examples they report include "*He's* a girl," and "*They* are putting *their* shoes on" (for *she* and *her*). Antony also had lexical problems with nouns and verbs. Curtiss and Yamada report a number of misuses including, "We saw them on the *birthday*" (for *cake*), "He's *cutting* the *mail*" (for *stamping* the *letter*), and "*What* is tape recorder?" (for *where*). They point out that it is striking that none of Antony's lexical errors involved violations of syntactic class or subcategorization features.

Finally, Curtiss and Yamada (1981) note several pragmatic deficits in Antony's speech. Semantic problems in presupposition and implicature often led to communication difficulties. Antony showed problems of topic maintenance and control. And while he appeared to have mastered the syntactic constraints on ellipsis (producing only well-formed elliptical structures), he rarely used ellipsis. Curtiss and Yamada argue that this suggests that he may not have control over the semantic and pragmatic constraints for the use of ellipsis.

This case has been quoted here in some detail for two reasons. First, it shows the level of analysis that is required if one is to get beyond the superficial descriptions of language that are the outcome of merely administering standardized language tests to groups of children with various kinds of mental retardation. Second, it illustrates clearly how a conceptual deficit can differentially affect specific subsystems of the grammar, affecting primarily the semantic component and those aspects of morphology and pragmatic use that are closely tied to meaning, while leaving the syntactic and phonological components relatively unaffected. Yamada (1981) has similarly presented the case of Marta, a hyperlinguistic, retarded adolescent, which also illustrates this approach.

By reviewing the work on language abilities in mentally retarded individuals, it has been possible to focus on known conceptual deficits and their effects on various subsystems of language. It is clear that only some subsystems of language are affected and that it is crucial that the term *language* be differentiated if one is going to study the effects of cognitive processes on it. But there are many differences in mentally retarded groups (and in individuals within those groups). Although most etiological differences in mental retardation do not differentiate later performance, there are conditions where specific cognitive impairments can be identified, and these may have specifiable effects on the particular subsystems of language. As was argued in the first part of this chapter, it is also necessary to differentiate the term *cognition*.

## Other Cognitive Impairments in Mental Retardation

It may not be only the conceptual system that is impaired in mentally retarded individuals. Other aspects of cognition and cognitive processing may be affected. For example, some researchers have hypothesized that memory deficits may limit the language in some individuals or groups. Graham (1968, 1974, 1980; Graham & Gulliford, 1968), in experiments with educationally subnormal children, found that repetition and comprehension scores on a number of different sentence types increased regularly with short-term memory assessed by a task of repeating words and digits. Graham concluded that children are unable to process sentence types that make demands on short-term memory that are beyond their capacity. Memory deficits have also been hypothesized to play a role in nonretarded language-disordered children (Menyuk, 1964, 1969). It is interesting to note that in Antony's battery of nonlanguage cognitive tasks, on only one did he perform age appropriately—auditory short-term memory. Yamada and Curtiss (1981) have reported details of a case study of a young girl,

Vivian, with Turner's Syndrome, a chromosomal abnormality in which there is pathological variation in or absence of the second x chromosome. This case also provides good evidence of poor conceptual abilities coupled with good language abilities in the syntactic component. On the battery of nonlanguage cognitive tests, there was only one nonlanguage area in which Vivian excelled—auditory short-term memory. It is tempting to suppose that adequate short-term memory capacity or processing ability is a cognitive prerequisite for language. However, Yamada (1981) reports that Marta, a hyperlinguistic adolescent who evidenced advanced syntactic ability in spite of limited conceptual abilities, scored poorly on auditory short-term memory tasks.

Most children diagnosed as autistic are severely retarded. Their language has often been characterized as bizarre and inappropriate. For those autistic children who have speech, a strong case can be made that a close analysis of their language reveals that it is the pragmatic component that is primarily affected. (See the careful linguistic analyses by Baltaxe, 1977; Baltaxe & Simmons, 1975, 1977; Chapter 9 in this volume by Baltaxe & Simmons; and Cromer, 1984, for a detailed review.) Particular cognitive or social/affective impairments may be responsible for the observed effects on this aspect of language.

It is possible to trace a number of other cognitive impairments in language-disordered individuals who are not mentally retarded. Such impairments include problems with rate of auditory processing (Tallal & Piercy, 1973a, 1973b, 1974, 1975, 1978), sequencing (Efron, 1963; Lowe & Campbell, 1965), hierarchical planning (Cromer, 1983), and "symbolic" capacities (Ricks & Wing, 1976). These studies have been reviewed elsewhere (Cromer, 1984).

## CONCLUDING NOTE

It should be clear that the old question of the relation between language and thought has been couched in terms that are no longer appropriate. The increase of knowledge about cognitive functioning accumulating from the cognitive sciences makes it naive to talk merely about "thought." There has been a growing concern with the underlying cognitive processes that make conceptual knowledge possible and with the representational capacities and abilities that affect the acquisition, growth, and use of those concepts. From advances in linguistics and psycholinguistics, it has become increasingly apparent that it is sterile to talk about "language." Language is a complex process that at present can be considered usefully in terms of a number of its subcomponents (phonology, syntax, morphology, and semantics) and in terms of its use (pragmatics).

This chapter has considered in some detail the differentiation of the term *language* and has noted some of the directions that differentiating *cognition* might take. By focusing on studies of language in mentally retarded individuals, it was possible to pinpoint those areas of language where conceptual limitations have important effects. Studies of children in whom the syntactic capacity of language is well developed in spite of those severe conceptual limitations not only reveal some surprising facts about capacities in mentally retarded individuals, but provide some intriguing hints about language and the processes that may be necessary for its acquisition.

## REFERENCES


Anderson, E. M., & Spain, B. (1977). *The child with spina bifida*. London: Methuen.

Aronoff, M. (1983). A decade of morphology and word formation. *Annual Review of Anthropology, 12*, 355–375.

Atkinson, M. (1982). *Explanations in the study of child language development*. Cambridge: Cambridge University Press.

Au, T. K. (1983). Chinese and English counterfactuals: The Sapir-Whorf hypothesis revisited. *Cognition, 15*, 155–187.

Baltaxe, C. A. M. (1977). Pragmatic deficits in the language of autistic adolescents. *Journal of Pediatric Psychology, 2*, 176–180.

Baltaxe, C. A. M., & Simmons, J. Q., III. (1975). Language in childhood psychosis: A review. *Journal of Speech and Hearing Disorders, 40*, 439–458.

Baltaxe, C., & Simmons, J. Q., III. (1977). Language patterns of adolescent autistics: A comparison between English and German. In P. Mittler (Ed.), *Research to practice in mental retardation: Vol. II. Education and training* (pp. 267–278). Baltimore: University Park Press.

Bartel, N. R., Bryen, D., & Keehn, S. (1973). Language comprehension in the moderately retarded child. *Exceptional Children, 39*, 375–382.

Bellak, L., & Bellak, S. S. (1974). *Children's Apperception Test*. Larchmont, NY: C.P.S.

Benton, A. (1965). *Visual Retention Test, Multiple Choice Forms*. Paris: Centre de Psychologie Appliquée.

Berko, J. (1958). The child's learning of English morphology. *Word, 14*, 150–177.

Bloom, A. (1981). *The linguistic shaping of thought*. Hillsdale, NJ: Lawrence Erlbaum.

Bloom, L. (1984). Review of M. Atkinson, Explanations in the study of child language development. *Journal of Child Language, 11*, 215–222.

Bradbury, B., & Lunzer, E. A. (1972). The learning of grammatical inflexions in normal and subnormal children. *Journal of Child Psychology and Psychiatry, 13*, 239–248.

Brown, R. (1973). *A first language*. Cambridge, MA: Harvard University Press.

Brown, R. (1977). In reply to Peter Schönbach. *Cognition, 5*, 185–187.

Brown, R. W. (1957). Linguistic determinism and the part of speech. *Journal of Abnormal and Social Psychology, 55*, 1–5.

Carey, S. (1978). The child as word learner. In M. Halle, J. Bresnan, & G. A. Miller (Eds.), *Linguistic theory and psychological reality* (pp. 264–293). Cambridge, MA: MIT Press.

Carroll, J. B. (Ed.). (1956). *Language, thought and reality: Selected writings of Benjamin Lee Whorf*. New York: MIT Press and John Wiley.

Chomsky, N. (1965). *Aspects of the theory of syntax*. Cambridge, MA: MIT Press.

Coggins, T. E., & Morrison, J. A. (1981). Spontaneous imitations of Down's syndrome children: A lexical analysis. *Journal of Speech and Hearing Research, 24*, 303–308.

Cromer, R. F. (1974). Receptive language in the mentally retarded: Processes and diagnostic distinctions. In R. L. Schiefelbusch & L. L. Lloyd (Eds.), *Language perspectives—Acquisition, retardation, and intervention* (pp. 237–267). Austin, TX: PRO-ED.

Cromer, R. F. (1981). Developmental language disorders: Cognitive processes, semantics, pragmatics, phonology, and syntax. *Journal of Autism and Developmental Disorders, 11*, 57–74.

Cromer, R. F. (1983). Hierarchical planning disability in the drawings and constructions of a special group of severely aphasic children. *Brain and Cognition, 2*, 144–164.

Cromer, R. F. (1984). *Language and cognition in relation to handicap.* Paper presented at the Spastics Society Medical Education and Information Unit conference, Language development and communication problems of the handicapped, Oxford, January 3–6, 1984.

Curtiss, S. (1981). Dissociations between language and cognition: Cases and implications. *Journal of Autism and Developmental Disorders, 11*, 15–30.

Curtiss, S., Fromkin, V., & Yamada, J. E. (1978). *The independence of language as a cognitive system*. Paper presented at the First International Congress for the Study of Child Language, Tokyo, August 7–12.

Curtiss, S., & Yamada, J. (1981). Selectively intact grammatical development in a retarded child. *UCLA Working papers in Cognitive Linguistics, 3*, 61–91.

Dever, R. B., & Gardner, W. I. (1970). Performance of normal and retarded boys on Berko's test of morphology. *Language and Speech, 13*, 162–181.

Efron, R. (1963). Temporal perception, aphasia, and déjà vu. *Brain, 86*, 403–424.

Fleming, C. P. (1968). The verbal behavior of hydrocephalic children. *Developmental Medicine and Child Neurology*, Supplement No. 15, 74–82.

Fodor, J. A. (1983). *The modularity of mind.* Cambridge, MA: MIT Press.

Fraser, C., Bellugi, U., & Brown, R. (1963). Control of grammar in imitation, comprehension, and production. *Journal of Verbal Learning and Verbal Behavior, 2*, 121–135.

Fraser, W. I., Agnew, J., & Grieve, R. (1975). The linguistic behaviour of the hydrocephalic mentally handicapped adult. *British Journal of Mental Subnormality, 21*, 38–42.

Fromkin, V., & Rodman, R. (1974). *An introduction to language*. New York: Holt, Rinehart and Winston.

Graham, J. T., & Graham, L. W. (1971). Language behavior of the mentally retarded: Syntactic characteristics. *American Journal of Mental Deficiency, 75*, 623–629.

Graham, N. C. (1968). Short term memory and syntactic structure in educationally subnormal children. *Language and Speech, 11,* 209–219.

Graham, N. C. (1974). Response strategies in the partial comprehension of sentences. *Language and Speech, 17,* 205–221.

Graham, N. C. (1980). Memory constraints in language deficiency. In F. M. Jones (Ed.), *Language disability in children: Assessment and remediation* (pp. 69–94). Lancaster, England: MTP Press.

Graham, N. C., & Gulliford, R. A. (1968). A psychological approach to the language deficiencies of educationally subnormal children. *Education Review, 20,* 136–145.

Griffiths, R. (1951). *Griffiths Mental Development Scales*. Sarasota, FL: Test Center.

Hadenius, A-M., Hagberg, B., Hyttnäs-Bensch, K., & Sjögren, I. (1962). The natural prognosis of infantile hydrocephalus. *Acta Paediatrica,* 51, 117–118.

Ingram, T. T. S., & Naughton, J. A. (1962). Paediatric and psychological aspects of cerebral palsy associated with hydrocephalus. *Developmental Medicine and Child Neurology, 4,* 287–292.

Jespersen, O. (1965). *A modern English grammar on historical principles* (1st ed., 1931). London: George Allen & Unwin.

Karlin, I. W., & Strazzulla, M. (1952). Speech and language problems of mentally deficient children. *Journal of Speech and Hearing Disorders, 17,* 286–294.

Kirk, S. A., McCarthy, J. J., & Kirk, W. D. (1969). *Illinois Test of Psycholinguistic Abilities*. Urbana, IL: University of Illinois Press.

Lackner, J. R. (1968). A developmental study of language behavior in retarded children. *Neuropsychologia, 6,* 301–320.

Lenneberg, E. H., Nichols, I. A., & Rosenberger, E. F. (1964). Primitive stages of language development in mongolism. In D. McK. Rioch & E. A. Weinstein (Eds.), *Disorders of communication* (Research publications of the Association for Research in Nervous and Mental Disease, Vol. XLII, pp. 119–137). Baltimore, MD: Williams & Wilkins.

Lieber, C. W. & Spitz, H. H. (1976). Inference of word meaning from syntax structure by normal children and retarded adolescents. *The Journal of Psychology, 93,* 3–12.

Lovell, K., & Bradbury, B. (1967). The learning of English morphology in educationally subnormal special school children. *American Journal of Mental Deficiency, 71,* 609–615.

Lovell, K., & Dixon, E. M. (1967). The growth of the control of grammar in imitation, comprehension and production. *Journal of Child Psychology and Psychiatry, 8,* 31–39.

Lowe, A. D., & Campbell, R. A. (1965). Temporal discrimination in aphasoid and normal children. *Journal of Speech and Hearing Research, 8,* 313–314.

McLeavey, B. C., Toomey, J. F., & Dempsey, P. J. R. (1982). Nonretarded and mentally retarded children's control over syntactic structures. *American Journal of Mental Deficiency, 86,* 485–494.

Menyuk, P. (1964). Comparison of grammar of children with functionally deviant and normal speech. *Journal of Speech and Hearing Research, 7,* 109–121.

Menyuk, P. (1969). *Sentences children use*. Cambridge, MA: MIT Press.

Miller, J. F., & Chapman, R. S. (1984). Disorders of communication: Investigating the development of language of mentally retarded children. *American Journal of Mental Deficiency, 88*, 536–545.

Moerk, E. L. (1976). Motivational variables in language acquisition. *Child Study Journal, 6*, 55–84.

Mooney, C. M. (1957). Age in the development of closure ability in children. *Canadian Journal of Psychology*, 11, 219–226.

Naremore, R. C., & Dever, R. B. (1975). Language performance of educable mentally retarded and normal children at five age levels. *Journal of Speech and Hearing Research, 18*, 82–95.

Newfield, M. U., & Schlanger, B. B. (1968). The acquisition of English morphology by normal and educable mentally retarded children. *Journal of Speech and Hearing Research, 11*, 693–706.

O'Connor, N., & Hermelin, B. (1963). *Speech and thought in severe subnormality.* Oxford: Pergamon Press.

*Oxford English dictionary*. (1933). J. A. H. Murray, H. Bradley, W. A. Craigie, & C. T. Onions (Eds.). Oxford: Clarendon Press.

Paris, S. G., Mahoney, G. J., & Buckhalt, J. A. (1974). Facilitation of semantic integration in sentence memory of retarded children. *American Journal of Mental Deficiency, 78*, 714–720.

Parsons, J. G. (1968). An investigation into the verbal facility of hydrocephalic children, with special reference to vocabulary, morphology and fluency. *Developmental Medicine and Child Neurology*, Supplement No. 16, 109–110.

Paul, R., Chapman, R. S., & Wanska, S. (1980). *The development of complex sentence use*. Paper presented at the annual meeting of the American Speech and Hearing Association, Detroit.

Pennington, B., Puck, M., & Robinson, A. (1980). Language and cognitive development in 47 XXX females followed since birth. *Behavior Genetics, 10*, 31–41.

Potter, M. C. (1979). Mundane symbolism: The relations among objects, names, and ideas. In N. R. Smith & M. B. Franklin (Eds.), *Symbolic functioning in childhood* (pp. 41–65). Hillsdale, NJ: Lawrence Erlbaum.

Potter, M. C., & Faulconer, B. A. (1975). Time to understand pictures and words. *Nature, 253*, 437–438.

Reynell, J. (1969). *Reynell Developmental Language Scales.* Windsor Berkshire, England: NFER-Nelson.

Rice, M. L. (1983). Contemporary accounts of the cognition/language relationship: Implications for speech-language clinicians. *Journal of Speech and Hearing Disorders, 48*, 347–359.

Rice, M. L., & Kemper, S. (1984). *Child language and cognition.* Austin, TX: PRO-ED.

Ricks, D. M., & Wing, L. (1976). Language, communication, and the use of symbols. In L. Wing (Ed.), *Early childhood autism* (2nd ed., pp. 93–134). Oxford: Pergamon Press.

Rosenberg, S. (1982). The language of the mentally retarded: Development, processes and intervention. In S. Rosenberg (Ed.), *Handbook of applied psycholinguistics* (pp. 329–392). Hillsdale, NJ: Lawrence Erlbaum.

Schiefelbusch, R. L., & Lloyd, L. L. (1974). *Language perspectives—acquisition, retardation, and intervention*. Austin, TX: PRO-ED.

Semmel, M. I., Barritt, L. S., & Bennett, S. W. (1970). Performance of EMR and nonretarded children on a modified Cloze task. *American Journal of Mental Deficiency, 74*, 681–688.

Spain, B. (1974). Verbal and performance ability in pre-school children with spina bifida. *Developmental Medicine and Child Neurology, 16*, 773–780.

Spitz, H. H. (1982). Intellectual extremes, mental age, and the nature of human intelligence. *Merrill-Palmer Quarterly, 28*, 167–192.

Spitz, H. H. (1983). Critique of the developmental position in mental-retardation research. *The Journal of Special Education, 17*, 261–294.

Spreen, O. (1965). Language functions in mental retardation: A review. I. Language development, types of retardation, and intelligence level. *American Journal of Mental Deficiency, 69*, 482–494.

Stone, M. H., & Wright, B. D. (1980). *Knox's Cube Test.* Chicago: Stoelting.

Swisher, L. P., & Pinsker, E. J. (1971). The language characteristics of hyperverbal, hydrocephalic children. *Developmental Medicine and Child Neurology, 13*, 746–755.

Tallal, P., & Piercy, M. (1973a). Defects of non-verbal auditory perception in children with developmental aphasia. *Nature, 241*, 468–469.

Tallal, P., & Piercy, M. (1973b). Developmental aphasia: Impaired rate of non-verbal processing as a function of sensory modality. *Neuropsychologia, 11*, 389–398.

Tallal, P., & Piercy, M. (1974). Developmental aphasia: Rate of auditory processing and selective impairment of consonant perception. *Neuropsychologia, 12*, 83–93.

Tallal, P., & Piercy, M. (1975). Developmental aphasia: The perception of brief vowels and extended stop consonants. *Neuropsychologia,* 13, 69–74.

Tallal, P., & Piercy, M. (1978). Defects of auditory perception in children with developmental dysphasia. In M. A. Wyke (Ed.), *Developmental dysphasia* (pp. 63–84). London & New York: Academic Press.

Taylor, E. M. (1959). *Psychological appraisal of children with cerebral defects*. Cambridge, MA: Harvard University Press.

Tew, B. (1979). The "cocktail party syndrome" in children with hydrocephalus and spina bifida. *British Journal of Disorders of Communication, 14*, 89–101.

Wechsler, D. *Wechsler Preschool and Primary Scale of Intelligence*. Cleveland, OH: Psychological Corporation.

Yamada, J. (1981). Evidence for the independence of language and cognition: Case study of a "hyperlinguistic" adolescent. *UCLA Working Papers in Cognitive Linguistics, 3*, 121–160.

Yamada, J., & Curtiss, S. (1981). The relation between language and cognition in a case of Turner's syndrome. *UCLA Working Papers in Cognitive Linguistics, 3*, 93–115.

Zigler, E., & Balla, D. (Eds.). (1982). *Mental retardation: The developmental-difference controversy*. Hillsdale, NJ: Lawrence Erlbaum.

# 6

# *Language and Cognition*

TERRY KIT-FONG AU

Once I was asked to translate *privacy* into Chinese. I stammered out several possibilities, happy with none, and decided that privacy was such a Western idea that there might be no simple expression for it in Chinese. When I later learned about the work of Edward Sapir and Benjamin Lee Whorf—the focus of this essay—I was reminded of this incident. While Sapir, Whorf, and I all observed some linguistic differences between English and unrelated languages, such as Hopi and Chinese, they believed that language determined one's way of thinking, and I thought it was the other way around. Both views presuppose that language and thought are related, but understanding how they may be related is a complex matter.

## THE SAPIR-WHORF HYPOTHESIS

Sapir and Whorf are associated with one of the best known hypotheses about the relation between language and cognition. Sapir (1949, p. 162) asserted, "Language is a guide to 'social reality'. . . . No two languages are ever sufficiently similar to be considered as representing the same social reality." Whorf (1956, p. 213) further argued, "The world is presented

This work was supported in part by a research assistantship from the Center for the Study of Language and Information. I thank Roger Brown, Richard Cromer, Elissa L. Newport, Karen E. Ravn, and Barbara Tversky for their helpful comments on the manuscript. To Herbert H. Clark, Susan A. Gelman, and Ellen M. Markman, I am especially grateful for their suggestions throughout the preparation of this chapter.

in a kaleidoscopic flux of impressions which has to be organized . . . largely by the linguistic systems in our minds." The Sapir-Whorf hypothesis has two tenets (cf. R. Brown, 1976; Whorf, 1956):

*Linguistic Relativity.* Structural differences between languages will generally be paralleled by nonlinguistic cognitive differences in the native speakers of the two languages.

*Linguistic Determinism.* The structure of a language strongly influences or fully determines the way its native speakers perceive and reason about the world.

Most empirical research on the Sapir-Whorf hypothesis has been devoted to testing linguistic relativity. The major findings, thus far, are in the domains of color terms, classifiers, and counterfactuals.

## Color Terms

Brown and Lenneberg (1954) reasoned that if there were parallels between language and cognition, they should exist within a language as well as across languages. For example, referents that are more easily named might be more memorable. With this hypothesis and some Munsell color chips, they proceeded to test linguistic relativity with English-speaking Americans. They first assessed the codability of various colors by asking their subjects to name the color of each chip. A color with greater consensus on its name was taken to be more codable. It also tended to be named more rapidly and given shorter names. In this study, a more codable color was predicted to be more memorable. When they gave a color recognition memory test to another sample of English speakers, the subjects in fact remembered the more codable colors better. In short, they found evidence for a parallel between language and cognition, although not necessarily for linguistic relativity.

In order to interpret Brown and Lenneberg's (1954) intralinguistic findings as evidence for linguistic relativity, one has to make two important assumptions about different languages (see also R. Brown, 1976). One has to assume that, for each color, the codability varies arbitrarily across linguistic communities, and that in each linguistic community, the codability scores will correlate with color recognition accuracy. In a study that did not require these assumptions, Lenneberg collaborated with Roberts (1956) to test linguistic relativity more directly. They noticed that monolingual speakers of Zuni, an American Indian language, had a color term, *lhupzʔinna*, that covered both yellow and orange. Bilingual Zunis who knew English tended to render *lhupzʔinna* as yellow; they often used a loan-word, *ʔolenchi* (from English *orange*), or its more common derivative,

*ʔolenchinanne*, for the orange color. When Lenneberg and Roberts tested the recognition memory of Zunis for yellow and orange, all four of their monolingual Zuni subjects failed miserably. Their eight bilingual Zuni subjects remembered the two colors better than the monolingual Zunis but not as well as the native English speakers in Brown and Lenneberg's study. Although the sample size was small, this study nonetheless yielded more direct support for linguistic relativity than Brown and Lenneberg's did.

Lenneberg and Roberts' (1956) findings, however, were confounded with subjects' age, schooling, and familiarity with Western culture and testing situation. According to Lenneberg and Roberts (1956, p. 31), "Unfortunately the monolingual subjects were elderly and on this basis alone were not representative of the general adult population." The monolingual Zunis' poor performance may have resulted from their poor memory due to old age, rather than their not having distinct color terms for yellow and orange. Lenneberg and Roberts (1956, p. 23) also noted, "Many [Zuni subjects] were somewhat apprehensive about participating in an unfamiliar test situation." In contrast, the native English speakers in Brown and Lenneberg's (1954) study were test-wise students at Harvard and Radcliffe colleges. The Zunis' relatively poor performance, then, may have reflected their feeling uneasy in the testing situation and their unfamiliarity with the stimulus materials (cf. Cole, Gay, Glick, & Sharp, 1971; Price-Williams, 1962). One way of dealing with these potential confounds in cross-linguistic data is to rely on measures other than subjects' absolute performance. This is exactly what Berlin and Kay did.

Berlin and Kay (1969) challenged linguistic relativity by studying the universality of basic color terms. They defined a term as "basic" if, among other criteria, it consisted of a single morpheme (e.g., *green* not *blue-green*); named a color that was not embodied by any other color terms (e.g., *red* not *magenta*); and was not restricted in use to a narrow range of objects (e.g., *yellow* not *blond*). Basic color terms were elicited from native speakers of 20 genetically diverse languages. The informants were also asked to map the focal point (i.e., the best, most typical instance) and the outer boundary of each of their basic color terms on an array of Munsell color chips varying in hue and brightness. Berlin and Kay found that although the variability in color boundaries was large and unreliable, the focal points of basic color terms were similar among their informants, and the variability across languages was no greater than that within a language.

The number of basic color terms also predicted surprisingly well which terms were encoded in a language. Berlin and Kay's (1969) findings based on 98 languages, with later emendations (e.g., Kay & McDaniel, 1978), are roughly as follows. When there are only two basic color terms in a language, they are *black* and *white*, or *dark* and *light*. When there are three, the third one is *red*. For a language with four to six basic color terms, the additional terms are drawn from *blue, green,* and *yellow*. When there are more than six terms, *brown, purple, pink, orange,* and *gray* are present in various combinations. Berlin and Kay's claim about the universality of basic color terms and focal points of color categories is a strong one. It directly challenges Sapir's notion that speakers of different languages live in distinct worlds and Whorf's idea that the world is presented to us in a kaleidoscopic flux of impressions that has to be cut up arbitrarily, and organized, by languages.

Yet Berlin and Kay's (1969) challenge to the Sapir-Whorf hypothesis has in turn been challenged on methodological grounds. For instance, in eliciting color terms from native speakers of 20 languages, Berlin and Kay often had only one informant for each language. For 18 of these languages, their informants lived in San Francisco and were bilingual in their native languages and English. The data on the additional 78 languages are also problematic. They were gathered from dictionaries, ethnographies, or other researchers through personal communication. The color lexicons so obtained were often incomplete; there was no independent verification that the color terms satisfied Berlin and Kay's criteria for basic color terms (see also Hickerson, 1971).

Here is where Heider (1972) stepped in. Heider began by testing Brown and Lenneberg's (1954) assumption that codability scores of colors would differ arbitrarily across languages. She put together an array of focal colors (e.g., blood red) and nonfocal colors (e.g., brick red), and asked native speakers of 23 genetically diverse languages to name the colors. The focal colors represented the centers of best-instance clusters of all basic color terms but *gray* found in Berlin and Kay's (1969) study. The nonfocal colors were either at the centers of the areas in which no chips had been chosen by Berlin and Kay's informants as the best instance of a basic color term, or in between one of these nonfocal colors and a focal color. Heider found that focal colors were named more rapidly and given shorter names than were the nonfocal colors. She did not report the codability scores language by language, but added later, "In twenty-three diverse languages . . . it was the same colours that were most codable" (Rosch, previously Heider, 1977, p. 512). Heider's findings showed that codability of colors does not differ arbitrarily across languages.

Heider went on to test the hypothesis that focal colors could be remembered more accurately than nonfocal colors, whether the focal colors were named in the language or not. She first asked some monolingual speakers of Dani, an Indonesian New Guinea language, to name an array of colors and found a sample who used only two color terms, *mili* (roughly *dark*) and *mola* (roughly *light*). She then tested the recognition memory of these Dani subjects and a sample of native English-speaking Americans for focal and nonfocal colors. The findings with the American sample were very similar to Brown and Lenneberg's (1954) results. That is, the more codable colors, in this case the focal colors, were more memorable. As in Lenneberg and Roberts' (1956) study, the English-speaking Americans in this study remembered color stimuli more accurately than speakers of a language with fewer basic color terms. This is hardly surprising. Here again, the superior performance of the test-wise American subjects was completely confounded with the subjects' experience in test-taking. But like the Americans, the Dani subjects also remembered the focal colors more accurately than the nonfocal ones. This result cannot be explained by codability because the Dani subjects used only two basic color terms, namely, *mili* and *mola*.

In short, while Lenneberg and Roberts' (1956) findings suggested that color naming might affect color memory, their findings were confounded with subjects' age, schooling, and familiarity with Western culture and the testing situation. Although clouded by methodological problems also, Berlin and Kay's (1969) findings were supported by Heider's (1972) experimental data. In fact, their findings converge with Heider's to suggest that color naming does not differ arbitrarily across languages, and that color naming can be tangential to color memory. Ironically, the research on color terms, as R. Brown (1976, p. 152) noted, "began in a spirit of strong relativism and linguistic determinism and has now come to a position of cultural universalism and linguistic insignificance."

## Classifiers

According to Whorf (1956), there are covert grammatical categories in every language that may affect how its speakers think. Consider what are called shape classifiers in Navaho. Whenever Navaho speakers talk about handling an object, they have to add a suffix called a classifier to the verb corresponding to the shape or some other important attribute of the object. For instance, they use one classifier for long flexible objects such as a piece of rope, another for long rigid objects such as a stick, and so forth. As a result, nouns are overtly classified by these suffixes of verbs, although the nouns themselves are not overtly classified as such. For any object that has a shape, the covert shape-class is consistent with the actual object's shape. It therefore seems possible that Navaho shape classifiers, as well as the covert shape-classes, have a perceptual basis. But Whorf (1956) did not think so. One of the counterexamples he gave was that, in Navaho, *sorrow* belongs to the round class, and this clearly can have no perceptual basis because *sorrow* is not a physical object. He therefore proposed that Navaho shape-classes were an example of covert grammatical categories dissecting and organizing nature in speakers' minds.

Carroll and Casagrande (1958) reasoned that if Whorf was right, the obligatory use of shape classifiers should render Navaho speakers more likely to group objects by shape than by, say, color and size. They tested this hypothesis with Navaho children who spoke only or predominantly Navaho, Navaho children who spoke only or predominantly English, and Caucasian children who spoke only English. The children were shown ten pairs of objects, one pair at a time, with the pair members differing from each other in two of the following aspects: shape, color, or size. For each pair, the children were asked which member went best with a third object that was similar to each pair member in one of the two contrasting features but that matched neither member exactly. The findings with the Navaho children were exactly as Carroll and Casagrande had predicted. The Navaho-dominant children preferred shape over color in grouping objects; the English-dominant Navahos preferred color over shape. Moreover, while in both groups the preference for shape increased with age, the former began to prefer shape over color around 3 to 4 years of age; the latter did not until 9 years of age.

These results would be straightforward evidence for a weak form of linguistic relativity if they were not complicated by the findings with the Caucasian English-speaking children. By 4 years of age, these children began to prefer shape over color in grouping objects, and their preference for shape was even stronger that that of the Navaho-dominant children. Carroll and Casagrande (1958) attributed the Caucasian children's preference to their experience with toys of various shapes, and argued that the shape-color preference could be affected by experience in handling objects of various shapes as well as covert shape-class in language. However, one can also argue that the Navaho-dominant children preferred shape over color because they had ample experience in handling objects of various shapes from their outdoor activities on the reservation, rather than because they spoke Navaho. Both Carroll and Casagrande's argument and the counterargument proposed here require very strong assumptions about these Navaho and Caucasian children's environments. Carroll and Casagrande did not report the home and school environments of these children in detail. It is therefore hard to interpret the difference in shape-color preference among these children.

Later research revealed that there might be a cognitive basis for shape classifiers. By surveying the semantics of classifiers in 37 Asian languages drawn from seven language families, Adams and Conklin (1973) revealed three recurring themes: round, long, and flat. These shape themes, alone or combined with properties such as rigidity and relative size, play an important role in the classifier systems of these languages. They are also common themes of classifiers in many American Indian languages (see E. Clark, 1976). Interestingly, young children also overextend word meanings based on properties of shape. For instance, they may use *ball* to refer to oranges, eggs, the moon, and other round objects. A survey of diaries kept of young children's speech revealed that the largest class of overextensions in word meanings was also based on shape, especially roundness and length (E. Clark, 1973). Because every object has both shape and color, if Whorf (1956) was right about languages dissecting the world arbitrarily, there should be color-classifiers as well as shape-classifiers in various classifier languages. Similarly, children's overextensions in word meanings should be based on color as well as shape. Yet while shape by itself has often been reported as a basis for both classifiers and children's overextensions, color has not (Adams & Conklin, 1973; Bowerman, 1977; E. Clark, 1973, 1976). Classifiers and children's overextensions, then, rather than dissecting the world arbitrarily as Whorf suggested, seem to have cognitive bases.

Because it has received so little convincing support from the research on color terms and classifiers, the Sapir-Whorf hypothesis has stimulated little research for almost a decade. Bloom (1981) proposed a promising research direction. He observed that previous studies focused almost exclusively on lexical schemata related to perceptual categorizations of the physical world. Since both linguistic and nonlinguistic schemata are adequate for coding perceptual experience, Bloom contended, it is no wonder that the research findings with color terms and shape-classifiers have been so inconclusive. As thought moves to higher levels of abstraction, Bloom argued, language may exert its most dramatic effects (see also R. Brown, 1977; Chase, 1956). In this new research direction, Bloom examined counterfactual reasoning in two unrelated languages, namely, English and Chinese.

## Counterfactuals

English, like other Indo-European languages, has a distinct counterfactual construction, the subjunctive, whereas other languages like Chinese do not. When talking about the present counterfactually (e.g., *If he were Sara's teacher, Sara would do better at school*), English speakers use *were to*, *was to*, or the past form of the verb in the *if* clause (the supposition) and *would*, *could*, or *might* in the main clause. When talking about the past counterfactually in English, one has to use the past perfect tense, and *would have*, *could have*, or *might have* (e.g., *If he had been Sara's teacher, Sara would have done better at school*). While the English subjunctive always unambiguously distinguishes a counterfactual sentence from an implicational one, Chinese offers only the "if-then" construction for both (Bloom, 1981). Consider this somewhat literal translation from Chinese: *He is not Sara's teacher. If he is, then Sara will do better at school*. To interpret a counterfactual statement like this in Chinese, Bloom reasoned, Chinese speakers have to integrate the negation of the premise (*He is not Sara's teacher*) and the premise (*if he is*) and implication (*then Sara will do better at school*) expressed by the "if-then" construction. This should require a greater cognitive effort than interpreting the subjunctive in English. Chinese speakers may therefore be less inclined than English speakers to think counterfactually.

To test his hypothesis, Bloom (1981) prepared a story with several counterfactual implications in both English and Chinese, followed by a question to test whether the subjects understood that the implications had never happened. The Chinese version of the counterfactual story was given to Chinese speakers in Hong Kong and Taiwan; the English version, to English speakers in the U.S. His findings were indeed dramatic. Only 7% of the Chinese-speaking subjects gave counterfactual interpretations to the story, whereas 98% of English-speaking subjects did so. Bloom argued that the counterfactual logic of the story was evident to English speakers because of the subjunctive and a correspondingly highly available counterfactual schema.

Bloom (1981) also asked Taiwanese subjects bilingual in Chinese and English to respond to a revised version of the story in English. Of these subjects, who had given only 6% counterfactual responses to the earlier version in Chinese, 86% this time gave counterfactual responses. This 86% rate is significantly higher than the 50% rate given by a comparable group of Taiwanese subjects to a revised Chinese version. Bloom concluded that the bilinguals' inclination to think counterfactually seemed to depend a great deal on whether the language they were using at that very moment had a distinct counterfactual marker.

Bloom's (1981) findings, if upheld, would be very important because they address the issue that Whorf was concerned with—grammar and thinking. I therefore tried to replicate his findings using an improved experimental design and both his revised story and a new counterfactual story (Au, 1983). Chinese and English versions of the two stories were given to Chinese bilinguals in Hong Kong. These subjects showed little difficulty in understanding the counterfactuals in these stories. In fact, they gave over 86% counterfactual responses to both stories in both languages. While there was a significant difference between the two stories in Chinese, favoring the new story over Bloom's story, the difference disappeared when Bloom's story was rewritten in more idiomatic Chinese. These findings suggest that the difficulty Bloom's Chinese subjects had with his counterfactual story was probably due to its unidiomatic Chinese, rather than to the counterfactual logic per se.

The English versions of both stories were also given to American English speakers. To Bloom's story, the American subjects gave fewer counterfactual responses in English than the Chinese bilinguals did in Chinese (72% vs. 97% counterfactual responses, respectively). Since the

American subjects had little difficulty in understanding the new counterfactual story, their low success rate for Bloom's story should probably not be interpreted as a lack of competence in counterfactual reasoning. Even so, some English speakers responded noncounterfactually to Bloom's story despite the distinct counterfactual construction in their native language.

As tests of the Sapir-Whorf hypothesis, the data of bilinguals are, unfortunately, difficult to interpret. In my research on counterfactuals, for instance, it is hard to know whether or not the success of the Hong Kong bilinguals on the Chinese versions was due to the subjects' mastery of the English subjunctive. They may have extended the counterfactual schema that was originally associated with the English subjunctive to their Chinese linguistic world. To address this issue, I asked some Chinese subjects in Hong Kong to translate a simple counterfactual statement from Chinese into English, and to respond to either Bloom's or my story written in idiomatic Chinese. While 98% of the 62 subjects responding to my story gave counterfactual responses, only one of them showed in her translation that she knew the English subjunctive (Au, 1983). To Bloom's story, 93% of the 42 subjects responded counterfactually, and only 12% of them knew the English subjunctive (Au, 1984). In short, the mastery of the English subjunctive seems to be quite tangential to counterfactual reasoning in Chinese; the lack of a distinct counterfactual construction in Chinese does not seem to hinder Chinese speakers from thinking counterfactually.

While research on color terms, classifiers, and counterfactuals initially yielded support for linguistic relativity, the weight of subsequent experimental and cross-linguistic evidence is in the other direction. Collectively, the findings in these domains give little convincing evidence for the Sapir-Whorf hypothesis at either the lexical or the syntactic level. On the contrary, the presence or absence of a distinct counterfactual marker has little effect on counterfactual reasoning. Moreover, color terms and shape classifiers, far from dissecting the perceptual world arbitrarily, may have cognitive bases.

## COGNITIVE BASES OF LANGUAGE

In Whorf's (1956) writings, a recurrent metaphor is that nature is a formless mass, or a kaleidoscopic flux of impressions, and each language cuts it up arbitrarily (cf. R. Brown, 1976). However, by virtue of being human, we tend to perceive, organize, and reason about the world in certain ways. To some extent, we seem to cut nature up and organize it by our nonlinguistic cognitive processes. This implies that languages may build upon our perceptual categories and conceptual organization. Evidence for this latter view is not directly against the Sapir-Whorf hypothesis, which merely states that languages differ and will affect thought differentially. Yet if certain language structures have cognitive bases, parallels between these language structures and cognition should be interpreted as cognition shaping language. This relationship between language and cognition is very different from what Sapir and Whorf proposed. In this section, I shall discuss several nonlinguistic cognitive processes that seem to constrain the structure of languages.

## Perceptual Space

Children are born into a flat world with gravity, and are endowed with eyes, ears, and eventually an upright posture. As a result, H. Clark (1973) noted, the human perceptual space has three important reference planes: the horizontal plane at ground level, the vertical plane separating the front and back, and the vertical plane separating the left and right. The first two are especially important because they are asymmetrical: Everything above ground level and in front of the perceiver is easily perceptible, and everything below ground level or behind a perceiver is not. When children acquire spatial terms, Clark proposed, they must learn to apply the terms to their prior knowledge about space. Hence, rather than cutting up perceptual space arbitrarily, the spatial terms should reflect the properties of perceptual space.

Consider verticality. Gravity pulls objects vertically downward; people normally walk, stand, and sit upright. A considerable portion of spatial terms also applies only to this dimension. Among them are adjectives such as *tall, short, high, low, deep, shallow* and prepositions such as *up, down, above, below, over, under, on top of, underneath,* and so forth. Some apply only to the part of perceptual space that is above ground level (e.g., *tall, short, high, low*); others often apply to the part below ground level (e.g., *deep, shallow*). Similarly, some prepositions apply only to the front-back dimension, falling into either the front or the back part of perceptual space. Some examples are *in front of, in back of, ahead,* and *behind*. For the left-right dimension, there are *beside, at the left of, at the right of,* and so forth. (For a more thorough discussion, see H. Clark, 1973.) In contrast, few spatial terms encode diagonality, or dimensions other than vertical, front-back, and left-right. When they do, they are often used with respect to the vertical dimension. For instance, a "tilted" object is usually seen as tilted with respect to the vertical dimension.

In light of various cross-linguistic findings on spatial terms (e.g., Bierwisch, 1967; Greenberg, 1966), the strong correspondence between perceptual space and spatial terms may also exist in languages other than

English. More importantly, perceptual space does not seem to be cut up and organized arbitrarily by language. It seems instead to depend largely on the properties of gravity and of the human perceptual apparatus. Its correspondence to spatial terms, then, suggests perception constraining language, rather than vice versa.

## Hue Perception

According to Hering (1920), every hue can be thought of either as one of the four primary hues—namely, red, blue, green, and yellow—or as a mixture of them. For instance, purple is thought to consist of red and blue, whereas red is not thought to be composed of different hues. Primary hues also seem to be more salient and easily identified than nonprimary hues. Bornstein (1975) found that 4-month-olds, when given a choice, spent more time looking at primary hues than at hues near the boundaries between them. Children between 2 and 3 years of age have been found to identify primary hues more accurately than nonprimary ones (Istomina, 1963). The macaque monkey's visual system, which is similar to the human's, also seems to be particularly sensitive to red, blue, green, and yellow (De Valois & Jacobs, 1968). These findings converge to suggest that the four primary hues are more fundamental and salient than nonprimary hues.

When the findings on hue perception are compared to Berlin and Kay's (1969) data on basic hue terms, a striking parallel emerges. Berlin and Kay's findings show that if a language has encoded fewer than five basic hue terms, it should include *red, blue, green,* and *yellow*. *Brown, pink, orange,* and *purple* are encoded only in languages that have encoded the four primary hues. This parallel between hue perception and basic hue terms cannot be accounted for by linguistic determinism because neither the infants in Bornstein's (1975) study nor the macaque monkeys in De Valois and Jacobs' (1968) research had any language. Instead, the encoding of basic hue terms seems to have a perceptual basis. (See also H. Clark & E. Clark, 1977; Kay & McDaniel, 1978; Miller & Johnson-Laird, 1976.)

## Similarity Perception

Striking perceptual or conceptual similarities between members of different object categories often play an important role in figurative language. Consider body part labels. A survey of 118 languages reveals that several figurative labels for body parts are present in many genetically diverse languages (C. Brown & Witkowski, 1981). These body parts are similar, in certain aspects, to the objects their figurative labels literally refer to. For instance, most of the figurative labels for the *pupil* of the eye literally mean "a small human" (e.g., baby, child, son, girl) or "a small humanlike entity" (e.g., doll, infant ghost). Among them, *pupil* in English means both "young student" and "pupil of the eye." These figurative labels, Tagliavini (1949) suggested, might result from the perceptual similarity between a small child and the minute reflections of an observer who looks into another person's eyes.

Another example is muscular body parts (e.g., thighs, biceps of the arm, calves of the leg). Their figurative labels often involve small animals such as mice, rats, toads, and lizards. In English, for instance, *muscle* comes from the Latin word *musculus*, literally "little mouse"; *calf* means both "a small cow" and "calf of the leg." These figurative labels, Brown and Witkowski (1981) noted, may have arisen from the perceptual similarity between the movements of small animals that hop or scurry about and the quick, tensing movements of muscle flexing.

Digits of hand or foot are also frequently equated with people, especially kinsmen. Thumbs and big toes, in particular, are often labeled as older relatives, usually parents; the remaining fingers and toes are often labeled as younger relatives, usually offspring. As Brown and Witkowski (1981) pointed out, the relationships among digits and those among kinsmen are conceptually very similar. Both digits and kinsmen are grouped: digits on hands and feet, and kinsmen in families. Moreover, parents are distinct from their children, so are thumbs and big toes from other digits. In short, the perceptual or conceptual similarities between members of different object categories seem to lead speakers of genetically diverse languages to come up with similar figurative labels for some object categories.

## Categorization

Categories defined by common or correlated attributes are generally quite useful for making inferences (Gelman & Markman, 1986), more so than are disjunctive categories such as "cat or story" (Bruner, Goodnow, & Austin, 1956). For instance, if I know that something is a cat, I know that it is likely to have fur, four legs, and a tail; that it is warm-blooded; that it has a four-chambered heart, and so forth. In contrast, if I am told that something is a "cat or story," I cannot be sure what it is like. One therefore should expect very few disjunctive categories encoded as single terms in languages. This is, in fact, the case. For instance, in theory, the continuum of brightness could be divided into "black or white" and "gray," but "black or white" has never been encoded as a single term (Witkowski & C. Brown, 1977). Instead, when a language has only two basic achromatic terms, they invariably are *black* and *white* (or *dark* and *light*). *Gray* has never been found in a language that has not encoded *black* and *white* (Berlin & Kay, 1969).

Another example involves folk botanical life-form terms such as *tree, grass, vine,* and *bush*. A survey of 105 languages reveals that for languages with only two botanical life-form terms, *tree* and *grerb* are invariably encoded. *Tree* refers to large and woody plants; *grerb* (a blend of *grass* and *herb*) refers to small herbaceous plants. While a language could have encoded "large or small plants" and "medium-size plants" as single terms, it never does (C. Brown, 1977). A similar argument can also be made with antonymous adjectives such as *long* and *short, hot* and *cold,* and so forth, which are present in many languages (Greenberg, 1966). In short, while both categories defined by common or correlated attributes and disjunctive categories can be encoded as single terms by languages, the former disproportionally outnumber the latter. Significantly, the former are also much more useful for making inferences.

Other categories that could have been, but rarely are, encoded by languages as single terms are categories of thematically related objects such as "a spider and its web," "a baby and its milk." (Some exceptions are *friends* and *roommates*; these terms refer to people who are related in certain ways.) While all languages may have a word for *baby*, they are unlikely to have a word referring to "a baby and its milk." Markman and Hutchinson (1984) have suggested that languages are organized in this way because object categories (e.g., "baby" and "milk") support inferences and can be used in various combinations to express thematic relations such as "a baby drinking its milk." In contrast, categories such as "a baby and its milk" support few inferences and cannot be used for talking about a baby and milk separately. Markman and Hutchinson have also found that children as young as 2 years begin to constrain the meaning of a count noun (e.g., *dog*) as referring to an object category, rather than to thematically related objects, although in other contexts they are generally more interested in thematic relations than in taxonomic relations. Taken together, these findings suggest that whether a category is encoded by languages depends in part on how useful it is for making inferences and for expressing ideas.

## Hierarchical Organization of Categories

A white pine is a pine, but it is also a tree, a plant, and a living thing. Organizing these categories into a hierarchy not only helps storing and retrieving information about them, but also is useful for making inferences. For instance, if I know something is a white pine, I can infer that it respires as all living things do; it produces carbohydrates by photosynthesis as all plants do; it is tall and woody as all trees are; it has needles and pine cones as all pines do, and so forth. One therefore may expect to find hierarchical organization of categories across cultures and linguistic communities. This certainly seems to be the case: Native speakers of over 100 languages have been found to organize biological categories hierarchically (Berlin, Breedlove, & Raven, 1973; C. Brown, 1977, 1979).

Learning to organize categories hierarchically, however, is not easy. Children generally learn to name objects first at what is known as the basic level (R. Brown, 1958; Rosch, Mervis, Gray, Johnson, & Boyes-Braem, 1976) and work their way up and down the hierarchy. Basic-level categories, to put it simply, are both informative and distinctive. Each of them captures many common attributes among its members and very few common attributes among members of different basic-level categories (Rosch et al., 1976; Tversky & Hemenway, 1984). To learn to organize categories hierarchically, children have to go beyond basic-level categories. They have to sort out the relation between categories at different levels of abstraction. Consider trees. Children usually learn the basic-level category label *tree* first.[1] When they acquire the labels of the superordinate categories for trees (e.g., *plant*) and those of the subordinate categories (e.g., *pine*), they often find it difficult to keep track of the inclusion relations among these categories, for example, that a tree is a plant (Inhelder & Piaget, 1964). On the other hand, children understand part-whole relations much more readily, for example, that a tree is part of a forest (Markman, Horton, & McLanahan, 1980; Callanan & Markman, 1982). Markman and her colleagues have suggested that collections such as *forest* and *army* have greater psychological coherence than do categories such as *trees* and *soldiers*, and therefore form hierarchies that are easier to represent.

If categories at a high level in a hierarchy were labeled by collective nouns, Markman (1985) reasoned, children might find them easier to learn. However, the relation expressed by a collective noun is a part-whole relation, and not true class-inclusion. Properties true of the whole (e.g., *forest*) may not be true of its parts (e.g., *trees*), whereas whatever is true of a superclass (e.g., *plant*) is always true of its subclass (e.g., *tree*). Collective nouns therefore cannot support inductive and deductive inferences in the way superordinate category terms do. Markman noted that mass nouns seemed to be a compromise between the two relations, and thereby could

---

1 There are two caveats. First, most city-dwellers may have "tree" as a basic-level category, but some botanists may have "oak," "pine," "elm," and so on as basic-level categories. That is, the basic level in a given hierarchy is not the same for everyone; it depends to some extent on how much each person knows about the categories in the hierarchy (see also Rosch et al., 1976; H. Clark & E. Clark, 1977). Second, young children do not always learn the basic-level category labels first. From their first words on, they also learn kin terms and proper names for significant persons, pets, and toy animals (cf. Katz, Baker, & Macnamara, 1974; Gelman & Taylor, 1984).

serve as superordinate terms. For instance, a piece of clay is part of the whole mass of clay, but is also clay in and of itself. Mass nouns, then, can both provide the stability of part-whole relations and serve as taxonomic categories that support inferences. Markman therefore predicted that children would find it easier to learn a superordinate category labeled by a mass noun (e.g., *fruit*) than one labeled by a count noun (e.g., *drinks*). When young children were taught some unfamiliar superordinate categories (e.g., *sports equipment*) labeled by nonsense words, they learned these categories more readily when the labels were mass nouns rather than count nouns.

This property of mass nouns is not confined to English. When Markman (1985) examined 19 genetically diverse languages with the mass-count distinction, she found that at least some superordinate categories of diverse and countable objects in each language were labeled by mass nouns (e.g., *fruit*). In contrast, the corresponding basic-level and subordinate categories (e.g., *apple, Delicious apple*) were almost always labeled by count nouns. The combination of part-whole and inclusion relations embodied in mass nouns, then, may help children grasp the class-inclusion relations between some basic and superordinate level categories, and organize categories hierarchically. It may also account for why only superordinate level but not lower-level categories of diverse and countable objects are encoded by mass nouns in various languages.

## Causal Attribution

According to the stimulus-response theory, stimuli elicit responses (e.g., Skinner, 1938). R. Brown and D. Fish (1983) have argued that this causal schema is perhaps also universally held and often used for making causal attributions of interpersonal events. To test this hypothesis, they asked people to specify the causes of various interpersonal events depicted by sentences such as "Ted amazes Paul" and "Ted pities Paul." They varied the depicted events by using different experiential verbs that fit this sentence frame and found that people consistently attributed the cause of the experience to the stimulus. For instance, in "Ted amazes Paul," Ted is the stimulus of the amazement, whereas Paul is the one who experiences the amazement. Ted, rather than Paul, is also generally viewed as the causal agent of this interpersonal event. Similarly, Paul is the stimulus of the pity, whereas Ted experiences the pity. In this case, Paul is also often seen as the cause of the event. These findings held up regardless of whether the stimulus named was the subject or the object of the sentence.

Brown and Fish (1983) have also found that there are far more adjectives, based on these verbs, that describe the disposition of the stimulus (e.g., *amazing, pitiful*) than that of the experiencer (e.g., *respectful, scornful*). This parallel between language (English word formation) and cognition (causal attribution) can be taken as evidence either for or against linguistic determinism. One may argue, for instance, that people attribute the causes of events to the stimulus rather than to the experiencer because there are more dispositional adjectives about the former than about the latter.

On the other hand, since English allows both types of derivational adjectives (e.g., *respectable* for the stimulus, *respectful* for the experiencer), why should the adjectives of one type outnumber those of the other type? Brown and Fish (1983) suggested that the basic causal schema—namely, that stimuli elicit responses—has brought the adjectives into line with the schema. They appealed to two sources of evidence. First, some adjectives that contradict the causal schema (e.g., *shockable, amazable, amusable*) were once in the English lexicon but have become obsolete. In contrast, their counterparts that are consistent with the causal schema (e.g., *shocking, amazing, amusing*) are now still widely used. Second, some adjectives that used to contradict the causal schema are now in line with the schema. Some examples are *delightful, wonderful, awful, dreadful, pitiful*. According to the *Oxford English Dictionary* (1933), these adjectives originally had the sense "full of . . ." as in *scornful* (i.e., an experiencer disposition). Today, however, all of these adjectives describe the stimulus that elicits delight, wonder, awe, and so forth. Both types of language change suggest that dispositional adjectives in English have a cognitive basis, namely, the causal schema of stimuli eliciting responses. Yet two important questions remain open. Presumably this causal schema has been operating in human beings rather far back in history. Why has it been only recently that adjectives contradicting the causal schema were brought into line with the schema, or dropped out of the English lexicon? Why have some adjectives in line with the causal schema (e.g., *thankworthy*) become obsolete, whereas others contradicting the schema (e.g., *thankful*) are still widely used?

To find out if dispositional adjectives in English have a cognitive basis, it seems necessary to go beyond observations of historical changes in these adjectives. One approach is to examine causal attributions cross-linguistically. If speakers of languages historically unrelated to English make causal attributions similar to those made by English speakers, the causal schema Brown and Fish (1983) proposed may be a human universal. That is, the causal schema is not language-specific. Research findings with Chinese and Japanese speakers show that this may be the case (R. Brown, 1983). Another approach is to study children's acquisition of dispositional adjectives and the causal schema. If children make causal attributions in line with the causal schema before they acquire the relevant dispositional adjectives, it would seem that the causal schema is not built on these adjectives. In a study using a procedure similar to Brown and Fish's (1983),

I (Au, 1986) found that English-speaking 5-year-olds and adults made causal attributions as predicted by Brown and Fish's causal schema. Moreover, the preschoolers did so even for verbs (e.g., *hate*, *worry*) for which they did not know the derived dispositional adjectives (e.g., *hateful*, *worrisome*). The development of this causal schema does not seem to depend on the knowledge of dispositional adjectives. Taken together, these findings suggest that the causal schema is not language-specific; the dispositional adjectives in English may have a cognitive basis.

The story of cognition shaping language certainly cannot be fully told here. The cognitive processes reviewed, nonetheless, seem to affect a variety of language structures (for more psychological constraints on language, see H. Clark & Malt, 1984). To understand better the relationship between language and cognition, let me tally the evidence for language shaping cognition, and vice versa.

## A TALLY: LANGUAGE VERSUS COGNITION

My attempt to find evidence for the Sapir-Whorf hypothesis was about as successful as my attempt to find a simple expression for *privacy* in Chinese. Thus far, there is little convincing evidence for linguistic determinism. What can be thought of as support for linguistic relativity shows little more than some parallels between language and cognition. But even the parallels, given the findings of hue perception, color terms, and classifiers, suggest that these aspects of language have cognitive bases. In short, there is little convincing evidence that structural differences among languages will make speakers of different languages perceive, and reason about, the world differently.

On the other hand, although not in the spirit of the Sapir-Whorf hypothesis, language seems to affect memory and reasoning. Labeling a figure, for instance, often leads people to remember it as being more similar to what the label refers to than it actually is (Carmichael, Hogan, & Walter, 1932). A problem becomes easier to solve when the required tools are labeled (Glucksberg & Weisberg, 1966). A question such as, "How fast was the car going when it passed the barn?" can lead people to believe that they have seen a barn in a film about the car, although there is in fact no barn in the film (Loftus, 1975). The generic use of *he*—that is, for human beings in general—is sometimes interpreted as referring to males only (Martyna, 1980).

These subtle effects on memory and reasoning all seem to be related to the cooperative use of language. According to Grice (1975), people generally try to be informative, truthful, relevant, and clear when they use language, and expect others to do the same. The subjects remembering the figures and solving problems, then, may have thought that the experimenters used the labels to help them do the task and were therefore affected by the labels. Similarly, the subjects answering questions may have been misled because they assumed that Loftus (1975) was truthful when she posed the question. Since the question implied that there was a barn, it was only natural for them to believe the implication to be true. When Martyna's (1980) subjects interpreted the generic *he* as the sex-specific *he*, they might also have thought that if Martyna had meant "he or she," she would have used *he or she* instead (cf. the discussion on pre-emption by E. Clark & H. Clark, 1979). In short, these findings may have been due to the subjects' faith that the experimenters were being fully cooperative. If so, the cooperative use of language, rather than the structure of language as Sapir and Whorf suggested, may be a domain where language is most likely to affect cognition.

The other half of the tally is rather easy: In domain after domain, cognition seems to constrain the structure of language. More importantly, investigations into the psychological reality of grammars (e.g., Bresnan, 1978), the learnability of language (e.g., Pinker, 1979), the M constraint on ontological category terms and predicates (e.g., Keil, 1979; Sommers, 1959, 1963; but see also Gerard & Mandler, 1983), and related topics may reveal more cognitive constraints on language. Another promising research direction is to find cognitive explanations for the language universals that Greenberg (1966) and others have uncovered.

An important question about cognitive constraints on language, however, remains unanswered. That is, via what mechanisms does cognition constrain language? One possibility is that when cognitive and linguistic structures are in conflict, the latter will eventually be abandoned by language users. Consider again Brown and Fish's (1983) findings of dispositional adjectives and the causal schema for interpersonal events. Some adjectives that used to contradict the causal schema either have become obsolete or have changed in meaning to fall in line with the schema. Yet, because not all dispositional adjectives derived from experiential verbs are now in line with the causal schema, the schema may be only a weak constraint on these adjectives. Moreover, this process of language change may be completed very slowly, if at all.

Another mechanism for cognition constraining language may lie in language acquisition. Various cognitive constraints on language may render some language structures easier to learn than others, thereby shaping the structure of languages.

As reviewed earlier in this essay, Markman (1985) has found that young children learn superordinate categories more readily when the category labels are mass nouns rather than count nouns. And for languages with the mass-count distinction, as Markman predicted, mass nouns name some categories of diverse and countable objects at the superordinate level (e.g., *furniture*) but almost none at the basic (e.g., *chairs*) and subordinate levels (e.g., *rocking chairs*). Young children also seem to constrain the meanings of count nouns to referring to object categories, rather than thematically related objects, although they usually find thematic relations more interesting than taxonomic relations (Markman & Hutchinson, 1984). It may not be a mere coincidence, then, that count nouns across languages also generally refer to object categories. In short, the way languages are structured may be partly determined by whether they can be readily learned by young children (cf. Pinker, 1979).

This tally of evidence for language shaping cognition, and vice versa, is hardly complete and will need updating as new findings accumulate. (See, e.g., some speculations about children formulating categories of meanings to fit certain language structures, in Bowerman, 1982.) A few tentative conclusions, however, can be drawn at this point. As Sapir and Whorf noted, languages differ arbitrarily in many aspects. Yet none of these differences has been convincingly shown to cause speakers of different languages to perceive and reason about the world differently. Quite the contrary, in a variety of domains, cognition seems to constrain the structure of language.

## REFERENCES


Adams, K. L., & Conklin, N. F. (1973). *Toward a theory of natural classification*. Papers from the Ninth Regional Meeting, Chicago Linguistic Society (pp. 1–10), Chicago Linguistic Society, Chicago.

Au, T. K. (1983). Chinese and English counterfactuals: The Sapir-Whorf hypothesis revisited. *Cognition, 15*, 155–187.

Au, T. K. (1984). Counterfactuals: In reply to Alfred Bloom. *Cognition, 17*, 289–302.

Au, T. K. (1986). A verb is worth a thousand words: The causes and consequences of interpersonal events implicit in language. *Journal of Memory and Language, 25*, 104–122.

Berlin, B., Breedlove, D. E., & Raven, P. H. (1973). General principles of classification and nomenclature in folk biology. *American Anthropologist, 75*, 214–242.

Berlin, B., & Kay, P. (1969). *Basic color terms: Their universality and evolution*. Berkeley and Los Angeles: University of California Press.

Bierwisch, M. (1967). Some semantic universals of German adjectivals. *Foundations of Language, 3*, 1–36.

Bloom, A. H. (1981). *The linguistic shaping of thought: A study in the impact of language on thinking in China and the West*. Hillsdale, NJ: Lawrence Erlbaum.

Bornstein, M. H. (1975). Qualities of color vision in infancy. *Journal of Experimental Child Psychology, 19*, 401–419.

Bowerman, M. (1977). The acquisition of word meaning: An investigation of some current conflicts. In P. N. Johnson-Laird & P. C. Wason (Eds), *Thinking: Readings in cognitive science* (pp. 239–253). Cambridge: Cambridge University Press.

Bowerman, M. (1982). Reorganizational processes in lexical and syntactic development. In E. Wanner & L. R. Gleitman (Eds.), *Language acquisition: The state of the art* (pp. 319–346). Cambridge: Cambridge University Press.

Bresnan, J. (1978). A realistic transformational grammar. In M. Halle, J. Bresnan, & G. A. Miller (Eds.), *Linguistic theory and psychological reality* (pp. 1–59). Cambridge, MA: MIT Press.

Brown, C. H. (1977). Folk botanical life-forms: Their universality and growth. *American Anthropologist, 79*, 317–342.

Brown, C. H. (1979). Folk zoological life-forms: Their universality and growth. *American Anthropologist, 81*, 791–817.

Brown, C. H., & Witkowski, S. R. (1981). Figurative language in a universalist perspective. *American Ethnologist, 8*, 596–615.

Brown, R. (1958). How shall a thing be called? *Psychological Review, 65*, 14–21.

Brown, R. (1976). Reference: In memorial tribute to Eric Lenneberg. *Cognition, 5*, 125–153.

Brown, R. (1977). In reply to Peter Schönbach. *Cognition, 4*, 185–187.

Brown, R. (1983). *Linguistic relativity*. Paper presented at the G. Stanley Hall Centennial Conference, October 12–13, Baltimore.

Brown, R., & Fish, D. (1983). The psychological causality implicit in language. *Cognition, 14*, 237–273.

Brown, R. W., & Lenneberg, E. H. (1954). A study in language and cognition. *Journal of Abnormal and Social Psychology, 49*, 454–462.

Bruner, J. S., Goodnow, J. J., & Austin, G. A. (1956). *A study of thinking*. New York: John Wiley.

Callanan, M. A., & Markman, E. M. (1982). Principles of organization in young children's natural language hierarchies. *Child Development, 53*, 1093–1101.

Carmichael, L., Hogan, H. P., & Walter, A. A. (1932). An experimental study of the effect of language on the reproduction of visually perceived forms. *Journal of Experimental Psychology, 15*, 73–86.

Carroll, J. B., & Casagrande, J. B. (1958). The function of language classifications in behavior. In E. E. Maccoby, T. M. Newcomb, & E. L. Hartley (Eds.), *Readings in social psychology* (pp. 18–31). New York: Holt, Rinehart and Winston.

Chase, S. (1956). Foreward. In J. B. Carroll (Ed.), *Language, thought, and reality: Selected writings of Benjamin Lee Whorf* (pp. v–x). Cambridge, MA: MIT Press.

Clark, E. V. (1973). What's in a word? On the child's acquisition of semantics in his first language. In T. E. Moore (Ed.), *Cognitive development and the acquisition of language* (pp. 65–110). New York: Academic Press.

Clark, E. V. (1976). Universal categories: On the semantics of classifiers and children's early word meanings. In A. Juilland (Ed.), *Linguistic studies offered to Joseph Greenberg on the occasion of his sixtieth birthday* (Vol. 3, pp. 449–462). Saratoga, CA: Anma Libri.

Clark, E. V., & Clark, H. H. (1979). When nouns surface as verbs. *Language, 55*, 767–811.

Clark, H. H. (1973). Space, time, semantics, and the child. In T. E. Moore (Ed.), *Cognitive development and the acquisition of language* (pp. 27–63). New York: Academic Press.

Clark, H. H., & Clark, E. V. (1977). *Psychology and language: An introduction to psycholinguistics*. New York: Harcourt Brace Jovanovich.

Clark, H. H., & Malt, B. C. (1984). Psychological constraints on language: A commentary on Bresnan and Kaplan and on Givon. In W. Kintsch, J. R. Miller, & P. G. Polson (Eds.), *Method and tactics in cognitive science* (pp. 191–214). Hillsdale, Lawrence Erlbaum.

Cole, M., Gay, J., Glick, J. A., & Sharp, D. W. (1971). *The cultural context of learning and thinking*. New York: Basic Books.

De Valois, R. L., & Jacobs, G. H. (1968). Primate color vision. *Science, 162*, 533–540.

Gelman, S. A., & Markman, E. M. (1986). Categories and induction in young children. *Cognition, 23*, 183–209.

Gelman, S. A., & Taylor, M. (1984). How two-year-old children interpret proper and common names for unfamiliar objects. *Child Development, 55*, 1535–1540.

Gerard, A. B., & Mandler, J. M. (1983). Ontological knowledge and sentence anomaly. *Journal of Verbal Learning and Verbal Behavior, 22*, 105–120.

Glucksberg, S., & Weisberg, R. W. (1966). Verbal behavior and problem solving: Some effects of labelling in a functional fixedness problem. *Journal of Experimental Psychology, 71*, 659–664.

Greenberg, J. H. (1966). *Language Universals*. The Hague: Mouton.

Grice, H. P. (1975). Logic and conversation. In P. Cole & J. L. Morgan (Eds.), *Syntax and semantics: Vol. 3. Speech Acts* (pp. 41–58). New York: Seminar Press.

Heider, E. R. (1972). Universals in color naming and memory. *Journal of Experimental Psychology, 93*, 10–20.

Hering, E. (1920). *Outlines of a theory of the light sense* (L. M. Hurvich & D. Jameson, Trans.). Cambridge, MA: Harvard University Press.

Hickerson, N. P. (1971). Review of "Basic color terms: Their universality and evolution." *International Journal of American Linguistics, 37*, 257–270.

Inhelder, B., & Piaget, J. (1964). *The early growth of logic in the child*. New York: Norton.

Istomina, Z. M. (1963). Perception and naming of color in early childhood. *Soviet Psychology and Psychiatry, 1*, 37–45.

Katz, N., Baker, E., & Macnamara, J. (1974). What's in a name? A study of how children learn common and proper names. *Child Development, 45*, 469–473.

Kay, P., & McDaniel, C. K. (1978). The linguistic significance of the meanings of basic color terms. *Language, 54*, 610–646.

Keil, F. C. (1979). *Semantic and conceptual development: An ontological perspective*. Cambridge, MA: Harvard University Press.

Lenneberg, E. H., & Roberts, J. M. (1956). The language of experience: A study in methodology. *International Journal of American Linguistics* (Memoir No. 13) (Suppl. 22), 1–33.

Loftus, E. F. (1975). Leading questions and the eyewitness report. *Cognitive Psychology, 7*, 560–572.

Markman, E. M. (1985). Why superordinate category terms can be mass nouns. *Cognition, 19*, 31–53.

Markman, E. M., Horton, M. S., & McLanahan, A. G. (1980). Classes and collections: Principles of organization in the learning of hierarchical relations. *Cognition, 8*, 227–241.

Markman, E. M., & Hutchinson, J. E. (1984). Children's sensitivity to constraints on word meaning: Taxonomic vs. thematic relations. *Cognitive Psychology, 16,* 1–27.

Martyna, W. (1980). The psychology of the generic masculine. In S. McConnell-Ginet, R. Borker, & N. Furman (Eds.), *Women and language in literature and society* (pp. 69–78). New York: Praeger.

Miller, G. A. & Johnson-Laird, P. N. (1976). *Language and perception*. Cambridge, MA: Harvard University Press.

*Oxford English Dictionary*. (1933). J. A. H. Murray, H. Bradley, W. A. Craigie, & C. T. Onions (Eds.). Oxford: Clarendon Press.

Pinker, S. (1979). Formal models of language learning. *Cognition, 7,* 217–283.

Price-Williams, D. R. (1962). Abstract and concrete modes of classification in a primitive society. *British Journal of Educational Psychology, 32,* 50–61.

Rosch, E. (1977). Linguistic relativity. In P. N. Johnson-Laird & P. C. Wason (Eds.), *Thinking: Readings in cognitive science* (pp. 501–519). Cambridge: Cambridge University Press.

Rosch, E., Mervis, C. B., Gray, W. D., Johnson, D. M., & Boyes-Braem, P. (1976). Basic objects in natural categories. *Cognitive Psychology, 8,* 382–439.

Sapir, E. (1949). In D. G. Mandelbaum (Ed.), *Selected writings of Edward Sapir in language, culture and personality*. Berkeley and Los Angeles: University of California Press.

Skinner, B. F. (1938). *The behavior of organisms*. New York: Appleton-Century-Crofts.

Sommers, F. (1959). The ordinary language tree. *Mind, 68,* 160–185

Sommers, F. (1963). Types and ontology. *Philosophical Review, 72,* 327–363

Tagliavini, C. (1949). Di alcune denominazioni della "pupilla." *Annali dell' Instituto Universitario di Napoli* (NS) 3, 341–378

Tversky, B., & Hemenway, K. (1984). Objects, parts, and categories. *Journal of Experimental Psychology*, General, *113*, 169–193.

Whorf, B. L. (1956). In J. B. Carroll (Ed.), *Language, thought and reality: Selected writings of Benjamin Lee Whorf*. Cambridge, MA: MIT Press.

Witkowski, S. R., & Brown, C. H. (1977). An explanation of color nomenclature universals. *American Anthropologist, 79,* 50–57.

# 7

# *Cognitive Processes in Written Language Dysfunction*

MARGARET J. SNOWLING AND
DOLORES PERIN

Dysfunction in using written language to read or to write is extremely inconvenient in a society that takes literacy for granted. Difficulty in reading or writing can pose serious problems in school, especially because, with advancing years, more and more material must be learned in written form. Children who fail to learn to read and spell adequately despite normal socioeconomic and educational opportunity are referred to as developmental dyslexics, and it is primarily with their functioning that this chapter is concerned.

Written and spoken English are related in complex ways (Gelb, 1963; Venezky, 1970). Therefore, it is remarkable that the majority of children master literacy skills with seemingly little effort. Nonetheless, the failure of a minority of children to learn to read and the sometimes intractable spelling problems of others are perplexing and have attracted a good deal of research attention for many years (see Benton & Pearl, 1978, for review). Most recently, there has been a move toward understanding dyslexia in terms of models available in cognitive psychology (Vellutino, 1979). It is the purpose of this chapter to review this approach, to identify the cognitive subskills that underlie reading and spelling, and to attempt to explain written language dysfunction in terms of deficiencies in these basic cognitive processes.

## WHAT IS MEANT BY WRITTEN LANGUAGE DYSFUNCTION?

Just as children vary considerably in the rate at which they acquire spoken language, there is enormous variation in the timing with which they learn to read (Francis, 1982). However, there is substantial correlation between reading age and mental age in the normal population. Thus, "bright" children learn to read more quickly than children of average intelligence, who in turn achieve written language skills before retarded children or slow learners. However, this is not meant to imply that low intelligence is a bar to literacy. Indeed, it is possible for severely subnormal persons to learn to read (Hermelin & O'Connor, 1967). In short, reading may develop slowly but normally in individuals of poor academic ability. The notion of delayed development can be applied.

Of more interest is the unexpected failure of otherwise intelligent children to read. The assumption is that dyslexia is a specific learning disability hindering the acquisition of written language skills, as distinct from a general retardation, which would manifest itself in a number of academic areas (Rutter, Tizard, Yule, Graham, & Whitmore, 1976). The term *developmental dyslexia* normally applies to individuals who have no known neurological or relevant physiological disorder. Both reading and spelling skills are affected, although serious spelling difficulties do occur in the absence of reading problems (Frith, 1978; Nelson & Warrington, 1974; Perin, 1981).

Finally, written language dysfunction may accompany other forms of language disorder. Reading and writing problems can occur in acquired dyslexia after brain damage (Coltheart, Patterson, & Marshall, 1980), and in childhood characteristic impairments of either reading or spelling are associated with developmental dysphasia (Cromer, 1980) and deafness (Dodd, 1980). In addition, specific difficulties with reading comprehension can occur even when normal decoding and spelling skills are intact in a condition known as *hyperlexia* (Frith & Snowling, 1983; Healy, 1982).

One of the problems in the literature is that studies have varied greatly in their criteria for subject selection (Mitchell, 1982; Taylor & Taylor, 1983). Terminology also varies widely across studies, so that subject samples may consist of "developmental dyslexics," "dyslexics," "poor readers," "backward readers," "reading retardates," or "poor spellers." In this chapter we will inevitably be drawing upon data from such samples. Furthermore, due to limitations of space, we will only be able to deal with English-speaking samples. However, readers interested in pursuing studies of dyslexia in other languages are referred to Kavanagh and Venezky (1980) and to Stevenson et al. (1982).

## COGNITIVE DEFICITS IN DYSLEXIC READERS

Various theories attempt to grasp the underlying difficulties that dyslexic readers experience when attempting to write. Possible explanations for such problems include deficits in visual perception and verbal memory, among others. The following sections address these theories.

### The Visual Perceptual Deficit Hypothesis

One of the earliest hypotheses was that written language disorders were caused by visual perceptual deficits (Benton, 1962; Orton, 1937). The problem of reversal errors (e.g., *b/d, p/q, was/saw*) in the reading and spelling of dyslexic individuals was accorded great significance—so much so that such errors became accepted as diagnostic signs (Critchley, 1964, 1970). Today, it is generally believed that the importance of reversals has been exaggerated; Fischer, Liberman, and Shankweiler (1978) have pointed out that only about 2% of disabled readers' errors are actually reversals, and many other sorts of confusion are present. Furthermore, if dyslexics are compared with normal readers equated for reading ability, the incidence of reversals in the two groups is similar. These findings do not rule out the possibility that reversals might be a persisting problem for individual children, but they do make the visual perceptual deficit theory less likely as an explanation for reading failure.

The same conclusion can be drawn from studies comparing dyslexics and normal readers on a variety of perceptual measures such as visual memory, figure-ground discrimination, and visual-motor integration. Very often dyslexics have fared worse than their peers, not because of the perceptual demands of the tasks but because they have been tested using verbal materials. Vellutino, Steger, Kaman, and DeSotto (1975) showed that when visual memory for English words was tested, dyslexics had more difficulty than normal readers. However, when the same words were presented in Hebrew orthography (an unfamiliar writing system for both groups), dyslexics performed at a level similar to controls. This experiment highlights the importance of equating the familiarity of groups with the materials used in an experiment before drawing inferences about processing differences between the groups. In short, if dyslexics have had less experience with printed words than controls, then they will inevitably process them less efficiently.

There is evidence that the "perceptual" deficits of dyslexic readers may in fact be traceable to verbal problems. For example, N. Ellis (1981) investigated the ability of dyslexic readers and chronological age controls to make judgments about the identity of simultaneously presented letter pairs. Using the Posner (1969) paradigm, subjects had to indicate whether the letters within a pair were the same or different. "Visual" pairs had the same shape (AA, bb), while "name" pairs contained letters having the same name but different shapes (Aa, Bb). Dyslexic readers took the same amount of time as controls to make visual matches. However, when items required a further stage of processing as with the name pairs, dyslexics were significantly slower than controls in comparing the letters. Thus, there was an important interaction between groups and conditions in this experiment. Ellis concluded that dyslexics were not subject to any visual perceptual deficit, but they had difficulties at a later stage of letter processing, namely, at the name-encoding stage. Ellis and Miles (1981) have developed this hypothesis further and suggested that dyslexics are subject to a lexical encoding deficiency. This hypothesis is an attractive one in the light of other studies, as will be seen.

## The Verbal Deficit Hypothesis

One of the most vehement critics of the perceptual deficit hypothesis has been Vellutino (1977), who has argued that previous findings can be interpreted in terms of verbal deficits. In a series of experiments on sequential processing, Bakker (1972) showed that dyslexics could not remember sequential information as well as mental age matched controls. However, Vellutino (1979) pointed out that their difficulty was restricted to memory for verbal materials, and there was little evidence for a more general deficit in temporal ordering. Since it is commonly held that an auditory-verbal code is by far the most efficient for the storage of material distributed over time, the dyslexics' difficulties in Bakker's experiments were probably attributable to their inability to make use of verbal memory codes. Thus, according to Vellutino, the majority of findings can be reinterpreted according to a verbal deficit hypothesis. Evidence for the verbal deficit hypothesis is presented in the following paragraphs.

***Speech and Language Difficulties.*** The verbal deficit hypothesis has become popular in recent years, not only because of empirical findings, but also because it fits well with what is known about the etiology of dyslexia. Almost all studies of clinical populations of reading-disabled children have identified a large proportion in whom there has been some speech and language disturbance (Mattis, French, & Rapin, 1975; Miles, 1983; Naidoo, 1972). It will be recalled that some children are poor readers due to low intelligence, whereas some children suffer from specific reading disability that does not reflect intellectual deficiency. Population studies that are not subject to sampling biases have found that children with specific reading retardation were primarily characterized by a history of speech and language delays, in contrast to generally backward readers, who exhibited a wide range of neurological "soft" signs such as visual perceptual problems and motor difficulties (Rutter & Yule, 1973).

Although the spoken language difficulties of dyslexic children are not immediately obvious during conversation, sensitive testing can bring these to the surface. Snowling (1981) and Miles (1983) have noted that dyslexic adolescents continue to have mild articulation difficulties and have particular problems with the pronunciation of polysyllabic words such as *preliminary* and *statistics*. In a similar vein, Montgomery (1981) found that dyslexics had more difficulty in accessing articulatory information than normal controls; they found it more difficult to decide upon the nature of the articulatory movements they themselves were making than did other children of the same age.

The word-finding difficulties of dyslexic children have also frequently been remarked upon (Critchley & Critchley, 1978; Miles & Ellis, 1981). A series of studies by Denckla and her associates have found dyslexic children to have more difficulties with object naming and to perform more slowly on rapid naming tasks than children of equivalent age and IQ (Denckla & Rudel, 1976; Denckla, Rudel, & Broman, 1981). In some cases, the performance of dyslexics was as poor as that of learning disabled children with brain damage. Furthermore, these difficulties have often been implicated to explain the memory difficulties characteristic of this group. For example, Spring and Capps (1974) argued that reduced naming speed could lead to ineffective rehearsal strategies and hence difficulties in learning information of a verbal nature.

Thus, the performance of dyslexic individuals on a variety of speech and language tasks points to the fact that they are subject to underlying verbal weaknesses. However, the majority of dyslexics appear to be able to "mask" their difficulties so that these are not detectable in normal conversation.

***Verbal Memory Difficulties.*** Agreement is virtually unanimous that dyslexic individuals are subject to a range of verbal memory difficulties. Reduced digit span is discernible on standardized intelligence tests (Naidoo, 1972; Rugel, 1974; Thomson, 1982), and this has been confirmed experimentally (Cohen & Netley, 1981). Furthermore, Nelson and Warrington (1980) showed that dyslexics have more extensive difficulties with verbal materials. For example, they had more difficulty than controls with a paired-associate learning task in which forenames and surnames had to be associated. It took them longer to learn the associations, and, once having learned them, longer to change the direction of these associations. These memory problems should make it more difficult for dyslexics to add new information to verbal semantic memory. To test this, Nelson and Warrington attempted to teach subjects the meanings of eight "new" words. In line with prediction, dyslexics took longer to learn these words than their age matched controls of the same intelligence. These findings have implications for the rate at which dyslexics might be expected to learn the names to associate with printed words as well as the rate at which they might add new spoken words to their existing vocabulary.

The memory codes utilized by dyslexic and nominal readers have also been investigated. If verbal material is to be retained over a short period of time, it is generally believed that a phonological code is used (Baddeley, 1979). Jorm (1983) discusses the relationship between the phonological information in memory and reading problems.

The use of a sound-based memory code is responsible for the phonemic similarity effect whereby sequences of letters in which the names of the letters rhyme (e.g., BDCTV) are remembered less well than sequences of letters in which the names are dissimilar (e.g., FHGIW). The effect holds regardless of whether presentation is auditory or visual. According to Conrad (1972) the phonemic similarity effect is first seen in children at around age 6. He speculated that its emergence at that time was associated with the child's learning to read. After that age, the phonemic similarity effect is present across age groups, indicating that subjects are making use of phonological code in memory. It is therefore striking that Liberman and colleagues have reported its absence in groups of disabled readers (Shankweiler, Liberman, Mark, Fowler, & Fischer, 1979). Disabled readers were unaffected by the phonological status of items to be remembered. They could remember sequences of rhyming letters just as well as nonrhyming sequences, and, furthermore, this effect extended to sequences of words and sentences (Mann, Liberman, & Shankweiler, 1980).

To rule out the possibility that the disabled readers in studies of this type were at a disadvantage because of their limited reading experience, Johnston (1982) compared the ability of dyslexic children to memorize sequences of phonologically confusable and nonconfusable items presented auditorily with the ability of normal readers of the same reading level. When matching children in this way, Johnston found that dyslexic children were just as susceptible to the phonemic similarity effect as reading age matched controls.

At first glance, this finding is difficult to reconcile with the existing literature. However, it should be noted that the normal readers in Johnston's (1982) study were much younger than the dyslexics (8 years old as compared to 12 years on average). Thus, to say that dyslexic readers are able to use a phonological code (for letters) as well as normal readers who are their juniors by four years is not to deny that it is difficult for them to utilize phonetic memory codes. The implication is still that dyslexics are less inclined to encode phonologically than other children of the same age.

If the phonological encoding deficit is causal, then the "non-availability" of phonological codes at critical times could have far reaching consequences for learning to read. At an early stage, children might be unable to memorize the spoken equivalents for printed words, and their ability to memorize the beginning of a sight vocabulary would be compromised. Later, when it is necessary to abstract and understand the intricate relationships between letters and the sounds embodied in spoken words, inordinate difficulty would be experienced. What Johnston's (1982) work shows is that the ability of dyslexics to make use of phonological codes may be inferior to that of normally developing children, but it does improve with age. Despite this improvement, there is evidence that dyslexics continue to utilize codes other than phonological ones in memory tasks, showing a preference for the use of visual or orthographic codes. Rack (1985) asked dyslexic subjects and reading age matched controls to decide whether or not pairs of words rhymed. There were four types of pairs, the most important for our purposes being words that rhymed (in British English) but were orthographically dissimilar (farm-calm) and words that did not rhyme but were orthographically similar (farm-warm). Having completed the rhyme judgment, subjects were unexpectedly asked to recall the words they had seen. One member of each pair was presented as a cue to recall, and the other had to be written down. These tasks were carried out in both visual and auditory modalities, the results being similar for both, as follows.

Significantly, the overall performance of the two groups was the same. However, there was a striking interaction between conditions and groups. Normal readers remembered more of the pairs that rhymed but were orthographically dissimilar (harm-calm) than dyslexics, but dyslexics remembered more of the pairs that did not rhyme but were orthographically similar (harm-warm). These findings add further support to the claim that dyslexics make less use of a phonological code in memory than normal readers, even though the use of this code may have been encouraged in Rack's experiments through a rhyming task. Instead, it seems that dyslexics might utilize an orthographic code (based on letters) when words are presented, regardless of whether presentation is through the auditory or visual modality.

***Segmentation Difficulties.*** So far, several verbal abilities have differentiated dyslexic from normal readers, but it is not clear how far these difficulties can account for their reading failure. The role of segmentation problems in written language dysfunction appears more direct and has received much research attention.

The seminal work of Liberman, Shankweiler, and colleagues showed that one of the best predictors of reading achievement was the ability of children at age 4 to segment spoken words into phonemic units (bat = [b] + [æ] + [t]) (Liberman & Shankweiler, 1977; Liberman et al., 1980).

Moreover, Gleitman and Rozin (1977) pointed to the importance of "phonemic" awareness in learning to read. Their argument was that, if children were to "crack the alphabetic code," it was crucial for them to understand that spoken words can be segmented into speech sounds (phonemes), which correspond to the divisible units of printed words (letters or graphemes). More recently, Bradley and Bryant (1983) have shown that the ability of 4-year-olds to segment auditorily presented materials in tests of rhyme and alliteration predicts reading and spelling but not mathematical attainment at age 8, even when the possible effects of intelligence and social class are partialed out.

Thus, segmentation ability is closely associated with written language skill, although whether it is a prerequisite of reading or a consequence of literacy remains a moot point (Morais, Cary, Alegria, & Bertelson, 1979; Snowling & Perin, 1983). Whatever the direction of this relationship, there is considerable evidence that dyslexic individuals do far worse on phoneme segmentation tasks than normal readers (Fox & Routh, 1980; Liberman & Shankweiler, 1977). Significantly, these differences persist even when reading experience is taken into account. Hence, Bradley and Bryant (1978) found that disabled readers performed less well than younger normal children, matched for reading age, when asked to detect the "odd one out" of four words presented auditorily (e.g., fun, gun, *bud*, sun). The older disabled readers also had more difficulty when asked to generate rhymes than their younger controls, again pointing to phonemic processing problems. Furthermore, a dyslexic student studied by Campbell and Butterworth (1985) was unable to complete an auditory acronym task in which the initial sounds of a series of words had to be segmented and then synthesized to make a new word. Presented with "green-eight-lamp," she could complete this task only by referring to the orthographic forms of the word presented. Therefore, she would arrive at the word "gel." In contrast, normal subjects would arrive at "gale" through phoneme segmentation.

In sum, a good deal of evidence is compatible with the verbal deficit hypothesis. More precisely, it appears that most developmental dyslexics have some kind of phonological impairment (see, e.g., Frith, 1981). We can speculate that early and even persistent speech problems are at least partly attributable to significant auditory processing and segmentation difficulties (see, e.g., Tallal, 1980). These difficulties might later impede the acquisition of literacy skills and may discourage the use of phonological codes in short-term memory.

## READING

The term *reading* can apply to many diverse activities from "barking at print" through speed reading to reading diligently for pleasure. For present purposes, discussion will be restricted to reading at the single-word level (i.e., the process of deriving pronunciation from print). Even at this level, reading is a complex activity, and experimental psychology has furnished us with a plethora of models to describe the processes involved (see Mitchell, 1982, and Henderson, 1983, for reviews).

## Models of Reading

Most authors postulate that there are at least two strategies available to the fluent reader who wishes to derive pronunciation for a printed word. The first strategy involves direct recognition of a word from its visual characteristics. Following recognition, the word's pronunciation is immediately accessed, and the word can be articulated. This strategy can be likened to the "look-say" approach to the teaching of reading. The second strategy is an indirect one, akin to the "phonic" teaching approach. Using this strategy, a word is read through a process of letter-sound or grapheme-phoneme translation. Hence, its phonology is assembled prior to recognition and pronunciation (Patterson, 1981). Coltheart's (1980) model provides a simple framework within which to discuss the processes underlying word recognition (Figure 7.1). Using the first strategy (pathway A in Figure 7.1), words are recognized directly. This route is particularly important for the recognition of irregular words such as *yacht* and *debt*, which cannot be read by letter-sound translation. In contrast, the second strategy (pathways B and C in Figure 7.1) uses phonological mediation. Pathway B is assumed to be involved in the reading of regular words (e.g., *fresh*, *boat*) in which letter-sound relationships are consistent. It would also be used to read words that, although known by the reader, had never been encountered in print—for example, the name of a new head of state whose name was known from radio announcements but was seen for the first time in a newspaper article. Pathway C accounts for the ability of fluent readers to read aloud nonwords (e.g., *blint*, *tegwop*) that they have neither seen nor heard before and for which there is therefore no lexical entry.

***The Homophone Effect.*** There has been some empirical support for the classical distinction between the direct, visual means of reading and the indirect, phonological strategy (Huey, 1908). Perhaps the most widely quoted evidence is the presence of a "pseudohomophone" effect in lexical decision experiments (Rubinstein, Lewis, & Rubinstein, 1971). In the lexical decision task, subjects are presented with a letter string, and they have to decide whether it is a word (e.g., *spade*) or a nonword (e.g., *blint*). Rubinstein et al. found that it took longer for subjects to respond "No" to a

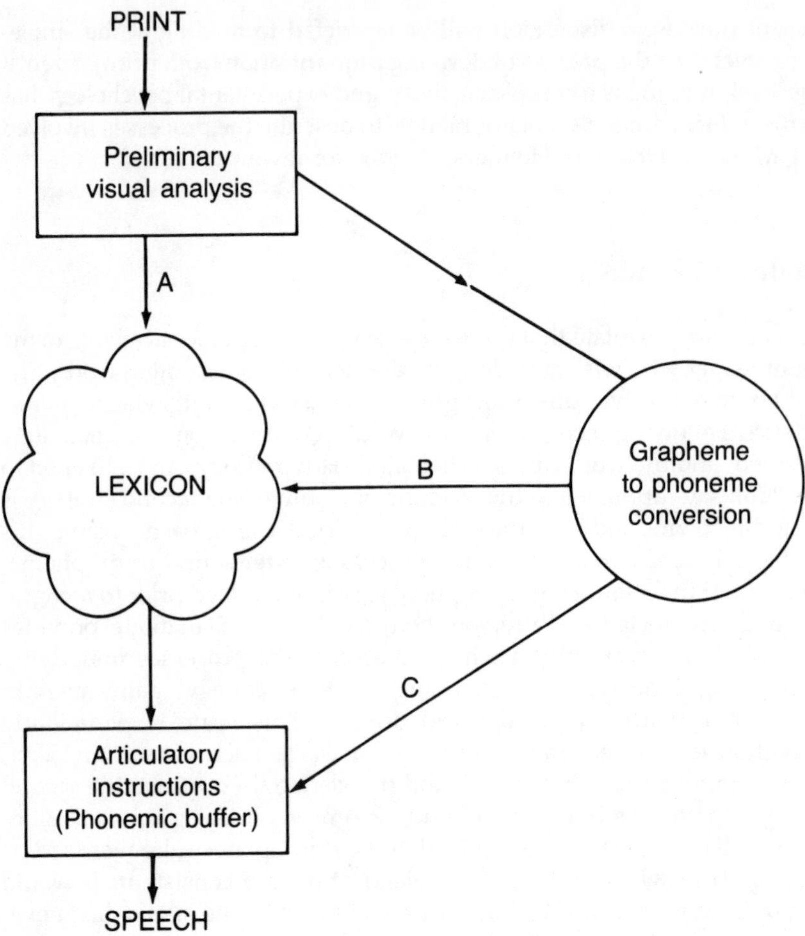


**Figure 7.1.** Model of reading. Adapted with permission from "Reading, Phonological Recoding and Deep Dyslexia" by M. Coltheart, 1980. In *Deep dyslexia* (p. 202), edited by M. Coltheart, K. Patterson, and J. Marshall, London: Routledge and Kegan Paul.

nonword if the nonword was homophonic with a real word (e.g., *brane*) than if it did not sound like a possible word (e.g., *bune*). Hence, the pseudohomophone effect. This effect was presumed to occur because subjects were using a system of grapheme-phoneme correspondence to translate the nonwords into sound before making their decision.

While this evidence has a bearing on how nonword decisions are made, it does not necessarily imply that real words are dealt with in the same way. In support of the claim that they are, Rubinstein et al. (1971) also showed that it took longer to say "Yes" (it is a word) to the lower frequency member of a pair of homophones (e.g., *sale*) than to other words of the same frequency that were not themselves homophones (e.g., *desk*). This finding supports the idea that real words are also translated into phonological form for the purposes of lexical decision. If the phonological form is ambiguous, as is the case with homophones, a spelling recheck may be necessary (Coltheart, Davelaar, Jonasson, & Besner, 1977)

In practice, the Rubinstein homophone effect has been difficult to replicate when adequate controls have been used, and the current view of this research is that the use of grapheme-phoneme translation in lexical decision tasks is under "strategic control." Thus, Davelaar, Coltheart, Besner, and Jonasson (1978) found that subjects took longer to respond to homophonic words than control words if the homophones were embedded within a list of words and nonwords that were not pseudohomophones (e.g., *blint, trist*). The effect disappeared when the homophones were embedded in a context of pseudohomophonic nonwords (e.g., *brane, caix*). In the first situation it would be advantageous for subjects to use a sound-based strategy to decide between words and nonwords. Therefore, decisions about homophones would be slowed because of their ambiguity. However, in the second situation a phonological strategy would be ineffective, because many of the nonwords would sound correct. Therefore, subjects apparently adopted a visual strategy of word/nonword decisions, and the homophone effect was consequently eliminated. In applying these results to normal reading, it can be argued that the direct visual route dominates and the phonological route is a back-up for new words (Patterson, 1981).

***Lexical Analogy Theory.*** The independent status of the phonological route (corresponding to pathways B and C, Figure 7.1) has been questioned (Glushko, 1979; Kay & Marcel, 1981; Marcel, 1980). For example, a nonlexical (phonological) account cannot sufficiently explain the process of nonword reading. Glushko (1979) showed that it took longer to read aloud nonwords like *heaf* than nonwords like *hean*. If these words were read by a straightforward process of grapheme-phoneme translation, then it would be impossible to explain this latency difference. He proposed that all words, whether regular or irregular, or nonsense, are read using one route. This route is based on an internal lexicon in which words are coded in terms of similarity of letter structure. Words containing many of the same letters in the same positions are termed *neighbors*. Words are of two types: *consistent*, where letter groups are always pronounced the same way (e.g., *-ean*), and *inconsistent*, where two or more pronunciations are possible (e.g., *-ave* as in *cave* vs. *have*).

As an alternative to grapheme-phoneme translation, Glushko (1979) proposed that nonwords are read through lexical "analogy" with real words. In brief, whenever a printed word is encountered, that word as well as all of its visually similar neighbors are activated within the orthographic lexicon. In the case of a nonword, word candidates that are orthographically similar to the nonword receive activation, and a pronunciation is synthesized from the available pronunciations of these real words. Exactly how this synthesis is brought about is not fully specified, but it is assumed to take longer for nonwords like *heaf*, which has neighbors with inconsistent pronunciations (*leaf*, *deaf*) than for nonwords like *hean*, whose neighbors are all consistently pronounced (*dean*, *bean*, *lean*). Furthermore, Kay and Marcel (1981) showed that the pronunciation of a nonword can be biased depending upon the current state of activation within the lexicon. Thus, they showed that a nonword like *yead* was more likely to be pronounced [jid] if it was preceded by the word *bead* than if it was preceded by the word *head*, in which case it would more likely be pronounced [jed].

***Reading Theories and Developmental Dyslexia***. The theory of reading that we accept does have a bearing upon how we understand developmental dyslexia. However, most of the research on this topic to date has been conceived of within the two-strategy framework. Further, the study of acquired dyslexia has utilized this approach (Coltheart et al., 1980; Patterson, 1981). It is possible that the two strategies are important developmentally, while the one-strategy theory best accounts for normal, fluent reading at higher levels.

Vygotsky (1934) insisted that to understand highly skilled cognitive operations, it is necessary to trace their development from the earliest stages. This seems important in understanding developmental dyslexia, where comparisons with reading age controls are often employed, if we wish to consider whether dyslexics are only developing more slowly than their age peers or whether cognitive processes are somehow qualitatively different (Seymour & Porpodas, 1980).

## The Development of Reading

The development of reading has been approached from a number of different angles, and the type of approach most useful for the study of dyslexia in children is debatable. Early theories conceived of reading development as the gradual accumulation of knowledge about grapheme-phoneme correspondences, spelling patterns, and orthographic rules, each stage in the reading process becoming automatized with increasing age and experience (Gibson, Osser, & Pick, 1963; LaBerge & Samuels, 1974). These ideas have now been superseded by theories that view the child as passing through a series of qualitatively different stages or phases before achieving full literacy. Marsh and his colleagues have argued for a stage theory of reading development, closely akin to the Piagetian theory of cognitive development (Marsh & Desberg, 1983; Marsh, Friedman, Welch, & Desberg, 1980). More recently Frith (1985) has argued for three phases in the development of literacy skills. In the first, the "logographic" phase, words are recognized on the basis of crude visual features (e.g., the double *ll* in *yellow*). When the child realizes that the letters of printed words are associated in some more or less predictable way with the sounds embodied in spoken words, he or she can break through to the "alphabetic" phase of reading. Here words are read utilizing knowledge of letter-sound correspondences in a somewhat piecemeal fashion. Finally, the child enters the "orthographic" phase. At this point, reading is totally independent of sound, and words are recognized according to orthographic features such as minimal cues concerning the position of letters within a word.

It would be interesting to consider whether Frith's ideas can be accommodated within our two-strategy framework. The simplest way of doing this would be to say that children begin to read by relying heavily upon a direct visual strategy (pathway A). If they have not yet achieved phoneme awareness, then a phonological strategy (pathways B and C) will not exist. Hence the logographic phase. Snowling and Perin (1983) argued that after setting up a small sight vocabulary, young children gradually develop the ability to segment words into phonemes. Having gained this insight and possibly encouraged through early attempts to spell, they begin to set up a system of grapheme-phoneme correspondences that they can subsequently use to decipher new and unfamiliar words. This constitutes a breakthrough to the alphabetic phase. There is evidence that, while skills of phonological translation continue to improve with increasing reading experience (Doctor & Coltheart, 1980; Perfetti & Hogaboam), children continue to prefer to use a visual strategy for reading for some time. This is consistent with Frith's (1985) concept of "phase," wherein earlier strategies may occasionally be utilized. Bryant and Bradley (1980) found that words that beginning readers at first found difficult could be read when embedded in lists of nonwords. In this situation, when a phonological strategy for reading was encouraged, the children were able to read the words they had previously failed.

To date, few experiments have been directed precisely toward orthographic processing in children. If lexical analogies are implicated, then Marsh et al. (1980) and Baron et al. (1980) do not see these emerging until an advanced stage of reading development. It is possible that children can recognize at least familiar words on the basis of orthographic cues at a much earlier stage. Barron and Baron (1977) investigated the use of phonological coding by asking young children to speak while carrying out a reading task ("concurrent articulation"). It was assumed that this technique would prevent recoding words to sounds. Since their young subjects were unaffected by this intervention, the authors argued that reading was taking place via the direct, visual route. While recent evidence suggests that concurrent articulation does not achieve disruption of phonological coding (Baddeley, Eldridge, & Lewis, 1981; Besner, Davies, & Daniels, 1981), research conducted by Snowling and Frith (1981) supports Barron and Baron's claim. Snowling and Frith (1981) found that 7-year-old beginning readers could read texts from which sound cues had been removed (by replacing letters with visually similar ones, e.g., e/c, f/t) easier than texts from which shape cues had been removed (by writing words phonetically, e.g., *taibul* for *table*). Furthermore, their evidence suggested that children are dependent more upon information about letter positions within words (orthographic cues) than upon the *overall* shape of words, because they found it easiest to read texts that were greatly distorted by writing each letter in a different typeface.

Hence, normal readers might quickly move through the phases of reading development to possess the two reading strategies available in fluent reading—the direct (visual or orthographic) strategy and the indirect (phonological or alphabetic) strategy. The phonological strategy might be particularly important in children's reading, as it can provide a technique for deciphering unfamiliar words and can therefore fuel the development of sight vocabulary (Baddeley, 1979; Jorm, 1983). The very earliest logographic and most fluent orthographic phases are dominated by a visual strategy. However, the latter is greatly enriched by and operates on the basis of word and sound knowledge which results from reading experience.

## Reading in Developmental Dyslexia

It will be recalled that dyslexic readers are subject to a variety of verbal deficits including verbal memory problems and naming and segmentation difficulties. The verbal learning that reading entails is naturally a great source of difficulty for these readers. However, as discussed earlier in this chapter, reading may proceed using one of at least two strategies. It is theoretically important to know whether dyslexic readers possess both visual and phonological strategies, as do normal child readers, or whether one or the other of these channels is deficient. Evidence from acquired phonological dyslexia suggests that the visual-orthographic strategy may be used effectively when a phonological strategy is inefficient. Thus, patients with this disorder can read real words well but are completely unable to read nonwords (Beauvois & Derouesne, 1979; Funnell, 1983). In contrast, patients with acquired "surface" dyslexia can read nonwords and regular real words perfectly, but they are unable to read irregular words (e.g., they might read "island" as *izland*, and "broad" as *brode*). It appears that these patients have normal use of the phonological strategy but their visual orthographic pathway is impaired (Coltheart, Masterson, Byng, Prior, & Riddoch, 1983; Marshall & Newcombe, 1973). Whether these particular dissociations are found in developmental form is a point of some controversy (Baddeley, Ellis, Miles, & Lewis, 1982; Ellis, 1979; Jorm, 1979a, 1979b; Snowling, 1983).

Relatively little attention has been paid to the early stages of reading acquisition in dyslexic children. There are several reasons for the dearth of literature in this area, primarily the fact that a child is not usually labeled dyslexic until well after the time when he or she has begun to fail in the endeavor to read. By then the child may already display a reading pattern that is contaminated by the use of strategies that have been partly taught or by habits that have been inappropriately learned. Moreover, since there is large variation in the rate and style with which children learn to read (Francis, 1982), it is difficult to discern what might be an abnormal pattern at this early stage. Nevertheless, evidence available from parents' remarks and teachers' reports suggests that many dyslexic children begin to read in a seemingly normal manner. They achieve some success in building a sight vocabulary (although function words, e.g., *for*, *the*, *where*, may be a problem), and they begin to encounter real difficulty only when phonics is introduced. While this evidence is anecdotal, it would fit with the picture of strengths and weaknesses seen in dyslexia.

If early reading is logographic, dyslexics should be able to learn some words on a visual basis, provided there are no visual-perceptual weaknesses. The acquisition of a sight vocabulary might be slow because of verbal labeling and memory demands, but this may go unnoticed, particularly if the child is bright and adept at using contextual or picture cues when reading stories. Furthermore, there is some empirical evidence that suggests that dyslexics have normal use of logographic strategies for reading. Thus, Rozin, Poritsky, and Sotsky (1971) found that disabled readers who had failed for many years to learn to read by traditional methods could be taught reading within a very short space of time using a Chinese pictogram system. Freed of the need to translate individual letters into sounds, the reading problems of the children diminished.

***Importance of Phonological Strategies.*** These findings suggest that for many dyslexics, poor reading is not the result of visual weaknesses but rather due to problems in the acquisition of phonological strategies. This is not surprising, given the verbal difficulties that have already been discussed. In order to break through to an alphabetic phase of reading, it is necessary to be aware of the links between spoken and written words. A dyslexic's knowledge of these links will be reduced because of difficulties with phoneme segmentation and auditory organizational skills. Moreover, even if phonics are explicitly taught, dyslexics may find it difficult to decode words in a piecemeal fashion because of limitations in auditory verbal short-term memory function. Accordingly, Frith (1985) has proposed that classic developmental dyslexia is characterized by a failure to break through to the alphabetic phase of reading development.

A number of studies provide direct evidence for Frith's (1985) theory. For instance, Snowling (1980) examined the development of grapheme-phoneme correspondence skills in dyslexic and normal readers. Children of reading ages 7 through 10 were tested. The subjects were matched according to the number of words they could read correctly on a standardized reading test. Since these words were recognized automatically, it was assumed that the two groups were equated for use of the visual route to reading. An examination of phonological strategies was made by asking children to decide whether pairs of nonwords presented successively were the same (*torp-torp*) or different (*birt-brit*). Four types of comparison were tested. In two, both words were presented in the same modality (auditory-auditory or visual-visual), while in the others, words were presented across modalities (auditory-visual or visual-auditory).

The comparison of most interest for present purposes is the one in which subjects first saw a nonword and then heard a nonword, because this is the condition that most closely mimics reading. The performance of normal children in this condition improved steadily as a function of reading age. In contrast, the performance of dyslexic children remained poor despite an increase in reading age. These results suggest that for normal children, the use of phonological strategies for reading develops alongside an increase in sight vocabulary (i.e., as their reading age increases, so does their alphabetic skill). However, an increase in reading age for dyslexics is predominantly attributable to an increased sight vocabulary; there is virtually no improvement in grapheme-phoneme translation skill. Evidence from a number of other studies is compatible with this interpretation (Jorm, 1981; Seymour & Porpodas, 1980; Snowling, 1981). Detailed case studies of dyslexic individuals carried out by Seymour and McGregor (1984) show that it is possible for a dyslexic reader to attain an adult reading level but still to exhibit major deficiencies whenever phonology must be "assembled" during reading (i.e., in order to decode nonwords or unfamiliar real words).

Now, if dyslexic reading is primarily logographic, it is possible to make a number of further predictions about its nature. First, dyslexic reading is likely to be rather inaccurate, and a tendency to make visual errors (e.g., *image* for *imagine* and *instruction* for *institution*) will be apparent. Second, dyslexic readers should not show any advantage for regular words (*treat, fresh*) over irregular words (*break, laugh*). This advantage in normal readers has usually been attributed to the fact that regular words can be read using either a visual or a phonological strategy whereas irregular words must be read by visual means (Baron & Strawson, 1976; Parkin, 1982). Thus, if phonological strategies are unavailable, then regular and irregular words must be treated similarly. There is a small amount of evidence upholding the prediction. For instance, Seymour and Porpodas (1980) asked dyslexic and normal readers to match letter arrays. These were either regular (e.g., *slint*) or irregular (e.g., *lntis*). While normal readers matched regular arrays faster than irregular arrays, this regularity effect was absent among dyslexics. Similarly, Frith and Snowling (1983) found that dyslexic readers could read irregular lists of words just as well as regular lists. However, normal readers of the same level of reading ability showed an advantage for regular words. The group by condition interaction was significant for both accuracy and time data.

Thus, there is considerable evidence consonant with the notion that dyslexic readers have specific difficulty with phonological reading strategies. In Gleitman and Rozin's (1977) terms, such readers are unable to crack the alphabetic code. This deficit has implications even for theories of reading that do not assume an independent phonological route.

***Explanations For Dyslexic Reading Difficulties***. If the one-strategy approach (Glushko, 1979; Marcel, 1980) is the correct conceptualization of the normal reading process, it is possible to understand problems dyslexics may have in becoming fluent readers. Although the lexical route is not based on grapheme-phoneme translation, it does have a phonological component—that is, "consistency" is determined by pronunciation of letter clusters. Bearing this in mind, we can propose an explanation for the poor nonword reading and the absence of the regularity effect in dyslexic reading.

It will be recalled that "one-route" ("analogy") theorists ascribe nonword reading to a process of lexical activation and synthesis. For example, presentation of the nonword *nean* would activate visually similar entries in the orthographic lexicon. The real words *bean*, *near*, *neat*, and so forth, would all receive partial activation. A pronunciation for the letter string n-e-a-n would be synthesized from an amalgamation of the evidence already active. A possible mechanism might be that the [ni-] from *near* overlaps with the [-in] from *bean* to give [nin]. As already mentioned, this synthesization process has not been fully specified, but whatever the exact details, it would presumably require phoneme segmentation as well as the assembly of phonological information for articulation. Thus, the dyslexic's difficulty could arise at either of these later stages, preventing nonword reading even in the face of normal lexical activation.

An alternative explanation might be that the internal lexicon of a dyslexic individual is arranged in a different manner from that of a normal reader. Analogy theory assumes that words are arranged in an orthographic lexicon, but Frith (1985) argues convincingly that dyslexics might never reach the orthographic phase of reading. Hence, their original logographic lexicon might extend according to visual similarities between entries rather than being reorganized according to phonological principles. The differences that would be entailed are not clear given our present state of knowledge, but it is likely that letter-order information would be represented in an orthographic lexicon whereas this would not be true of a logographic system.

If the internal lexical arrangement characteristic of dyslexia is logographic, it follows that a system of activation and synthesis would not work as successfully as it would if the lexicon were orthographic. There would be a far greater number of potential neighbors for any real word if the neighborhood were based on broad visual similarity and not upon similarity of orthographic features. Thus, whenever a nonword were presented, there would be more activation within the system and greater competition if a single pronunciation had to be derived. Difficulties with nonword reading would be particularly marked, as no one pronunciation would readily win out.

A similar explanation might also account for the lack of regularity effect in dyslexic reading. Glushko (1979) accounts for the so-called "regularity" effect by the fact that most regular words possess orthographic neighbors that are pronounced in a consistent way. For example, the pronunciation of *boat* is consistent with the pronunciation of its neighbors *coat*, *moat*, and *stoat*. In contrast, irregular words usually have neighbors that are inconsistently pronounced— the pronunciation of *broad* is inconsistent with *road*, *toad*, and *load*. If a dyslexic's internal lexicon is arranged according to the overlap of visual features regardless of letter order, regular words could have as many inconsistent neighbors as irregular words. For instance, the regular consistent word *make* would be represented similarly to the word *meat* (because of shared letters) and therefore would have *great* (an exception word) as a neighbor. This being the case, the regularity effect would be eliminated.

Therefore, it seems possible to account for the phonological deficits in dyslexic reading without having to retain a two-strategy framework. In any case, it may not be appropriate to utilize a static model of the reading process (one-strategy or two-strategy) to account for a developmental reading disorder. Theories of the type proposed by Frith (1985), which account for the disorder in terms of failure to move from one phase to the next during reading acquisition, may provide a more fruitful way to proceed in the future.

To conclude, it seems that dyslexics are forced to rely upon logographic strategies for an extended time because of poor development of phonological skills. However, this does not mean that reading development will be arrested, although novel words (e.g., names) may present a persisting problem (Campbell & Butterworth, 1985). Fortunately, in most instances, unfamiliar words are encountered in a context of familiar words. Therefore, to the extent that dyslexic individuals can use semantic and syntactic cues to guide their reading, they will derive assistance. Indeed, Frith and Snowling (1983) found that dyslexic readers made better use of context in tests of reading comprehension than normal readers of the same reading age. Thus, dyslexics might be able to use "top-down" comprehension strategies to compensate to some extent for their specific decoding difficulty.

***An Interactive Model of Reading.*** Based on two major lines of evidence, Stanovich (1980) and Stanovich, West, and Freeman (1981) have proposed an "interactive-compensatory" model of reading. First, subjects can respond faster to a target word (e.g., *nurse*) if it is preceded by a semantically related word (e.g., *doctor*) than if it is preceded by an unrelated word (e.g., *bread*). This is known as the semantic context effect (Meyer, Schvaneveldt, & Ruddy, 1975). It is well established that the size of the context effect is increased if the target word is visually degraded—probably because by making a word harder to read, subjects have to attend more to contextual cues to decipher it (Posner & Snyder, 1975; Stanovich & West, 1981). Second, several investigations have found that both young normal and poor readers display larger context effects than older or more proficient readers (Schvaneveldt, Ackerman, & Semlear, 1977; Schwantes, Boesl, & Ritz, 1980; West & Stanovich, 1978). Again there is the suggestion that higher order processes are being used to compensate for difficulties with lower level processing. Children as well as adults make use of top-down processing strategies whenever the stimuli they are decoding are difficult to decipher and bottom-up processes are slowed. Placing the findings of Frith and Snowling (1983) in the context of this interactive approach, it can be said that deficiencies in bottom-up processing can be compensated for by top-down processing. It may even be possible to become highly literate using a combination of logographic and top-down (semantic) strategies.

It thus appears that the prognosis for reading in dyslexia is relatively good, provided the affected individuals have intact visual skills and particularly if they can make use of semantic strategies. However, the prognosis for spelling is considerably worse.

## SPELLING

It is much easier to recognize and identify objects one has seen before than it is to reconstruct precise details in their absence. If fluent spelling is conceptualized as producing strings of letters based on words one has seen previously, it is not surprising that it is more difficult than reading and that even highly literate people occasionally spell incorrectly. To model spelling production is not merely to reverse models of reading, and understanding cognitive dysfunction underlying poor reading skill will not necessarily explain dysfunctions underlying the poor spelling almost always found in developmental dyslexia. Although, as in reading, phonological and lexical codes are used in spelling, their procedures are as different as reconstruction is from recognition.

## Models of Spelling

Spelling production has been researched much less than reading. However, many theorists have made use of a two-route framework when modeling spelling. Thus, all spellers possess a number of automatic spelling routines. These can be directly accessed (cf. the *direct* route to reading). Spelling can also make use of certain procedures for spelling unfamiliar words (cf. the indirect or *phonological* route to reading). According to a model proposed by Personke and Yee (1966), "kinesthetic bypass" was effected when a spelling was automatically available and no cognitive effort was required to retrieve component letters. When this was not possible, the speller would use a "memory channel" and consciously retrieve the needed letters from memory. This could take place on a visual or phonological basis, the latter requiring the use of generalized rules. Interestingly, this model, cognitive in nature, allows for external aids such as a dictionary when kinesthetic bypass and memory fail (although, of course, memory for the first few letters of a word is needed in order to find it in a dictionary). This model also allows for "checking" and "proofreading" so that the speller can monitor his or her production.

Simon and Simon (1973) presented a similar model, although they considered the use of "generalizations," or phoneme-grapheme correspondences, in greater depth. Their model, expanded in Simon (1976), was developed in the course of a computer simulation of the spelling (and spelling errors) of 9-year-old children. The model is in the form of a hierarchy where the highest level is automatization and the lowest is phoneme-grapheme conversion. As in Personke and Yee's (1966) model, a word can be made available automatically. While this is similar to the direct, lexical route in reading, more information must be produced than is normally needed for reading. While word recognition can be accurate on the basis of only a few letters, accurate spelling requires precise, letter-by-letter specification (Frith & Frith, 1980). Further, an important component for spelling is its expression through a motor program for writing (Luria,

1966), typing, or speech for oral spelling (Henderson, Chard, & Clark, 1981; Sternberg, Monsell, Knoll, & Wright, 1978).

Simon and Simon (1973) suggest that if an automatic specification is not available, the speller makes a conscious search for specific component letters (i.e., engages in a "generation" process). A first step is to consult a visual representation in memory, which is then copied. More recently, Smith and Sterling (1983) have argued that spelling relies more on construction of separate morphemic elements than on direct retrieval of letters from memory.

According to Simon and Simon (1973), when a copying strategy does not result in a letter string that the speller considers correct, the word is syllabified. When a syllable cannot be spelled adequately, recourse is made to a tedious phoneme-grapheme translation procedure. While spelling by phoneme-grapheme conversion seems similar to the phonological route in reading, phoneme-grapheme rules are not grapheme-phoneme rules in reverse (Hanna, Hodges, & Hanna, 1971; Henderson & Chard, 1980). For example, the phoneme /f/ can be spelled in four ways (*f*, *ff*, *ph*, and *gh*), but the grapheme *gh* can map to the phoneme /f/, /g/, or /ø/ (the latter representing "silent" letters in the word *through*). In general, there are many more phoneme-grapheme correspondences for a speller to consider than there are grapheme-phoneme relationships. This means that a process of phoneme-grapheme translation does not guarantee a correct English spelling. It does, however, provide a basis for generating plausible graphemic segments which can then be tested against visual memory for accuracy.

Several authors have discussed the importance of "checking" procedures in spelling. Simon and Simon (1973) emphasized the use of visual memory to monitor production, a "generate and test" procedure. In this case, the speller is assumed to have in memory a stored list of "graphemic options" from which the most plausible choice is made. The speller examines what has been written and, with any luck, decides that the word is correctly spelled, terminating the generation procedure.

In a similar vein, "monitoring" has been emphasized by Tenney (1980) and by Sterling (1983). While Tenney was concerned with the role of matching produced spelling with stored visual characteristics, Sterling referred to a "lexical monitor." This would serve as a "word recognizer," and its mechanism could be visual or orthographic; in the latter case, the monitoring mechanism operates on the basis of letter rather than visual information. An interesting characteristic of the monitor is that it can operate in an overt or covert way. In covert monitoring, an error is detected before it is output. Sterling argues that this is frequent in spelling, so most errors are detected and corrected before they are even written. Spelling, being a language production system, is similar in many ways to speech; hence, it is useful to compare mechanisms for monitoring speech (Laver,

1980) with those for monitoring spelling. Ellis (1982) draws attention to the importance of inner speech in the evaluation of spelling. Here, the phonological route may serve as a back-up, as it can in reading.

*A Two-Route Model.* Ellis (1982) has offered a model of spelling that is similar to those discussed above, although it is couched in terms of Morton's (1979) "logogen" model of word recognition. Ellis also conceptualizes spelling as being possible on the basis of two independent routes (see Figure 7.2). When a word is to be spelled, component letters may be directly available through the "graphemic output logogen system" (route A). Failing this, the "phonemic buffer" would isolate phonemes to be converted to graphemes (route B). Although the syllable phase, specified by Simon and Simon (1973), and the construction of separate morphemes, suggested by Sterling (1983), are not specified, these would require only small additions to Ellis' model.

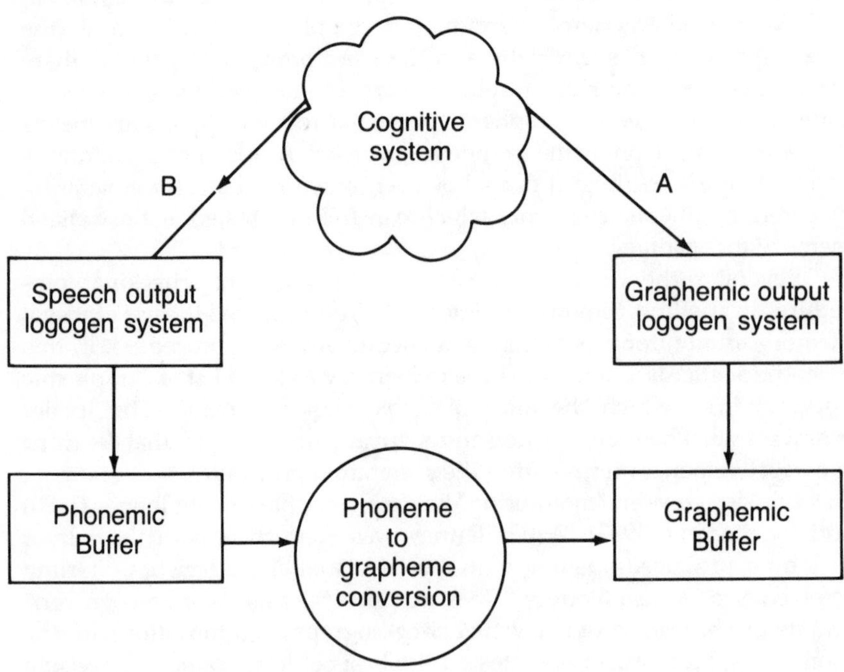


**Figure 7.2.** Model of spelling. Adapted with permission from "Spelling and Writing (and Reading and Speaking)" by A. W. Ellis, 1982. In *Normality and pathology in cognition functions* (p. 117), edited by A. W. Ellis, London: Academic Press.

According to Ellis (1982), the more often a word is spelled, the more automatic is its availability (via route A). This is akin to the operation of the direct route in reading, which is based on familiarity. Brown (1970) found that frequency was more important than regularity in spelling. If the speller is not entirely familiar with a word, Ellis argues that there may be an interaction between lexical and phonological strategies for production.

Smith (1980) reports an experiment where adults were asked to spell nonsense words embedded in otherwise meaningful sentences that were presented aurally. Stimuli included nonwords ending in a single consonant preceded by a tense vowels. Such words (e.g., a word pronounced /nodu:d/) could in principle be spelled using a vowel letter plus marker *e* (e.g., nodude) or a vowel digraph (e.g., nodood). It was found that subjects had a small but significant tendency to use the marker *e* spellings for stimulus words that served the syntactic function of verb, while for nouns the digraph was used. Smith attempts to account for this result with reference to the distribution of marker *e* spellings in real words. He states that such spellings are not more frequent for verbs than nouns. However, verbs derived from Latin and Greek do tend to be spelled with the final *e*. Smith argues that his subjects ascribed a "non-Latin foreign quality" to noun nonsense words and a Latin quality to verbs, which resulted in different orthographic choices. Frith (1980), in her investigations of spelling, has also noted "preferred" spellings for nonsense words. Therefore, spelling new words, or words with which the subject is partly or wholly unfamiliar, will not be based solely on a mechanical phoneme-grapheme translation process. This process is supplemented and influenced by knowledge about words' syntactic functions and derivations stored in the internal lexicon. While these interactions characterize normal spelling, models of spelling raise the issue of whether in principle the lexical and phonological routes could operate independently in spelling.

If there are two routes available for spelling, it would be expected that relatively regular spellings would depend more on a phonological route where phoneme-grapheme translation could be employed, while relatively irregular spellings would require the lexical route (routes B and A respectively, Figure 7.2). Nonsense words, for which in principle there is no one correct spelling, could be spelled using the phonological route. There exist syndromes of acquired dyslexia where spelling is impaired selectively, which can be shown by varying the nature of the stimulus word. Beauvois and Derouesne (1981) report on a patient whose spelling was excellent for nonsense words although very poor for irregular real words. The patient's brain damage appeared to have had consequences for the lexical route (A), leaving the phonological route (B) relatively unimpaired. The spelling performance of another acquired dyslexic, reported by Shallice (1981), seems to involve impairment of the phonological route (B) with relative sparing of the lexical route (A). This patient found it extremely difficult to spell nonsense words, although spelling of regular and irregular real words was good, except for functors (which may, according to Shallice, require the phonological route). The dissociations found in spelling by Beauvois and Derouesne and by Shallice suggest that, indeed, two routes are available in spelling. However, in normal spelling, the lexical route seems to dominate, with the phonological route performing a back-up function in cases of doubt and for checking purposes including covert monitoring.

***Processes of Excellent Spelling.*** Error analyses have shed light on processes employed when spelling is less than perfect. More difficult to explain is the production of the flawless spelling of which many people are capable. A plausible hypothesis is that visual images for words are activated automatically in spelling and that rapid reference is made to these as the speller proceeds letter by letter. Sloboda (1980) made an interesting attempt to investigate the use of visual imagery in spelling among adults. Subjects, both excellent and average spellers, were allocated to groups on the basis of introspective reports concerning whether they thought they used visual imagery for spelling. The subjects' use of imagery was also tested more objectively in the following way: A word was spoken aloud, and subjects were required to indicate how many letters it contained. Words were either "transparent," where there was a one-to-one relationship between grapheme and phoneme (e.g., *stands*), or "opaque," where there were more graphemes than phonemes (e.g., *yellow*). If visual imagery were available for spelling, reaction time for the two types of words should not differ, while if visual imagery were not being used, opaque words should take longer. Results showed that "visualizers" were equally fast for both word types, while "nonvisualizers" were slower for opaque words. Therefore, the introspective accounts were borne out by the data. However, visualizers were not necessarily better spellers. Sloboda proposed that excellent spellers use *letter* information, while merely average spellers are somewhat dependent on phoneme-grapheme rules. In other words, he proposed that visual imagery cannot account for perfect spelling. The letter information accessed by the excellent speller appears to be of an abstract nature, transcending the strictly visual level (Frith, 1978). Ehri's (1980) account of spelling is compatible with this. She postulates "orthographic images" that incorporate aspects of phonological and lexical information.

In fluent, accurate spelling, output from the graphemic output logogen system (Figure 7.2) should be coded in terms of letters rather than phonemes or syllables. In other words, production should proceed without explicit reference to the phonological structure of the word. Observing where pauses occur in spelling gives important information as to the underlying unit of organization, because it is during pauses that planning takes place. Farnham-Diggory and Nelson (1983) studied pauses in the on-line spelling production of adults and children. Output tended to be based on clusters of three letters. Many written syllables in English comprise three letters, so these findings might suggest phonological organization of spelling. However, Farnham-Diggory and Nelson reported that three-letter clusters occurred even when syllable conventions were contravened, as in the production *chi-ldr-en*. This supports the hypothesis that fluent spelling takes place on an orthographic (letter) basis.

Models of spelling describe the process as it exists in the fully developed state. In the development of spelling, there is a qualitative change in the internal organization of the orthography before fluency and automatic production of spelling are possible.

## The Development of Spelling

Luria (1966) emphasized the importance of analysis of words' constituent sounds at the beginning stages of spelling. Read (1975) and Bissex (1980) have examined spelling errors of preschoolers who spontaneously attempt to write messages on the basis of little alphabetic information before they learn to read. Analysis of the errors these children make suggests that the very early stages of spelling are based partly on articulatory information and partly on phonetic information. With only minimal knowledge of phoneme-grapheme correspondence to aid them, these precocious spellers seemed to be reflecting on the articulatory patterns contained in words and in the names of alphabetic letters they knew. For example, for *dragon*, "jagin" was produced; for *smaller*, "smolr"; and for *fishing*, "feheg" (Read, 1975). In the first example, the sound and place of articulation of initial *d* followed by *r* is /ʤ/, which is plausibly represented by *j*; in the second, the sound /ɔː/ and the letter name "o" have the same place of articulation; and in the third example, the fricative /ʃ/ is similar in articulation to the affricate in the letter name "h."

Cognitive processes underlying these early attempts to spell are markedly different from the earliest attempts to read. Written word production seems to be directly related to speech, while written word recognition is apparently influenced to a greater extent by visual characteristics of words (Frith, 1985). When formal instruction in the two skills begins, spelling and reading do not immediately become tied to each other. Rather, they appear to have separate development and only later do they merge and come to rely on similar cognitive processes.

Bradley and Bryant (1979) found that children aged 7½ who were progressing normally in school were sometimes unable to read words that they could spell correctly, and unable to spell words that they knew how to read. The words that could be spelled but not read tended to be regular (e.g., *bun*), while the words that could be read but not spelled tended to be irregular and visually distinctive (e.g., *school*). This finding is in line with the supposition that at the beginning of literacy acquisition, reading proceeds visually, with the child building a sight (reading) recognition vocabulary often without reference to phonological characteristics of words. However, Bradley and Bryant's results strongly suggest the importance of phonological strategies in early spelling.

Frith's (1985) phase theory of literacy acquisition, mentioned earlier for its phases of reading, also postulates phases in spelling development. The earliest phase of spelling is hypothesized to involve copying either from a concrete model or from memory. This is referred to as the logographic phase, because the basic unit is the word, with no analysis of smaller components. In the alphabetic phase, spellings are generated on the basis of articulatory and then phonological information. As the alphabetic principle becomes more ingrained, words can be spelled by means of phoneme-grapheme translation. When the spelling of a word is not overlearned, it is often produced on the basis of pronunciation. Indeed, Sterling (1983) reported that nonphonetic errors may be based on faulty articulation. In the last phase of spelling, the orthographic phase, the specific letter-by-letter structure of a word can be produced.

A number of suggestions have been provided to account for the development of the highest levels of spelling skill. Marsh et al. (1980) suggest that advanced spellers often use analogy to help them spell. For example, *criticize* would be generated on the basis of *critical*. C. Chomsky (1970) has suggested that the use of analogy is an important instructional tool. Perin (1983) found that cueing adolescents with lexically related words which nevertheless differed in pronunciation led to significant improvement in spelling. For example, a subject might originally spell *strategy* as "stratigy" on the first try but, after being cued with *strategic*, would then spell the word correctly.

However, there are many words that cannot be spelled by analogy (although, in line with Glushko's, 1979, theory of reading, it is certainly possible to spell parts of words by analogy). Sloboda (1980) has suggested that excellent spellers somehow learn the many words in their spelling vocabularies by rote. This may be an implicit process based on a reading strategy where attention is paid to all rather than just a few letters in the string (Frith, 1985). Thus, the phase of spelling where words are generated on the basis of orthographic rather than alphabetic information characterizes normal spellers who read well. The spelling of developmental dyslexics is quite different.

## Spelling in Developmental Dyslexia

Models of spelling suggest that when a word cannot be spelled automatically or by visual means, recourse is made to the phonological code, where sounds are mapped with letters so that spelling is "by ear" (Frith, 1979). Phonetic errors are often taken as evidence that a phonological code has been employed.

Analysis of spelling error patterns has been considered useful in studying cognitive dysfunction underlying spelling difficulty. Naidoo (1972) found that some dyslexics tended to make phonetic errors. However, Boder (1973) used errors diagnostically to categorize various types of dyslexia: "Dysphonetic" dyslexics tended to make nonphonetic errors, seeming to prefer a visual approach to the printed word, while "dyseidetic" dyslexics tended to rely on a phonological code, making many phonetically acceptable errors. Other authors have differentiated groups according to whether they were impaired in both reading and spelling or in spelling only (Frith, 1978, 1980; Jorm, 1981; Nelson & Warrington, 1974; Sweeney & Rourke, 1978). Perin (1981) has also employed this method with adults. In these studies it was the good readers who made proportionately more phonetically accurate spelling errors, suggesting that they make more use of a phonological code in spelling than do poor readers (Frith, 1980). In contrast, poor readers made phonetically inaccurate spelling errors. Nelson and Warrington (1974) argued that these were related to a general language deficit, and, according to Rourke (1983), this deficit becomes more serious with increasing age.

***Need for Caution in Error Analysis.*** However, there has been some inconsistency in the criteria used for error analysis. This has led to competing claims in the literature. For example, Barron (1980) studied phonetically accurate spelling errors of good and poor readers as a function of orthographic regularity. He concluded that there was no difference in the phonological process employed by the two groups. Instead, poor readers were reported to be deficient in a "visual-orthographic" strategy. (This conclusion would have been more convincing had the nonphonetic error data been reported.) Holmes and Peper (1977) and Goyen and Martin (1977) have also claimed no difference between good and poor readers in the incidence of phonetic errors. Carpenter (1983) found that poor readers and younger controls made similar numbers of phonetic errors. Moats (1983) reports a similar finding, although this would be entirely in line with expectation, since many of her dyslexics had received intensive training in phonic techniques. Thus, the literature on spelling errors has revealed a good deal of inconsistency. Nelson (1980) has pointed out several important weaknesses in the use of errors for studying spelling processes. Perin (1983) suggested that error patterns could be experimentally manipulated rather easily by word context.

Snowling (1983) has drawn attention to the need to distinguish between tutored and untutored dyslexics when conducting research in this field, and the study reported by Moats (1983) can be criticized on similar grounds. Therefore, while error analysis is a useful diagnostic tool for suggesting remedial procedures (Carpenter, 1983; Ganshow, 1981; Pollack, 1977), caution is needed in using errors as the sole method for investigating cognitive processes underlying spelling dysfunction.

***Spelling and Phonemic Segmentation.*** There are other reasons to expect dyslexics to have difficulty using a phonological code when in fact it would be appropriate for spelling. Since many dyslexics have severe segmentation problems, they are unable to analyze words into phonemes, which would seriously hinder phoneme-grapheme translation. Children with a history of speech problems are particularly prone to make nonphonetic spelling errors, and the errors of children with marked articulation difficulties are of a similar type (Robinson, Beresford, & Dodd, 1982; Snowling & Stackhouse, 1983; Stackhouse, 1982). Therefore, it seems that inadequate access to the structure of speech—whether metalinguistically, through phonemic segmentation, or on the level of production through pronunciation—decreases the ability to employ the phonological route for spelling.

The relation between speech and spelling development has been discussed by Marcel (1980) and Snowling (1982). A type of spelling error quite common among dyslexics is the omission or misplacement of letters representing nasal and liquid phonemes when they occur in initial and final consonant clusters. Marcel argued that the incidence of this type of error, even in adults who appear to produce and comprehend speech normally, suggests a subtle abnormality in the way speech has developed. He suggests that such individuals have not developed an awareness of phonemic units of speech. However, Snowling (1982) found no difference in the ability to spell liquid and nasal consonants when she compared dyslexics and reading age controls. She argued that spelling knowledge plays an important part in phonemic awareness.

Phonemic awareness was investigated in relation to spelling skill by Perin (1983). Subjects were divided into groups according to reading and spelling skills and were aurally presented with stimulus names comprising two words which were to be "Spoonerized." To carry out this task, it was necessary to segment the initial phonemes of each of the names and then transpose them (*Bob Marley*—› "Mob Barley"). The group of good spellers performed the task well, while the poor spellers experienced difficulty. It was argued that there was a close association between phonemic segmentation skills and spelling: Not only could poor phonemic skills hinder the development of spelling, but spelling skills also seemed to have an effect on specific responses subjects made in the task. Words where initial phonemes were spelled with grapheme clusters tended to produce errors that were orthographically rather than phonetically based (*Ray Charles*—› "Kay Rarles"). Thus, even poor spellers might possess some isolated orthographic knowledge. In a second task, the relationship between spelling and phonemic awareness was investigated further. Subjects were aurally presented with individual words and asked to indicate how many sounds each contained. Stimuli were regular words and nonsense words (one letter–one phoneme) and irregular words (more letters than phonemes). It was found that all groups, regardless of reading or spelling skill, tended to be misled by orthographic information in analyzing the phonemic structure of the stimulus words. Thus, it appears that phonemic awareness and spelling have a complicated relationship, even among poor spellers, so that as each skill develops, there is a mutual influence and possibly a mutual facilitation. It is difficult to envisage the initial stages of spelling in the lack of phonemic awareness, although presumably it would be possible to learn, by rote, spellings according to letter names. Indeed, the developmental dyslexic R. E. studied by Campbell and Butterworth (1985) was a good speller but had extreme difficulty generating Spoonerisms and carrying out other tasks requiring phonemic analysis. In this case, there was an enormous amount of compensation, which is unusual among developmental dyslexics, who are almost always poor spellers.

***Importance of the Alphabetic Phase in Spelling.*** According to Frith (1985), the explanation for poor spelling in dyslexia lies in the failure to operate competently in the alphabetic phase. There is no basis for the move to the higher (orthographic) phase, even though as Perin's results (above) show poor spellers can possess "islets" of orthograhic knowledge.

The characteristic of true orthographic spelling is that precise letter-by-letter structure can be recalled at will. Good evidence that dyslexics do not spell in this way is offered by Farnham-Diggory and Nelson (1983), who studied spelling in 11-year-old dyslexics, chronological and reading age matched controls, and adults. All subjects tended to produce "chunks" of three letters. However, dyslexics took particularly long to produce a chunk, similar to younger reading age controls. It was suggested that the dyslexics were organizing spelling information in an immature way and that they had difficulties with auditory representation, which hindered access to orthographic information (i.e., component letters).

Perin recently investigated pauses in the oral spelling of adult fluent readers who were good or poor spellers. Preliminary results indicate that syllable structure plays an important role in spelling production. However, while 80% of good spellers' unfilled pauses were at syllable breaks, only 65% of poor spellers' pauses were. This suggests that syllable structure is important but that poor spellers are inefficient at using it. There was an interaction between regularity and spelling ability so that good spellers paused significantly more often at syllable boundaries in regular than in irregular words. The poor spellers displayed the same percentage of pauses regardless of regularity of target words. These preliminary results indicate that, for good spellers, there is an executive process whereby words are "sifted" according to regularity. Syllabic analysis seems to be applied when possible so that when words are known to be irregular, letter information supersedes syllable information and dominates spelling. Poor spellers do not seem to use regularity in this way, relying on syllable structure indiscriminately as far as word structure is concerned. These findings offer further support for Frith's three-phase model of spelling development. As spelling ability develops, orthographic information becomes increasingly important but never completely replaces alphabetic (syllabic) information.

***An Analysis of Dyslexic Spelling.*** In accounting for the poor spelling of dyslexics, it is necessary to analyze the way they read. Although they may reach a level where they can read as quickly and understand as much as normal individuals, it is probable that cognitive processes underlying performance will be qualitatively different. Frith (1985) carried out an experiment with adolescents that suggests that poor spellers do not read for detail. As in an earlier study (Frith, 1979), subjects were allocated to groups according to reading and spelling skills. An *e*-cancellation task was employed requiring subjects to cross out each *e* in connected but meaningless text consisting of phrases. Target words were of two types, containing either "important" or "unimportant" *e*'s. Important *e*'s are crucial for word recognition, as in the word *left*, while words with unimportant *e*'s are easily identified without actually seeing the *e* (e.g., the word *lifted*). While important *e*'s are found in stressed syllables and are usually at the beginning or in the middle of a word, unimportant *e*'s usually represent schwa or are silent and occur toward the end of a word. If one is paying attention to detail when reading, all letters, regardless of their importance in a word, should be noticed, even if only fleetingly. Frith hypothesized that poor spellers do not pay attention to all letters when reading, which has consequences for their spelling skills. Results of the experiment support her claim. While good and poor spellers were equally able to cancel important *e*'s, poor spellers missed significantly more unimportant *e*'s. It thus seems that poor spellers attend mostly to the more salient letters that occur earlier in the word or have an explicit relationship to pronunciation. When it comes to recalling unimportant *e*'s for spelling, they are therefore at a disadvantage. An important test of this hypothesis would be a spelling error analysis in terms of "important" and "unimportant" letters.

Although spelling is highly valued in school, it is rarely explicitly taught. Teachers often expect pupils to learn lists for spelling tests, but strategies for learning are not suggested. It seems that in most cases, spelling is learned implicitly through reading experience. The dyslexic is disadvantaged in this process, since reading strategies are not providing a basis whereby the specific letter-by-letter structure is noticed. While comprehension is not hindered by this approach, spelling cannot develop to the highest (orthographic) level.

From our discussion of cognitive processes in written language dysfunction, it is clear that reading and spelling can be analyzed as separate sets of functions. In particular, spelling skill is not guaranteed by a high level of reading ability. However, investigations of spelling suggest that to achieve an adequate understanding of the *production* of written language, it is necessary to study the means by which words are *recognized*. Moreover, an understanding of developmental dyslexia requires an appreciation of the ways in which emerging visual-perceptual and phonological skills interact in the acquisition of literacy.

## REFERENCES

Baddeley, A. (1979). Working memory and reading. In H. Bouma, P. A. Kolers, M. E. Wrolstad (Eds.), *The processing of visible language* (pp. 355–370). New York: Plenum.

Baddeley, A., Eldridge, M., & Lewis, V. (1981). The role of subvocalisation in reading. *Quarterly Journal of Experimental Psychology, 33A*, 439–454.

Baddeley, A., Ellis, N., Miles, T. R., & Lewis, V. J. (1982). Developmental and acquired dyslexia: A comparison. *Cognition, 11*, 185–199.

Bakker, D. J. (1972). *Temporal order in disturbed reading*. Rotterdam: University Park Press.

Baron, J., & Strawson, C. (1976). Use of orthographic and word specific knowledge in reading words aloud. *Journal of Experimental Psychology: Human Perception and Performance, 2*, 386–393.

Baron, J., Treiman, R., Wilf, J. F., & Kellman, P. (1980). Spelling and reading by rules. In U. Frith (Ed.), *Cognitive processes in spelling* (pp. 159–194). London: Academic Press.

Barron, R. W. (1980). Visual-orthographic and phonological strategies in reading and spelling. In U. Frith (Ed.), *Cognitive processes in spelling* (pp. 195–214). London: Academic Press.

Barron, R. W., & Baron, J. (1977). How children get meaning from printed words. *Child Development, 48*, 587–594.

Beauvois, M. F., & Derouesne, J. (1979). Phonological alexia: Three dissociations. *Journal of Neurology, Neurosurgery and Psychiatry*, *42*, 1115–1124.

Beauvois, M. F., & Derouesne, J. (1981). Lexical or orthographic agraphia. *Brain*, *104*, 21–49.

Benton, A. L. (1962). Dyslexia in relation to form perception and directional sense. In J. Money (Ed.), *Reading disability: Progress and research needs in dyslexia* (pp. 81–102). Baltimore: Johns Hopkins Press.

Benton, A. L., & Pearl, D. (Eds.). (1978). *Dyslexia: An appraisal of current knowledge*. New York: Oxford University Press.

Besner, D., Davies, J., & Daniels, S. (1981). Reading for meaning: the effects of concurrent articulation. *Quarterly Journal of Experimental Psychology*, *33A*, 415–437.

Bissex, G. L. (1980). *GNYS at work: A child learns to write and read*. Cambridge, MA: Harvard University Press.

Boder, E. (1973). Developmental dyslexia: A diagnostic approach based on three atypical reading-spelling patterns. *Developmental Medicine and Child Neurology*, *15*, 663–687.

Bradley, L. (1983). The organization of visual-perceptual and motor strategies in reading and spelling. In U. Kirk (Ed), *Neuropsychology of learning, reading and spelling* (pp. 235–254). New York: Academic Press.

Bradley, L., & Bryant, P. (1978). Difficulties in auditory organization as a possible cause of reading backwardness. *Nature*, *271*, 746.

Bradley, L., & Bryant, P. E. (1979). Independence of reading and spelling in backward and normal readers. *Developmental Medicine and Child Neurology*, *21*, 504–514.

Bradley, L., & Bryant, P. E. (1983). Categorizing sounds and learning to read: A causal connexion. *Nature*, *301*, 419.

Brown, H. D. (1970). Categories of spelling difficulty in speakers of English as a first and second language. *Journal of Verbal Learning and Verbal Behavior*, *9*, 232–236.

Bryant, P. E., & Bradley, L. (1980). Why children sometimes write words which they do not read. In U. Frith (Ed.), *Cognitive processes in spelling* (pp. 355–372). London: Academic Press.

Campbell, R., & Butterworth, B. (1985). Phonological dyslexia and dysgraphia in a highly literate subject: A developmental case with associated deficits of phonemic processing and awareness. *Quarterly Journal of Experimental Psychology*, *37A*, 435–475.

Carpenter, D. (1983). Spelling error patterns of able and disabled readers. *Journal of Learning Disabilities*, *16*, 102–104.

Chomsky, C. (1970). Reading, writing and phonology. *Harvard Educational Review*, *40*, 287–309.

Cohen, R. L., & Netley, C. (1981). Short-term memory deficits in reading disabled children in the absence of the opportunity for rehearsal strategies. *Intelligence*, *5*, 69–76.

Coltheart, M. (1980). Reading, phonological recoding and deep dyslexia. In M. Coltheart, K. Patterson, & J. Marshall (Eds.), *Deep dyslexia* (pp. 197–226). London: Routledge and Kegan Paul.

Coltheart, M., Davelaar, E., Jonasson, J., & Besner, D. (1977). Access to the internal lexicon. In S. Dornic (Ed.), *Attention and performance VI* (pp. 535–555). Hillsdale, NJ: Lawrence Erlbaum.

Coltheart, M., Masterson, J., Byng, S., Prior, M., & Riddoch, J. (1983). Surface dyslexia. *Quarterly Journal of Experimental Psychology, 35A*, 469–496.

Coltheart, M., Patterson, K., & Marshall, J. (Eds.). (1980). *Deep dyslexia*. London: Routledge and Kegan Paul.

Conrad, R. (1972). Speech and reading. In J. F. Kavanagh & I. G. Mattingly (Eds.), *Language by ear and by eye: The relationship between speech and reading* (pp. 205–240). Cambridge, MA: MIT Press.

Critchley, M. (1964). *Developmental dyslexia*. London: Heinemann.

Critchley, M. (1970). *The dyslexic child*. London: Heinemann Medical Books.

Critchley, M., & Critchley, E. A. (1978). *Dyslexia defined*. Great Britain: R. J. Acford.

Cromer, R. F. (1980). Spontaneous spelling by language disordered children. In U. Frith (Ed.), *Cognitive processes in spelling* (pp. 405–422). London: Academic Press.

Davelaar, E., Coltheart, M., Besner, D., & Jonasson, J. T. (1978). Phonological recoding and lexical access. *Memory and Cognition, 6*, 391–402.

Denckla, M. B., & Rudel, R. G. (1976). Rapid "automatized" naming (R.A.N.). Dyslexia differentiated from other learning disabilities. *Neuropsychologia, 14*.

Denckla, M. B., Rudel, R. G., & Broman, M. (1981). Tests that discriminate between dyslexic and other learning disabled boys. *Brain and Language, 13*, 118–129.

Doctor, E. A., & Coltheart, M. (1980). Children's use of phonological encoding when reading for meaning. *Memory and Cognition, 8*, 195–209.

Dodd, B. (1980). Spelling in deaf children. In U. Frith (Ed.), *Cognitive processes in spelling* (pp. 423–442). London: Academic Press.

Ehri, L. (1980). Reading and spelling in beginners: The development of orthographic images as word symbols in lexical memory. In U. Frith (Ed.), *Cognitive processes in spelling* (pp. 311–338). London: Academic Press.

Ellis, A. W. (1979). Developmental and acquired dyslexia: Some observations on Jorm 1979. *Cognition, 7*, 413–420.

Ellis, A. W. (1982). Spelling and writing (and reading and speaking). In A. W. Ellis (Ed.), *Normality and pathology in cognition functions* (pp. 113–146). London: Academic Press.

Ellis, N. (1981). Visual and name coding in dyslexic children. *Psychological Research, 43*, 201–218.

Ellis, N. C., & Miles, T. R. (1981). A lexical encoding deficiency II. In G. Th. Pavlidis & T. R. Miles (Eds.), *Dyslexia research and its applications to education* (pp. 177–216). Cambridge, MA: MIT Press.

Farnham-Diggory, S., & Nelson, B. (1983). Microethology of spelling behaviors in normal and dyslexic development. In D. A. Rogers & J. A. Sloboda (Eds.), *The acquisition of symbolic skills* (pp. 109–122). New York: Plenum Press.

Fischer, F. W., Liberman, I. Y., & Shankweiler, D. (1978). Reading reversals and developmental dyslexia: A further study. *Cortex, 14*, 496–510.

Fox, B., & Routh, D. K. (1980). Phonemic analysis and severe reading disability in children. *Journal of Psycholinguistic Research, 9*, 115–120.

Francis, H (1982). *Learning to read. Literate behavior and orthographic knowledge.* London: Allen and Unwin.

Frith, U. (1978). Spelling difficulties. *Journal of Child Psychology and Psychiatry, 19,* 279–285.

Frith, U. (1979). Reading by eye and writing by ear. In H. Bouma, P. A. Kolers, & M. E. Wrolstad (Eds.), *The processing of visible language* (pp. 379–390). New York: Plenum.

Frith, U. (1980). Unexpected spelling problems. In U. Frith (Ed.), *Cognitive processes in spelling* (pp. 495–516). London: Academic Press.

Frith, U. (1981). Experimental approaches to developmental dyslexia. *Psychological Research, 43,* 97–103.

Frith, U. (1984). *Specific spelling problems.* NATO Advanced Study Institute, Dyslexia: A global issue, Oct. 10–22, Maratea.

Frith, U. (1985). Beneath the surface of developmental dyslexia. In J. C. Marshall, M. Coltheart, & K. E. Patterson (Eds.), *Surface dyslexia and surface dysgraphia* (pp. 301–330). London: Routledge and Kegan Paul.

Frith, U., & Frith, C. (1980). Relationships between reading and spelling. In J. F. Kavanagh & R. L. Venezky (Eds.), *Orthography, reading and dyslexia* (pp. 287–295). Austin, TX: PRO-ED.

Frith, U., & Snowling, M. (1983). Reading for sound and reading for meaning: A comparison of autistic and dyslexic reading. *British Journal of Developmental Psychology, 1,* 329–342.

Funnell, E. (1983). Phonological processes in reading: New evidence from acquired dyslexia. *British Journal of Psychology, 74,* 159–180.

Ganschow, L. (1981). Discovering children's learning strategies through error pattern analysis. *The Reading Teacher, 34,* 676–680.

Gelb, I. J. (1983). *A study of writing.* Chicago: University of Chicago Press.

Gibson, E. J., Osser, H., & Pick, A. D. (1963). A study of the development of grapheme-phoneme correspondences. *Journal of Verbal Learning and Verbal Behaviour, 2,* 142–146.

Gleitman, L. R., & Rozin, P. (1977). The structure and acquisition of reading. I. Relations between orthographics and the structure of language. In A. S. Reber & D. L. Scarborough (Eds.), *Toward a psychology of reading* (pp. 1–54). Hillsdale, NJ: Lawrence Erlbaum.

Glushko, R. J. (1979). The organization and activation of orthographic knowledge in reading aloud. *Journal of Experimental Psychology: Human Perception and Performance, 5,* 674–691.

Goyen, J. D., & Martin, M. (1977). The relation of spelling errors to cognitive variables and word type. *British Journal of Educational Psychology, 47,* 278–273.

Hanna, P. R., Hodges, R. E., & Hanna, J. S. (1971). *Spelling: Structure and strategies.* New York: Houghton Mifflin.

Hanson, V. L. (1981). *When a word is not the sum of its letters: Finger spelling and spelling.* Proceedings of the 3rd National Symposium on Sign Language, Research and Teaching.

Healy, J. M. (1982). The enigma of hyperlexia. *Reading Research Quarterly, 17,* 319–338.

Henderson, L. (1983). *Orthography and word recognition in reading.* London: Academic Press.

Henderson, L., & Chard, J. (1980). The reader's implicit knowledge of orthographic structure. In U. Frith (Ed.), *Cognitive processes in spelling* (pp. 85–116). London: Academic Press.

Henderson, L., Chard, M. J., & Clark, A. (1981). Preparation and speech programming in rapid reading and reciting. *Canadian Journal of Psychology, 35*, 224–243.

Hermelin, B., & O'Connor, N. (1967). Remembering of words by psychotic and subnormal children. *British Journal of Psychology, 58*, 213–218.

Holmes, D. L., & Peper, R. J. (1977). An evaluation of the use of spelling error analysis in the diagnosis of reading disabilities. *Child Development, 48*, 1708–1711.

Huey, E. B. (1908). *The psychology and pedagogy of reading*. New York: Macmillan.

Johnston, R. S. (1982). Phonological coding in dyslexic readers. *British Journal of Psychology, 73*, 455–460.

Jorm, A. F. (1979a). The cognitive and neurological basis of developmental dyslexia. A theoretical framework and review. *Cognition, 7*, 19–33.

Jorm, A. F. (1979b). The nature of the reading deficit in developmental dyslexia. A reply to Ellis. *Cognition, 7*, 421–433.

Jorm, A. F. (1981). Children with reading and spelling retardation: Functioning of whole-word and correspondence-rule mechanisms. *Journal of Child Psychology and Psychiatry*, 22, 171–178.

Jorm, A. F. (1983). Specific reading retardation and working memory—a review. *British Journal of Psychology, 74*, 311–342.

Kavanagh, J. F., & Venezky, R. L. (1980). *Orthography, reading and dyslexia*. Austin, TX: PRO-ED.

Kay, J., & Marcel, A. (1981). One process, not two, in reading aloud: Lexical analogies do the work of nonlexical rules. *Quarterly Journal of Experimental Psychology, 33A*, 397–413.

LaBerge, D., & Samuels, S. J. (1974). Toward a theory of automatic information processing in reading. *Cognitive Psychology, 6*, 293–323.

Laver, J. D. M. (1980). Monitoring systems in the neurolinguistic control of speech production. In V. A. Fromkin (Ed.), *Errors in linguistic performance: Slips of the tongue, ear, pen and hand* (pp. 287–306). New York: Academic Press.

Liberman, I. Y., & Shankweiler, D. (1977). Speech, the alphabet and teaching to read. In L. B. Resnick & P. A. Weaver (Eds.), *Theory and practice of early reading* (pp. 109–132). Hillsdale, NJ: Lawrence Erlbaum.

Liberman., I. Y., Shankweiler, D., Liberman, A. M., Fowler, C., & Fischer, F. W. (1977). Phonetic segmentation and recoding in the beginning reader. In A. S. Reber & D. L. Scarborough (Eds.), *Toward a psychology of reading. The proceedings of the CUNY conference* (pp. 207–226). Hillsdale, NJ: Lawrence Erlbaum.

Liberman, I. Y., Liberman, A. M., Mattingley, I. G., & Shankweiler, D. (1980). Orthography and the beginning reader. In J. Kavanagh & R. Venezky (Eds.), *Orthography, reading and dyslexia* (pp. 137–189). Austin, TX: PRO-ED.

Luria, A. R. (1966). *Higher cortical functions in man*. New York: Basic Books.

Mann, V. A., Liberman, I. Y., & Shankweiler, D. (1980). Children's memory for sentences and word strings in relation to reading ability. *Memory and Cognition, 8*, 329–335.

Marcel, T. (1980). Phonological awareness and phonological representation: Investigation of a specific spelling problem. In U. Frith (Ed.), *Cognitive processes in spelling* (pp. 373–404). London: Academic Press.

Marsh, G., & Desberg, P. (1983). The development of strategies in the acquisition of symbolic skills. In D. A. Rogers & J. Sloboda (Eds.), *The acquisition of symbolic skills* (pp. 149–154). New York: Plenum Press.

Marsh, G., Friedman, M., Welch, V., & Desberg, P. (1980). The development of strategies in spelling. In U. Frith (Ed.), *Cognitive processes of spelling* (pp. 339–354). London: Academic Press.

Marshall, J. C., & Newcombe, F. (1973). Patterns of paralexia: A psycholinguistic approach. *Journal of Psycholinguistic Research, 2,* 175–199.

Mattis, S., French, J. H., & Rapin, I. (1975). Dyslexia in children and young adults: Three independent neurological syndromes. *Developmental Medicine and Child Neurology, 17,* 150–163.

Meyer, D. E., Schvaneveldt, R. W., & Ruddy, M. G. (1975). Loci of contextual effects in visual word recognition. In S. Dornic & P. M. A. Rabbitt (Eds.), *Attention and performance V* (pp. 98–118). London: Academic Press.

Miles, T. R. (1983). Dyslexia: *The patterns of difficulties*. Suffolk, England: Granada.

Miles, T. R., & Ellis, N. C. (1981). A lexical encoding deficiency II. Clinical observations. In G. Th. Pavlidis & T. R. Miles (Eds.), *Dyslexia research and its applications to education* (pp. 217–244). New York: John Wiley.

Mitchell, D. C. (1982). *The process of reading. A cognitive analysis of fluent reading and learning to read*. New York: John Wiley.

Moats, L. C. (1983). A comparison of the spelling errors of older dyslexic and second grade normal children. *Annals of Dyslexia, 33,* 121–140.

Montgomery, D. (1981). Do dyslexics have difficulty accessing articulatory information? *Psychological Research, 43,* 235–244.

Morais, J., Cary, L., Alegria, J., & Bertelson, P. (1979). Does awareness of speech as a sequence of phones arise spontaneously? *Cognition, 7,* 323–331.

Morton, J. (1979). Word recognition. In J. Morton & J. C. Marshall (Eds.), *Psycholinguistics series* (Vol. 2, pp. 107–156). London: Elek.

Naidoo, S. (1972). *Specific dyslexia*. The research report of the ICAA Word Blind Centre for Dyslexic Children. London: Pitman.

Nelson, H. E. (1980). Analysis of spelling errors in normal and dyslexic children. In U. Frith (Ed.), *Cognitive processes in spelling* (pp. 475–494). London: Academic Press.

Nelson, H. E., & Warrington, E. K. (1974). Developmental spelling retardation and its relation to other cognitive abilities. *British Journal of Psychology, 65,* 265–274.

Nelson, H. E., & Warrington, E. K. (1980). An investigation of memory functions in dyslexic children. *British Journal of Psychology, 71,* 487–503.

Orton, S. T. (1937). *Reading, writing and speech problems in children*. New York: Norton.

Parkin, A. J. (1982). Phonological recoding in lexical decision: Effects of spelling to sound regularity depend upon how regularity is defined. *Memory and Cognition, 10,* 43–53.

Patterson, K. E. (1981). Neuropsychological approaches to the study of reading. *British Journal of Psychology, 72,* 151–174.

Perfetti, C. A., & Hogaboam, T. (1975). Relationship between single word decoding and reading comprehension skill. *Journal of Educational Psychology, 67*, 461–469.

Perin, D. (1981). Spelling, reading and adult illiteracy. *Psychological Research, 43*, 245–257.

Perin, D. (1982). Spelling strategies in good and poor readers. *Applied Psycholinguistics, 3*, 1–14.

Perin, D. (1983). Phoneme segmentation and spelling. *British Journal of Psychology, 74*, 129–145.

Personke, C., & Yee, A. H. (1966). A model for the analysis of spelling behaviour. *Elementary English, 43*, 278–284.

Pollack, C. (1977). Of reading disabilities, ability testing and the urban school. *The Learning Disabilities Newsletter, III*, 1–6.

Posner, M. I. (1969). Abstraction and the process of recognition. In J. T. Spencer & G. Bower (Eds.), *The psychology of learning and motivation* (Vol. 3, pp. 44–100). London: Academic Press.

Posner, M. I., & Snyder, C. R. R. (1975). Attention and cognitive control. In R. L. Solso (Ed.), *Information processing and cognition: The Loyola Symposium* (pp. 55–85). Hillsdale, NJ: Lawrence Erlbaum.

Rack, J. (1985). Orthographic and phonetic encoding in normal and dyslexic readers. *British Journal of Psychology, 76*, 325–340.

Read, C. (1975). Lessons to be learned from the preschool orthographer. In E. Lenneberg (Ed.), *Foundations of language development—a multidisciplinary approach* (Vol. 2, pp. 329–346). Paris: UNESCO.

Robinson, P., Beresford, R., & Dodd, B. (1982). Spelling errors made by phonologically disordered children. *Spelling Progress Bulletin, 22*, 19–20.

Rourke, B. P. (1983). Reading and spelling disabilities: A developmental neuropsychological perspective. In U. Kirk (Ed.), *Neuropsychology of language, reading and spelling* (pp. 209–234). New York: Academic Press.

Rozin, P., Poritsky, S., & Sotsky, R. (1971). American children with reading problems can easily learn to read English represented by Chinese characters. *Science, 171*, 1266–1267.

Rubinstein, H., Lewis, S. S., & Rubinstein, M. A. (1971). Evidence for phonemic recoding in visual word recognition. *Journal of Verbal Learning and Verbal Behaviour, 10*, 645–657.

Rugel, R. P. (1974). WISC subtest scores of disabled readers. *Journal of Learning Disabilities, 7*, 57–64.

Rutter, M., Tizard, J., Yule, W., Graham, P., & Whitmore, K. (1976). Research report. Isle of Wight Studies, 1964–1974. *Psychological Medicine, 6*, 313–332.

Rutter, M., & Yule, W. (1973). Specific reading retardation. In L. Mann & D. Savatino (Eds.), *The first review of special education*. Philadelphia: Buttonwood Farms.

Schvaneveldt, R., Ackerman, B. P., & Semlear, T. (1977). The effect of semantic context on children's word recognition. *Child Development, 48*, 612–616.

Schwantes, F. M., Boesl, S. L., & Ritz, E. G. (1980). Children's use of context in word recognition: A psycholinguistic guessing game. *Child Development, 51*, 730–736.

Seymour, P. H. K., & McGregor, C. J. (1984). Developmental dyslexia: A cognitive experimental analysis of phonological, morphemic, and visual impairments. *Cognitive Neuropsychology, 1*, 43–82.

Seymour, P. H. K., & Porpodas, C. D. (1980). Lexical and nonlexical processing of spelling in developmental dyslexia. In U. Frith (Ed.), *Cognitive processes in spelling* (pp. 443–474). London: Academic Press.

Shallice, T. (1981). Phonological agraphia and the lexical route in writing. *Brain, 104*, 413–429.

Shankweiler, D., Liberman, I. Y., Mark, L. S., Fowler, C. A., & Fischer, F. W. (1979). The speech code and learning to read. *Journal of Experimental Psychology: Human Learning and Memory, 5*,531–545.

Simon, D. P. (1976). Spelling—a task analysis. *Instructional Science, 5*, 277–302.

Simon, D. P., & Simon, H. A. (1973). Alternative uses of phonemic information in spelling. *Review of Educational Research, 43*, 115–137.

Sloboda, J. (1980). Visual imagery and individual differences in spelling. In U. Frith (Ed.), *Cognitive processes in spelling* (pp. 231–250). London: Academic Press.

Smith, F. (1973). Alphabetic writing: A language compromise? In F. Smith (Ed.), *Psycholinguistics and reading* (pp. 116–130). New York: Holt, Rinehart and Winston.

Smith, P. T. (1980). Linguistic information in spelling. In U. Frith (Ed.), *Cognitive processes in spelling* (pp. 33–50). London: Academic Press.

Smith, P. T., & Sterling, C. M. (1983). Factors affecting the perceived morphemic structure of written words. *Journal of Verbal Learning and Verbal Behaviour, 21*, 704–721.

Snowling, M. J. (1980). The development of grapheme-phoneme correspondence in normal and dyslexic readers. *Journal of Experimental Child Psychology, 29*, 294–305.

Snowling, M. J. (1981). Phonemic deficits in developmental dyslexia. *Psychological Research, 43*, 219–234.

Snowling, M. J. (1982). The spelling of nasal clusters by dyslexic and normal children. *Spelling Progress Bulletin, 22*, 13–18.

Snowling, M. J. (1983). The comparison of acquired and developmental disorders of reading. *Cognition, 14*, 105–118.

Snowling, M., & Frith, U. (1981). The use of sound, shape and orthographic cues in early reading. *British Journal of Psychology, 72*, 83–88.

Snowling, M., & Perin, D. (1983). The development of phoneme segmentation skills in young children. In D. R. Rogers & J. A. Sloboda (Eds.), *Acquisition of symbolic skills* (pp. 155–162). New York: Plenum Press.

Snowling, M., & Stackhouse, J. (1983). Spelling performance of children with developmental verbal dyspraxia. *Developmental Medicine and Child Neurology, 25*, 430–437.

Spring, C., & Capps, C. (1974). Encoding speed, rehearsal and probed recall of dyslexic boys. *Journal of Educational Psychology, 66*, 780–786.

Stackhouse, J. (1982). An investigation of reading and spelling performance in speech disordered children. *British Journal of Disorders of Communication, 17*, 53–60.

Stanovich, K. E. (1980). Toward an interactive-compensatory model of individual differences in the development of reading fluency. *Reading Research Quarterly, 16*, 32–71.

Stanovich, K. E., & West, R. F. (1981). The effect of sentence context on ongoing word recognition: Tests of a two process theory. *Journal of Experimental Psychology: Human Perception and Performance, 7*, 658–672.

Stanovich, K. E., West, R. F., & Freeman, D. J. (1981). A longitudinal study of sentence context effects in second grade children: Tests of an interactive compensatory model. *Journal of Experimental Child Psychology, 32*, 185–199.

Sterling, C. M. (1983). Spelling errors in context. *British Journal of Psychology, 74*, 353–364.

Sternberg, S., Monsell, S., Knoll, R. L., & Wright, C. E. (1978). The latency and duration of rapid movement sequences: Comparisons of speech and typewriting. In G. Stelmach (Ed.), *Information processing in motor control and learning* (pp. 118–152). New York: Academic Press.

Stevenson, H. W., Stigler, J. W., Lucker, G. W., & Lee, S. Y. (1982). Reading disabilities: The case of Chinese, Japanese and English. *Child Development, 53*, 1164–1181.

Sweeney, J. E., & Rourke, B. P. (1978). Neuropsychological significance of phonetically accurate and phonetically inaccurate spelling errors in younger and older retarded spellers. *Brain and Language, 6*, 212–225.

Tallal, P. (1980). Auditory temporal perception, phonics and reading disabilities in children. *Brain and Language, 9*, 182–198.

Taylor, I., & Taylor, M. M. (1983). *The psychology of reading*. New York: Academic Press.

Tenney, Y. J. (1980). Visual factors in spelling. In U. Frith (Ed.), *Cognitive processes in spelling* (pp. 215–230). London: Academic Press.

Thomson, M. E. (1982). The assessment of children with specific reading difficulties (dyslexia) using the British Ability Scales. *British Journal of Psychology, 73*, 461–478.

Vellutino, F. R. (1977). Alternative conceptualizations of dyslexia: Evidence in support of a verbal deficit hypothesis. *Harvard Educational Review*, Special Issue on Reading and Language, *47*, 334–354.

Vellutino, F. R. (1979). *Dyslexia: Theory and research*. Cambridge, MA: MIT Press.

Vellutino, F. R., Steger, J. A., Kaman, M., & Desotto, L. (1975). Visual form perception in deficient and normal readers as a function of age and orthographic linguistic familiarity. *Cortex, 11*, 22–30.

Venezky, R. L. (1970). *The structure of English orthography*. The Hague: Mouton.

Vygotsky, L. S. (1934). *Thought and language*. Translated by E. Haufmann & G. Vakar. Cambridge, MA: MIT Press.

Vygotsky, L. S. (1962). *Thought and language*. Cambridge, MA: MIT Press.

West, R. F., & Stanovich, K. E. (1978). Automatic contextual facilitation in readers of three ages. *Child Development, 49*, 717–727.

SECTION IV

# *Communicative Function and Language*

JAMES E. McLEAN, EDITOR

# 8

# *Pragmatics and Child Language Disorders*

LYNN S. SNYDER AND
JAN SILVERSTEIN

A problem faces professionals engaged in assessment and intervention with children whose pragmatic development may be delayed. It is the effects that different assumptions about pragmatics can have on clinical practice. To determine the pervasive impact that such assumptions can have, it is necessary to look at what we mean by *pragmatics*.

## DEFINING PRAGMATICS

Defining pragmatics is like challenging five master bakers to bake the perfect chocolate cake. They all agree that the cake must contain flour, eggs, sugar, chocolate, and so forth. The precise proportions of these ingredients, however, vary from baker to baker. Training and experience lead each one to a different combination. Each baker will have an argument to defend a particular recipe and to demonstrate why it results in the best cake.

Just as we may turn to a master baker for guidance, speech and language professionals turn to the thinking of master linguists, psychologists, language philosophers, or anthropologists for guidance. Just as master bakers tend to agree on the ingredients for the cake, thinkers about pragmatics tend to agree about communicative behavior. They agree that pragmatics involves how people use language in a variety of situations to achieve personal and societal social goals. And just as several master bakers' different training and experience lead them to different proportions and combinations of ingredients, the different orientations of the thinkers about language lead them to focus upon and emphasize different aspects of pragmatic behavior.

Four orientations or areas of study have made significant contributions to our knowledge of pragmatics. These include the philosophy of language, linguistics, cognitive psychology, and social anthropology.

## Philosophically Influenced Points of View

Philosophers of language concern themselves with the truth value and meaning of language. The first ideas about pragmatics came from this tradition and were expressed by John L. Austin during his presentations in the William James lecture series at Harvard University in 1955. His lectures were posthumously published in two books: *How to Do Things with Words* (Austin, 1962) and *J. L. Austin's Philosophical Papers* (Austin, 1970).

Austin turned from the traditional philosophical concern of how meaning or sense is made with language to more dynamic and practical—hence, pragmatic—concerns of how things get accomplished with language. He looked at language functionally by distinguishing between the *constative* or content aspects of language and its *performative* or functional aspects. Specifically, he suggested that many utterances cannot have content that reports or describes something true or false. Rather, their very production performs an action (Austin, 1962). An example is a priest who christens a child by saying, "I christen thee Tobias." The utterance actually performs the action of christening the child. Thus, some utterances are performative.

After outlining his concept of performative utterances, Austin presented his classification of *infelicities*. These are the ways context or circumstances surrounding the utterance may or may not conform to social conventions or other conditions. For example, although an utterance making a false promise in fact performs a promise, it violates social convention. Thus, he considered it "unhappy" or "infelicitous."

A more scrupulous analysis of the performative/constative distinction and the notion of infelicities led Austin to realize that these distinctions broke down. He abandoned them and examined the problem in a more generic manner. He then distinguished between the force of an utterance and its meaning. The *illocutionary force* of an utterance was the act that the speaker performed with the utterance (Austin, 1962). He distinguished between illocutionary acts, or acts performed by utterances or speech acts that contain an illocutionary force, and *locutionary* and *perlocutionary* acts.

Locutionary acts are the production of sentences that contain a particular sense and reference. Perlocutionary acts are consequences of the act, the effect of the utterance. These notions form the cornerstone for the functional aspect of language, its pragmatic aspect.

In the year following his Harvard lecture series, Austin reviewed these concepts (Austin, 1970). He challenged philosophers to pursue the identification and classification of all possible forces of utterances. Among those philosophers accepting this challenge was John Searle, who developed what is perhaps the most comprehensive theory of speech acts to date (Searle, 1965, 1969). He reasoned that to speak language is to perform speech acts and that linguistic rules regulate such acts. Thus, he viewed the speech act as the basic unit of communication. He delineated four basic types of speech acts and corresponding sets of rules that govern them. Such rules are conditions that must be met if a particular act (e.g., promising) within a basic speech act category is to be performed. The comprehensive and detailed nature of Searle's speech act theory makes it an ideal basis for many approaches to the analysis of children's speech acts.

As philosophers began to explore these notions, they realized that once one began to consider the circumstances surrounding an utterance, one had to consider the discourse or conversation in which it occurred. Consequently, some philosophers of language turned their attention to discourse. They attempted to identify rules governing the way discourse is conducted. One such thinker was Herbert Grice. He specified sets of rules that regulate conversations (Grice, 1975). Like Austin, he thought about language in a practical way. His postulates reflect his common-sense approach to the problem. For example, one of his conversational postulates is to be polite. This rule may be simply stated, but it can have a far-reaching effect on utterances. At the level of discourse, it implies that you greet someone at the outset of a conversation. At the level of the utterance or speech act, it implies that you should be indirect. Consequently, you would more appropriately ask, "Can you reach the sugar?" at a dinner table instead of saying, "Give me the sugar."

The philosophers of language, then, set the stage for viewing language functionally. Their delineation of categories of speech and of rules constraining speech acts and discourse provide a rich basis for taxonomies to analyze these aspects of children's communicative language.

## Linguistically Influenced Points of View

In contrast to the philosophical point of view, thinkers more heavily influenced by linguistics were sensitive to the subtleties of linguistic form as it accomplished its social objective. This is not to suggest that they did not also recognize the function performed by the utterance or the role of cognition and concepts in pragmatics. Rather, these thinkers delineated the formal structure that could be used to accomplish a variety of functions.

We see the first evidence of this fine-tuned attention to linguistic form in the later work of John Dore (1977, 1978, 1979). Dore, a linguist by training, was one of the first to study the emergence of speech acts in children (1973, 1975). His early work on the emergence of primitive speech acts was heavily influenced by the philosophical point of view, identifying the general intentions carried by children's one-word utterances. He emphasized how context can override the literal meaning of an utterance.

Subsequently, Dore (1977, 1978, 1979) explored the speech acts performed by preschool children. In refining his taxonomy of communicative acts, he indicated that the propositional content, the function of the utterance, the context of the situation in which it occurred, and some specific aspects of grammatical form must be considered. This introduction of specific aspects of formal structure into the classification of speech acts demonstrates a shift toward more comprehensive theories of pragmatic behavior.

It is natural that this increased consideration of syntactic form came from the work of linguists examining child language. As Halliday (1975) observed and demonstrated, the number of functions achieved by speech acts increases with the number of syntactic forms the child can produce. Thus, how functions were related to specific syntactic forms became more apparent.

Perhaps the most explicit consideration of the role played by linguistic form can be seen in the later work of Lois Bloom and her colleagues (Bloom & Lahey, 1978; Bloom, Lightbown, & Hood, 1975; Bloom, Rocissano, & Hood, 1976). Bloom's particular contributions were that she sensitized us to the ways children learn rules that govern the choice of linguistic forms in a given context as well as how children produce utterances in discourse that are *linguistically* contingent with the preceding utterance. Bloom et al. (1975) documented how children learn to use the alternative nominal or pronominal form in reference according to the context of the situation. Bloom et al. (1976) examined the development of discourse between 2 and 3 years of age. They described the linguistic strategies children used to produce linguistically contingent utterances (i.e., utterances that share the same topic) in discourse. Bloom et al. (1976) defined such topic-sharing in linguistic terms, that is, as utterances sharing the same verb relation. Further, the strategies they described were linguistic (e.g., addition or modification of subject-verb complements). Thus, Bloom's work focused on the child's growing control over intentional manipulation of the linguistic form of the message in response to pragmatic constraints.

These thinkers directed our attention to how the linguistic form of the utterance relates to communicative functions and the structure of discourse. In addition, they observed the ways in which children developed control over the precise manipulation of these linguistic forms in response to the needs imposed by the context or situation.

## Cognitively Influenced Points of View

Bloom and her colleagues explicitly stated that children's cognitive development is important to their language development and what they can do with words. However, apart from Bloom's (1973) study that tied the acquisition of first words to the development of Piaget's (1963) stage six object permanence, she made no further attempt to specify the nature of the cognitive developments related to developments in child language. The more direct influence of cognitively oriented points of view can be seen in the work of the psychologists and psycholinguists Parisi and Antinucci (1978) and Elizabeth Bates (1976).

Parisi and Antinucci, Italian psychologists and psycholinguists, developed a grammar that is uniquely pragmatic in nature (Parisi & Antinucci, 1978). They postulated a system in which the underlying structure of every utterance is its performative. The performative, as they defined it, is the speaker's communicative intention. Their grammar also specified the underlying structure of the speaker's presuppositions about the context of the situation. These *presuppositions*, which provide input into the speaker's utterance, are attitudes, beliefs, experiences, and expectations the speaker thinks he or she shares with the listener. In this theory, the speaker's concepts and thinking about a situation influence what he or she says.

Parisi and Antinucci's (1978) grammar indicates that the content of the utterance is dependent upon the underlying communicative intention. The propositions mapped by speakers reflect the underlying performative. Parisi and Antinucci are generative semanticists. Their grammar presents the predicate and argument relations mapped by various sentences. Thus, they do not concern themselves specifically with syntactic forms.

Bates' (1976) contribution to pragmatics is different. She studied the emergence of various pragmatic skills in children during the first 6 years of life. She examined the relationship between milestones in the child's acquisition of pragmatic structures and corresponding advances in cognitive development. Two of the relationships between pragmatic and cognitive development documented by Bates are the child's acquisition of sensorimotor or gestural performatives and later acquisition of polite forms. Bates, Camaioni, and Volterra in Bates (1976), and in a subsequent larger study (Bates, Benigni, Bretherton, Camaioni, & Volterra, 1979), documented that the emergence of intentional communicative gestures such as giving, showing, and pointing coincides with the development of sensorimotor stage five tool use in which a new or novel tool is used to accomplish a familiar goal. Bates' (1976) treatment of the child's acquisition of polite forms suggests that children's ability to construct indirect speech acts in which the goal is never mentioned (i.e., hints) develops in correspondence with the child's development of role-taking ability. Role taking is the ability to assume the other person's point of view. Thus, Bates (1976) sees cognitive development as an important developmental corollary of pragmatic development.

Those thinkers influenced by cognition then directed our attention to the speaker's cognitive understanding of the context or situation in which he or she finds himself. Parisi and Antinucci's (1978) grammar turned our attention to the speaker's presupposition and its effect on the utterance. Bates (1976), because she was looking at children's development of pragmatics, drew our attention to their developing understanding of the context.

## Socially Influenced Points of View

A last major influence upon thinking in pragmatics comes from social anthropologists, sociolinguists, and psychologists interested in social development. This approach attends to aspects of social life that interact with language in communication. These aspects are diverse and include such far-ranging considerations as societal systems for interaction, verbal and nonverbal regulations of exchanges, the social role and dominance of the interlocutors, and the nature and synchrony of the interaction. The contribution of socially influenced researchers and thinkers has been significant. We will confine our discussion to a few contributors whose work exemplifies the different types of information that have come from this area.

One of the most notable contributions from socially influenced thinkers is the work of Dell Hymes. An anthropologist and a linguist by training, he was able to bring together his knowledge of the societal structure of social interaction and his knowledge of language theory in a dynamic view of communication. He directed everyone's attention away from the idea of "linguistic" communication and linguistic competence (Hymes, 1971). In addition, he outlined its dimensions and developed a taxonomy of features that must be addressed by any theory or model of the interaction between language and social life (Hymes, 1972). These include consideration of the speech community as the social unit of analysis, because it shares a common set of rules for conducting spoken interactions. Hymes distinguished between speech events and speech acts. The former are whole activities (e.g., a party, a memorial service, or parts of activities such as a conversation that occurs during a party). The latter is consistent with Austin's notion and occurs at the sentence level. In addition, speech style and the components of speaking are introduced as important features. Hymes firmly rooted the components of speaking in a broader perspective than traditional linguistic description. The components include the message form, its content, the setting, the scene (e.g., formal or informal), the speaker, addresser, hearer, addressee, conventionally recognized outcomes, goals, key, channel of communication, genre, and the normative character of the interaction and interpretation. Hymes then introduced a new set of considerations to pragmatics. He provided an organizational framework that describes the social as well as the linguistic aspects of the context.

Of a related nature but more narrow in scope than Hymes' work, we find the work of Emmanuel Schegloff (1971, 1972). Schegloff, a sociologist, described the social rules that structure conversations. One of his best-known contributions characterized general rules that underlie question and answer and summons and answer sequences in conversations. These rules consider both verbal and nonverbal elements of the exchange. He drew attention to something he called the distribution rule. For example, in a phone conversation, the answerer speaks first. The caller provides the topic of conversation. He followed this distribution rule in a wide variety of telephone conversations. Schegloff also identified rules that set expectations for summons-answer sequences, that is, what is involved when one is required to answer. The features of these sequences that bear particular relevance are whether the sequence is nonterminal (i.e., it prefaces additional conversation or activity) and whether the answer has conditional relevance or is expected from such a summons. In addition to studying the temporal ordering of conversational activity, Schegloff (1972) explored the nature of conversational openers and how locative information is formulated within the conversational structure (Schegloff, 1971). Thus, he drew our attention to regular constraints that structure or set a format for the larger unit of communication, conversation. In addition, he integrated nonverbal communication into the structure of his analysis.

A linguist interested in children's development of pragmatic forms, Elaine Andersen (1977, 1978) reflects the thinking and methodology of socially influenced theorists. She studied children's production of indirect requests during different symbolic play episodes. The children assumed roles that had different dominance or social power characteristics (e.g., doctor or nurse and patient, mother or father and child). She observed that the children were able to change to a register associated with each role (Andersen, 1977). For example, little girls would use a deeper pitched voice when they assumed a male role. More interestingly, the directness of the children's requests was influenced by dominance characteristics associated with each role. By contrast, they produced higher proportions of indirect requests when they assumed socially nondominant—and often, female—roles (e.g., the nurse). Thus, a direct interaction could be observed between societal features and pragmatic forms.

Thinkers influenced by social issues incorporated a number of social and societal parameters into their models. This can be seen in the work discussed in this section and can be observed in the child language research of linguists such as Elaine Andersen (1977, 1978) and psycholinguists such as Susan Ervin-Tripp (1977).

## Implications for the Speech and Language Pathologist

The four orientations briefly outlined here have distinct effects on pragmatic analysis. This analysis can examine the speaker's communicative intention, selection of topic, initiation, continuation and change of topic, revision behavior, selection of speaking style, use of turn taking, and the speaker's adherence to truth values and politeness rituals. The pragmatic processes are transactions that may occur on the utterance level. More frequently, they are examined within a conversational exchange. If one thinks about it, these 10 processes can be viewed as primarily philosophical, linguistic, cognitive, or social in motivation or nature. This presents 40 possible effects, a rather unwieldy task to consider at this time.

To efficiently allocate resources, this chapter focuses on three pragmatic processes that appear most frequently in the literature on normal language development and in current models and taxonomies used by clinicians—specifically, communicative intentions, revisions, and topic continuation in discourse. Popular taxonomies are described, and the influence of one or more of the four basic theoretical orientations are identified and examined. The implications or effect of each taxonomy or model and its theoretical bias on clinical language assessment and intervention are discussed. Finally, a model for clinical decision making in the assessment and remediation of the pragmatics of language is presented.

## INFERRING COMMUNICATIVE INTENTIONS

The impact of different assumptions or points of view is felt when the professional must infer the communicative intent of a child's utterance. Take, for example, the utterance, "Can you tell me why you said that?"

Dore's (1979) taxonomy would characterize this utterance as in the requestive conversational class because it solicits information. It is classified as a process question conversational act (RQPC), because it seeks an extended explanation of something. By contrast, Ervin-Tripp's (1977) taxonomy would characterize it as an embedded imperative, because the actor, verb, and object of the desired act are explicit. A cognitively influenced point of view such as that of Bates (1976) would suggest that the utterance is metapragmatic in nature. A more socially influenced system such as Schegloff's (1972) might classify it as a conversational gambit. The different assumptions upon which these systems are based generate obviously different characterizations of the communicative intent. The eclecticism of some thinkers, however, or the simple necessity to find ways of classifying intentions that seem to be substantially different from one another, often result in taxonomies whose different categories represent different points of view.

## Methodological Differences

Taxonomies or classification systems for communicative intentions that reflect more than one theoretical bias seem to be more the rule than the exception. If we look at the systems used most frequently by clinicians, we begin to observe the effect of different assumptions. We will see that we are judging the child's utterances by one metric at one point, and by a very different metric at yet another point in our analysis of one language sample.

***Ervin-Tripp's Levels of Directives.*** Focusing on the category of intentions, Ervin-Tripp (1977) developed a developmentally ordered classification of directives. She chose this type of speech act because it makes up the greatest proportion of children's utterances, is readily identified, and reflects the interpersonal rather than the linguistic aspects of the situational context. Drawing on data from studies of non-English–speaking as well as American-English–speaking children, Ervin-Tripp described five levels of development in children's mapping of directives (see Table 8.1). At the first level, that of telegraphic directives, we see seven such forms: vocatives that specify the child's wants in the situation, rising intonation, statements of desire, mention of desired objects or goal locations, possessive statements, imperatives, and problem statements. The majority of these classifications rely upon judgments about the intended meaning of the utterance as it is mapped by its semantic relations (e.g., possessives and locatives). However, the directive mapped solely by rising intonation relies upon a judgment about suprasegmental form. Thus, six of those directive categories are influenced by semantic linguistic notions, while one category is influenced by attention to a formal structural or linguistic system concept.

Taking another of Ervin-Tripp's (1977) developmental levels, her attention shifts—with the children's burgeoning syntactic skills—to a more linguistically influenced basis for decision. The level of embeddings and

**TABLE 8.1**

**Ervin Tripp's Levels of Development of Directive Forms**

| Forms of Directives | Examples |
|---|---|
| 1. *Telegraphic Directives* (found prior to age 2 years) | |
| Vocatives (situation specific) | |
| Rising intonation | |
| Desire statements | More. I want dolly. |
| Goal objects or locations | More juice. More up. Here, |
| Possessives | That mine. |
| Imperatives | Gimmie. Book read. Apple me. |
| Problem statements | Carol hungry. |
| 2. *Limited Routines* | Where is the shoe?<br>What's that? |
| 3. *Embeddings and Structural Modifications* (interrogatives, inflected forms, modal embeddings, tense contrast, permission forms) | Can you give me one car, please?<br>You could give one to me.<br>Don't forget to smoke your pipe. |
| 4. *Hints Without Explicit Imperatives* | He made sand go in my eyes.<br>Jean, we didn't have a snack. |
| 5. *Elaborate Oblique Strategies* (desired object typically mentioned) | That house is nice inside.<br>We haven't had any candy for a long time. |
| (desired object not mentioned; child may embed several moves) | Six-year-old in supermarket: "Can I have a penny?"<br>Mother (surprised at small request): "Why, yes."<br>At another stop, child deposits penny in gum machine. |

Reprinted with permission from "Wait for Me Roller-Skate" by S. Ervin-Tripp, 1977, in *Child Discourse* (pp. 173-178), edited by S. Ervin-Tripp & E. Mitchell-Kernan, New York: Academic Press.

structural modifications of directives is characterized by the children's use of interrogative forms, model embeddings, tense contrasts, permission forms, and inflected forms. However, when the clinician must decide whether an utterance such as, "Can I have a penny?" is an oblique question directive or an embedded directive, the linguistically influenced metric must be abandoned. The clinician must turn to the semantic or philosophical distinction of the child's underlying motive or intent.

Finally, a number of the elaborate oblique strategy directives of the final developmental level involve negotiations about rules and roles. To classify some directives into this more advanced category requires consideration of social features. Thus, Ervin-Tripp's (1977) categories are based upon some different systems. Sometimes, as in the case of telegraphic directives, the basis for a categorization decision can vary within the category itself.

***Dore's Classification of Conversational Acts.*** Another taxonomy frequently used by clinicians is Dore's (1979) classification of conversational acts. Initially described in 1977 and revised subsequently (Dore, 1978, 1979), Dore's taxonomy is one of the most comprehensive available. He distinguished among three hierarchical levels of communicative intent expressed by children conversationally. These are the levels of primary conversational *function*, general conversational *class*, and particular conversational *act*. At the most general or highest level of the hierarchy, we find three primary conversational functions: the communication of content, the regulation of the conversation, and the expression of attitudes. The communication of content can either be an initiation or a response in the conversation. Initiations include requestive, assertive, and performative conversational classes, while responses include responsive classes. A number of particular conversational acts fall within each conversational class. For the most part, Dore's taxonomy appears to be based upon highly semantic linguistic and philosophical criteria (e.g., "tease, annoy, taunt, or playfully provoke a hearer" and "descriptions predicate events, properties, locations, etc., of objects or people" (Dore, 1979, p. 355). However, within the requestive class, product questions are defined by more linguistic criteria; they seek information, often with the use of *wh-* interrogative pronouns. By contrast, within that same conversational class, action requests attempt to move the hearer to action. The function of the regulative class is to regulate the flow of conversation. Almost all these conversational acts are defined by socially influenced criteria. Speaker selection regulatives indicate the person who will take the next speaking turn. Boundary marker regulatives mark conversational openings, closings, and topic shifts. Thus, Dore, too, was influenced by more than one point of view in developing his taxonomy.

***Garvey's Philosophical Taxonomy.*** Garvey's (1975, 1977) taxonomy was developed to examine children's requests, responses, and contingent questions in their conversations with other children. Of the classification systems, Garvey's is most heavily and consistently influenced by the philosophical point of view and, additionally, by the cognitive point of view. She analyzes requests for action and queries in relationship to the speech act that immediately precedes them in the conversation and in relationship to the obligations, rights, intentions, abilities, and so forth, of the speaker and/or hearer. The latter were based upon Searle's (1969) work. In addition, Garvey also considers what the child understands and interprets as requests and responses, reflecting the effect of some more cognitively oriented considerations. Although she acknowledges that the linguistic operation that most frequently maps contingent queries in conversations is embedding, she does not use the structural form as the basis for decision making in her system. This represents an approach different from Bloom et al. (1976), who define children's contingent utterances in conversation in terms of the linguistic forms in the utterances. Garvey does, however, make use of phrase final intonation, but only in conjunction with other criteria. Thus, her taxonomy is heavily influenced by the philosophical point of view.

***Taxonomies for School-Aged Children.*** The three taxonomies just discussed were designed primarily for preschool children. A somewhat different system can be observed in Tough's (1977) taxonomy for children between $5^1/_2$ and $7^1/_2$ years of age. This taxonomy considers four major functions of language: directive, interpretive, projective, and relational. As Chapman (1981) observed, this system categorizes communicative intentions in terms of the way language behaves in problem solving and thinking. For example, the four strategies identified in imagining, a projective function in Tough's taxonomy, are (a) renaming objects and people in pretend play, (b) commentary on a pretend situation, (c) the development of a scene through language, and (d) language associated with a particular role. Thus, Tough's taxonomy is heavily influenced by the cognitive point of view, one that considers language a tool of cognition. And its influence appears to be consistent throughout the system.

Another taxonomy frequently used with school-aged children is by Wiig and Semel (1984). They focus on the ritualizing, informing, controlling, and feeling functions of communication. Ritualizing includes common forms of greeting, parting, telephone calls, and so forth. The informing function includes describing and asking. Describing is examined in terms of referentiality and adaptation to listener needs, which represent a cognitive influence. By contrast, asking is described with a linguistic bias, focusing on the linguistic interrogative form as opposed to declarative statements that function as questions. Wiig and Semel's controlling function includes directives and politeness forms. Some directives are determined by form (e.g., direct requests take the form of the imperative), while other types are heavily weighted by semantic or cognitive content (e.g., state-of-affairs requests are defined by a mention of the event occurring). Categorization of an utterance as a politeness form is based primarily upon the presence of politeness features. Finally, the feeling function of utterances includes disputing and action disagreement forms. The criteria for determining that a disputing form is being used are socially dominated, with occasional use of linguistic form (e.g., "inversion" of a string) and of semantic or cognitive information (e.g,, the expression of imagined states and self-beliefs). The basis for determining whether an utterance is an action disagreement involves cognitive (e.g., statement of reason and perspective taking) and social criteria.

We see Wiig and Semel (1984) dealing with the same biases reflected in Ervin-Tripp's (1977) taxonomy. Like Ervin-Tripp's taxonomy, the bias for decision making—social, cognitive, or linguistic—changes even within functional categories. (See Table 8.2 for a depiction of this taxonomy.)

Another model for school-aged children was developed by Simon (1984). While she has developed a "functional-pragmatic" evaluation (Simon, 1984, p. 83), it covers more than pragmatic skills. It includes syntactic comprehensive, vocabulary comprehension, and syntactic and morphological description. She applies Halliday's (1973) seven pragmatic functions as an organizational frame for assessing semantic, metalinguistic, cognitive, and philosophical considerations to determine the "functional flexibility" of a child's communication. Eight of the 18 tasks address children's expression of communicative intent (see Table 8.3). Simon's task for assessing the regulatory function requires the child to provide sequential directions. With this task, she evaluates the philosophical aspect of the effect upon the listener and explores verbal sequencing, a more cognitive consideration. The instrumental function tasks, the description of an object that appears in different contexts, emphasizes both philosophical and semantic dimensions. The heuristic function is explored with two productive questioning tasks: a barrier game and a mystery question game. Here the focus is both cognitive and linguistic in evaluating the function of questions to formulate hypotheses as well as to examine question types used. The description and explanation tasks used by Simon to evaluate the informative function relate to cognitive and social role-taking dimensions. The tasks within her evaluation are designed for an array of cognitive and metalinguistic dimensions more peculiar to the older school-aged child.

***Sensorimotor Classification.*** A final taxonomy to consider is by Coggins and Carpenter (1981). It is for very young children, those in the sensorimotor period of development. The eight categories of communicative

**TABLE 8.2**

**Patterns in the Acquisition of the Informing, Controlling, and Feeling Functions of Communication**

| Informing | Controlling | Feeling |
|---|---|---|
| *Describing* | *Directives* | *Disputing* |
| Ability to use referential statements that are specific and adapted to listener needs improves from grades K-9. Ninth graders do not perform up to adult standards. | Controlling by use of directives progresses from<br>1. Direct requests (Give me . . .; Get . . .)<br>2. Indirect requests (Can I have/take . . .), polite requests (Please, can I . . .), indirect negative requests (Can't you . . .)<br>3. State-of-affairs requests (Must you . . .)<br>4. Pretend directives (Pretend you're . . .; Tell me . . .)<br>5. Subtle directives (Just give me . . . and I'll . . .) | Third and fourth graders rely on threats, bribes, insults, and praise in settling disputes. They repeat feelings of self-beliefs, escalate the imaginative component (tear eyes out), or invert the statement pattern (no, I'm not . . .). |
| *Asking* | *Politeness Forms* | *Action Disagreement* |
| Question-asking behaviors proceed from yes/no to *wh-* questions in the order from what, where, why, how, to when. *Wh-* questions are interpreted on the basis of verb meaning by preschoolers. | Judgment of relative degree of politeness of requests increases from ages 3 to 7. Performances at age 7 do not differ from those of adults.<br>Expression of directives, with increasing politeness features, improves from ages 3 to 7. Performances at age 7 do not differ from those of adults.<br>Both judgment and expression of politeness forms relate positively to a perspective-taking for preferences. | 7- to 8-year-olds ask others to stop action if they disagree (Don't erase/rip out . . .).<br>9- to 10-year-olds state their reasons for disagreeing (Don't erase/rip out . . .; I liked the drawing/sweater . . .).<br>11- to 12-year-olds provide reasons that involve the other's perspective (Your husband will like the sweater/ The teacher thought it was great). |

Reprinted with permission from *Language Assessment and Intervention for the Learning Disabled* (p. 507) by E. Wiig & E. Semel, 1984, Columbus, OH: Charles E. Merrill. Drawn from research by Brenneis & Lein (1977), Glucksberg & Kraus (1967), Kraus & Glucksberg (1967), Leonard, Wilcox, Fulmer, & Davis (1978), Mitchell-Kernan & Kernan (1977), Nippold, Leonard, & Anastopoulas (1982), Tyack & Ingram (1977), Wiig (1982), and Wood & Gardner (1980).

intention include request for an object, comment on an object, request for action, comment on an action, acknowledgment, protest, answer, and request for information. These categories have well-defined propositions and are semantic-linguistic and philosophical in their criteria. Moreover, Coggins and Carpenter (1981) report good reliabilities on interrater agreement. Thus, Coggins and Carpenter's taxonomy is consistent in its bias, and that is reflected in the reliability of its application by clinicians.

***Conclusions.*** Each of the taxonomies discussed reflects a different underlying point of view. Some, like that of Ervin-Tripp (1977), Dore (1979), and Wiig and Semel (1984), shift from one set of underlying assumptions to another within the taxonomy itself. Others reflect greater consistency. Two of the three taxonomies for preschool-aged children are influenced by semantic-linguistic and philosophical assumptions as well as structural or formal syntactic-linguistic considerations. Tough's (1977) model, which focuses on the school-aged child, was developed in an educational milieu. Because this milieu has a well-defined purpose, the model has a consistent focus. Similarly, Coggins and Carpenter's (1981) taxonomy, which focuses on the very young child, was developed in a clinical milieu—another milieu with a well-defined purpose—and therefore also has a consistent focus. In addition, the limited repertoire of speech acts of the very young child may limit the need for multiple points of view. A simple system may require a simpler taxonomy.

## Clinical Assumptions

The assumptions upon which the criteria for making taxonomic decisions about a child's expressed communicative intention are based can have a far-reaching effect for the practicing clinician. They can influence the clinical impression of the child's underlying strengths and weaknesses. They can also help determine the content and the form that the child's intervention program will take.

***Assessment.*** Most of the taxonomies for assessing communicative intent apply to normal child language development. Coggins and Carpenter's (1981) taxonomy was developed for both language normal and language delayed children. None of the taxonomies have been normed developmentally or scaled for order of emergence or, apart from Coggins and Carpenter's (1981), for frequency of use. Although Chapman (1981) describes some general developmental guidelines for the emergence of speech acts, the practicing clinician is never quite sure where the expression of a particular pragmatic intent really lies on the developmental continuum. Nor does he or she know whether the failure of a particular intent to emerge is an

**TABLE 8.3**

## Simon's Application of Halliday's Communicative Functions

I. Regulatory (Do as I tell you.): Control the behavior of others.

| *Task 11* | *Purpose* |
|---|---|
| Provide sequential directions for the use of a telephone at home | Assess quality of the regulatory function of language when it is used to relate directions or game instructions so that the listener is able to perform the task |

II. Instrumental (I want.): Satisfy material needs.

| *Task 13* | *Purpose* |
|---|---|
| Description of an object depending on the context in which it appears | Assess the student's situational skills; an instrumental function task to see if a student can get the exact object desired |

III. Interactional (me and you): Get along with others.

(No particular task designated for purpose of exploring interactional function)

IV. Personal (Here I come.): Express self-identity.

| *Task 18* | *Purpose* |
|---|---|
| Expressing an opinion and a justification for the opinion | Assess the use of the personal function of language to assert one's individuality verbally |

V. Heuristic (Tell me why.): Learn and explore reality.

| *Task 15* | *Purpose* |
|---|---|
| Barrier game—listener role | Assess ability to use the heuristic function to ask clarification questions |
| *Task 16* | *Purpose* |
| Using questions to systematically gather identifying characteristics about a mystery item. | Assess ability to use productive questioning to form an hypothesis |

VI. Imaginative (Let's pretend.): Create reality.

| *Task 17* | *Purpose* |
|---|---|
| Formulating a creative story | Assess the imaginative function of language and the ability to coherently structure a story that has a beginning, several events, and a conclusion |

**TABLE 8.3.** Continued

| | |
|---|---|
| VII. Informative: Communicate content. | |
| *Task 12* | *Purpose* |
| Description | Assess ability to feature some and subordinate other details; an informative function |
| *Task 14* | *Purpose* |
| Explanation of why two objects belong together (role-playing with kindergarten children) | Assess the student's ability to take the role of a teacher and use the informative language function |

Adapted from the 18 tasks to assess "functional flexibility" included within C. Simon's (1984) "Functional Pragmatic Evaluation of Communication Skills in School-Aged Children" in *Language, Speech and Hearing Services in the School*, *15*, 89-91.

important or critical consideration. Further, apart from Coggins and Carpenter's (1981) effort, extensive studies have not been conducted on the reliability and validity of the taxonomies.

In addition, Chapman (1981) points out that it is important to know at which level you are analyzing—at the level of the utterance or at the level of discourse. Tough (1977), for example, analyzes intention in relationship to the discourse in which it is embedded. Chapman (1981) suggests that it is important to know the child's level of cognitive development. Such information would be helpful in determining the child's meaning for a particular intention.

It is important to know when a taxonomy decision is based upon semantic, syntactic, social, or cognitive criteria. This will let you know whether the child's success or failure is being influenced by his or her linguistic, social, or cognitive skills or by delays in development. It is not unusual to observe a child who fails to produce communicative intentions that require more advanced syntactic formulation skills but who can produce intents that require social formulaic forms. The taxonomies discussed here offer the practicing clinician a variety of choices. However, we suggest that they be used wisely and judiciously.

***Intervention.*** Once the child's production of communicative intentions has been assessed, the determination of whether he or she has difficulty with those intents (characterized by linguistic, cognitive, or social criteria) has a direct effect on the child's intervention program. If the child's deficits appear to be related more to linguistic form, it is likely that intervention can focus on the development of syntactic structures, particularly those most frequently used to express a targeted intention. If the child's deficits appear to reflect a delay in a specific cognitive development (e.g., symbolic play), intervention would likely focus on the child's achievement of the nonverbal cognitive milestone as well as the form that maps it. If the child's deficits appear to be related to a failure to perceive social roles and relations, intervention might focus on creating contexts that highlight and mark the targeted social role or relation.

The determination of the underlying deficit inferred from the criteria used can also affect the remediation. By definition, some taxonomies (e.g., Garvey, 1975, 1977) are concerned with the child's expressed intent relative to prior utterances. Consequently, intervention will need to take place at the level of discourse. By contrast, other taxonomies form their categorization judgment only at the level of the utterance. In such cases, intervention can proceed at the utterance level.

# JUDGING REVISIONS

Another pragmatic skill is the ability to revise or repair an utterance when the listener indicates that he or she does not understand. Since the pragmatic purpose of speaking is to achieve an intended goal, it is in the speaker's best interests to ensure that messages are understood. The ability to revise one's utterances includes (a) the perception that the listener seeks some clearer statement of intention and (b) strategies that can be mobilized to "fix up" the message. Normal and language delayed children seem to acquire these skills. A description of the language delayed or disordered child's revision strategies offers the clinician additional insight into the child's pragmatic development.

## Methodological Differences

A few researchers have examined children's revision strategies. Tanya Gallagher (1977) examined how normal children at Brown's (1973) Stages I, II, and III revise their utterances in response to listener feedback. Her system for analyzing the children's revisions categorized their responses into repetition, revision, and no-response categories. Within the revision category, Gallagher classified four strategies: phonetic change, constituent elaboration, constituent reduction, and constituent substitution. Phonetic change was characterized by any change made in the phonetic shape of the child's utterance. Constituent elaboration was marked by the presence of an additional morpheme that did not appear in the original utterance. Constituent reduction was characterized by the deletion of a morpheme from the original utterance. Constituent substitution occurred when the child replaced words in the original utterance while preserving the major syntactic and semantic characteristics of the original utterances. In addition, Gallagher analyzed the parts of speech and syntactic constituents that were revised.

Gallagher's (1977) taxonomy of revision strategies is based on concern for linguistic form or structure. Thus, a child's failure to engage or develop these strategies reflects difficulty in manipulating syntactic structures.

In contrast to this more structurally biased taxonomy of Gallagher (1977), we find the work of Keenan and Schieffelin (1976). They talked of revisions as repair responses in a social interactive framework. They distinguished between self-initiated and other-initiated repairs. Self-initiated repairs are those the speaker immediately proceeds to repair, often within the same turn in conversation. Other-initiated repairs are performed because the conversational partner indicates some misunderstanding or mishearing of the speaker's utterance. Such repairs may take several turns in the conversation. Other-initiated repairs may be performed by the speaker or, in some cases, his or her conversational partner. According to Keenan and Schieffelin's (1976) model, repairs or revisions occur when one of the following steps has not been satisfied by a speaker.

1. The speaker gains the hearer's attention.
2. The speaker speaks with sufficient intelligibility and loudness for the listener to hear the utterance.
3. The speaker identifies the conversational referents in the discourse topic.
4. The speaker maps the semantic relations of the referents contained in the discourse topic.

Keenan and Schieffelin (1976) observed that children, at an age similar to that studied by Gallagher, often make repairs (in utterances that fail the second condition) by increasing their speaking volume and by trying to articulate the lexical items more clearly. When repairs are needed because the conversational referent has not been sufficiently identified for the listener, young children can meet the listener's needs by pointing to or locating the referents if they are present in the physical context. Keenan and Schieffelin suggest that children will probably not revise by referring to referents not perceptually present nor by repairing their syntactic formulation of semantic relations until their language development is somewhat more advanced. Keenan and Schieffelin's view of revisions appears to reflect a strong social point of view as well as the semantic-linguistic notion of topic.

Schegloff, Jefferson, and Sacks (1977) take an approach to conversational revisions of repairs somewhat like Keenan and Schieffelin's (1976). Schegloff et al., too, distinguish between self- and other-initiated repairs. They differ from Keenan and Schieffelin in that their system for repairs is organized around some hierarchy of preferences (Levinson, 1983). They propose that revisions or repairs are organized with two components. The first component involves a sequence of opportunities when the repair may be made; the second component is a rank-ordered set of preferences of those opportunities.

The sequence of repair opportunities proposed by Schegloff et al. (1977) contains a number of slots systematically spaced across at least three turns in a conversation. The first turn contains the item that needs revision and presents itself as the first opportunity for self-initiated self-repair. They proposed that a transition space occurs between the first and second turn. This is the second chance for the speaker to perform a self-initiated revision. The second turn, taken by the conversational partner, is the third opportunity for revision. This turn, however, provides the chance for the conversational partner to revise (i.e., an other-initiated repair) or to prompt the first speaker to repair (i.e., other-initiated self-repair). The third turn in the conversation provides a fourth chance for revision after the other partner's prompt, an other-initiated self-repair.

Schegloff et al.'s (1977) analyses suggest that speakers have preferences among these opportunities. Their first preference is to revise (perform a self-initiated self-repair during the first opportunity) in their own turn. Their next preference is to revise during the transition space. Their third preference is to have the conversational partner prompt the first speaker to repair during the next turn. The last preference is for the conversational partner to revise the utterance during the third opportunity. This system is highly social. Unlike Keenan and Schieffelin's (1976) approach, it does not attend to semantic linguistic aspects such as the topic of conversation. Nor is it similar to Gallagher's (1977) attention to the linguistic form of the revision.

A somewhat different approach is provided by Meline (1978), who focused upon different aspects of revision. Looking at more advanced children whose average MLUs were 5.0, Meline observed children use two revision strategies in response to a screened listener asking the child to tell him more. He considered one a "naming" strategy in which the child tried to suggest one object or thing to which the target object was similar. The other strategy was an "attribute" strategy in which the child described a physical feature of the target object in greater detail. Meline's categories seem to be predominantly cognitive, revealing more of what the child knows about the world. Consequently, any attempt to characterize a child's revisions with his approach would speak to the strengths and weaknesses of the child's world schemes.

Hoar (1977) looked at normal and language-impaired children's ability to paraphrase sentences. She viewed paraphrases as an important communicative tool. She analyzed the paraphrases of her school-aged subjects and separated them into four categories: lexical paraphrase, syntactic paraphrase, combination lexical-syntactic paraphrase, and nonparaphrase. Lexical paraphrase is characterized by the substitution of words into the same syntactic structure. Syntactic paraphrase involves the rearrangement of the sentence structure. The combination lexical-syntactic paraphrase is characterized by both the substitution of different words and reformulation of the syntactic structure. The nonparaphrase category represents a repetition of the original sentence. Hoar seemed to have some specifically linguistic biases about the nature of paraphrase. Unlike Meline (1978), who characterized revisions in terms of the types of information the child provided, Hoar attended to the linguistic form and units the children mobilized in their efforts.

## Clinical Implications

*Assessment.* The revisions or repairs that children make in conversations can be analyzed from a number of different approaches. Each approach reflects different underlying assumptions. Based upon the methodology employed to describe a child's success and failure at revisions or the strategies mobilized to make repairs, the clinician may be assessing the child's syntactic or semantic linguistic skills, his or her knowledge of the social system, or some specific items of cognitive development.

In addition, a child may be less successful with Gallagher's (1977) approach because he or she is unable to syntactically revise an utterance. This same child, however, may be successful if one applies Meline's (1978) criteria for supplying specific types of additional information, regardless of syntactic form. Or the child may be less successful with Schegloff et al.'s (1977) approach because the child does not initiate self-revision but is prompted by his or her conversational partner. Thus, the clinician's impression of the adequacy of the child's revision skills can be affected by the methodological approach.

*Intervention.* If a clinician's impression of a child's communicative adequacy can be influenced by the choice of methodological approach employed, intervention will be influenced more strongly. If the clinician uses Gallagher's (1977) or Hoar's (1977) approach to characterize the child's revision strategies, intervention may focus on the development of syntactic forms that can be mobilized in the revision process. By contrast, in Keenan and Schieffelin's (1976) approach, intervention may stress the development of topic marking in discourse and the mapping of semantic relations. If Schegloff et al.'s (1977) approach is employed, intervention may focus on the timing of the child's revision attempts and increased self-monitoring of utterances. Or if Meline's (1978) criteria are used, intervention may emphasize the provision of attribute information for the topic of concern. Thus, each analysis will identify different goals and content for intervention. All can be traced back to the different points of view in each analytic method.

## INFERRING DISCOURSE SUCCESS: TOPIC CONTINUATION

The child who has just learned to talk does not seem to be much of a conversationalist. As a beginner in this communicative art, the child's conversation might sound something like this:

> Adult: Who's watching Daddy?
>
> Carol: Shaving (Ervin-Tripp, 1970, p. 85)

This exchange does not meet our speech community's criteria for a well-formed conversation, and it makes the child a dubious conversational partner. Yet, within a few years, by the time the child enters school, he or she has developed into a communicative partner who can participate in, orchestrate, and develop a conversation over successive turns. This developing pragmatic skill is of interest to the practicing clinician (Rees, 1978).

Research in child language acquisition has examined some of the skills mobilized in the maintenance and development of conversations. Of particular interest is the child's ability to contribute or add a piece of information to the topic of conversation. A conversational topic is the idea or concept about which the communicative partners are exchanging information. Each partner may request or provide new information about the topic.

### Methodological Approaches.

In a very early study of conversational exchanges in child-child discourse, Mueller (1972) looked at an eclectic array of dimensions in the child's communication. These included the following:

1. Clarity of the spoken message.
2. Completion of the grammatical forms.

3. Adaptation to the perspective of the listener.
4. Attentional devices.
5. Content relevant to the listener's or speaker's activities or interests.
6. Grammatical form of the utterance.
7. Utterance as a reply to a query or summons.
8. Speaker securing listener's attention.
9. Listener visually monitoring the speaker.
10. Physical distance between the partners.

Although these categories appear eclectic, socially influenced categories predominate. There are two distinctly cognitive categories: adaptation to the listener's perspective and partner-relevant content. While these are introduced here, they are not specified, nor does Mueller offer well-developed criteria for judging them.

***Analysis of Contingent Queries.*** Another taxonomy, also designed for analyzing child-child discourse, is Garvey's (1977, 1979) approach to analyzing contingent queries. Part of her 1979 taxonomy was discussed earlier with reference to aspects of communicative intent. Her 1979 paper expanded her analysis, describing how discourse cohesion is achieved in children's contingent queries. Garvey (1979) considers a contingent query sequence to be a two-party component containing a query and its response. It can occur anywhere within discourse: It may follow any type of discourse content, function, or formula. The cohesion of this two-party component is determined by the relationship among the occasional message, the utterance that precedes the query, and the query itself and between the query and its response.

Garvey (1979) specified the following types of queries:

1. Nonspecific requests for repetition.
2. Specific requests for repetition.
3. Specific requests for confirmation.
4. Specific requests for specification.
5. Potential requests for confirmation.
6. Potential requests for elaboration.

While these all appear to be influenced by the philosophical point of view, Garvey's expanded work (1979) describes a number of the linguistic devices that map these query types. For example, both the specific request for confirmation and the specific request for specification select a noun phrase component from the preceding occasion message and use specified intonation patterns. Thus, Garvey places the structural syntactic-linguistic component at the service of the philosophical functional component as children construct contingent query sequences. The coding decision is made first on the basis of the philosophical point of view.

***Identification of Discourse Topic.*** Keenan and Schieffelin (1976) take a different approach in their language acquisition research on child-child and child-adult discourse. Their basic premise is that conversational partners must direct their utterances to a specific proposition or idea in order to construct discourse. They point out that discourse may evolve or grow through collaboration on a common discourse topic or integration with a shared discourse topic. In collaboration, the partners produce utterances that develop or continue a common idea or shared topic. In integration, a series of somewhat different discourse topics may be integrated or linked. This sequencing or integration occurs when a shared claim or assumption upon which the preceding discourse was based is used as the new topic for discourse. Thus, Keenan and Schieffelin (1976) suggest that discourse is continued or maintained through topic collaboration and topic incorporation.

One problem for children learning to construct discourse sequences, then, is how to determine the discourse topic. They suggest that children do this by picking up clues from both the verbal and nonverbal contexts. They feel that successful collaboration on a discourse topic requires sufficiently intelligible utterances, a strongly established discourse topic, and the partner's attention. Keenan and Schieffelin (1976) claim that much of young children's difficulty in collaborating on discourse is related to difficulty in these three areas. A subsequent study of child-child discourse (Keenan, 1974, 1977) indicated that preschool-aged children often used the repetition of a whole or a part of a partner's utterance as a vehicle for collaborative discourse. Thus, they took their conversational turn repeating the prior utterance using intonation and vocal quality contrasts or substituting some words in the utterance (Keenan, 1974). In doing so, they can continue the discourse. Keenan (1977) observed that partial and whole repetitions are used to answer questions, comment, affirm, self-inform, query, imitate, make counter-claims, return a greeting, reverse orders and information questions, and request clarification. These repetitions serve to continue discourse because they usually contain the established topic. Keenan (1974) also observed that young children use sound play as a means of producing collaborative talk.

Keenan (1974, 1977) and Keenan and Schieffelin's (1976) work stresses the notion of identifying topic in terms of its proposition, a semantic linguistic notion. They do use, however, some cognitive considerations such as nonverbal reference (e.g., pointing to or touching objects) and linguistic formal considerations in characterizing the child's strategies for cooperative discourse.

***Other Approaches.*** Other methodological approaches are found in the child language acquisition research on child-adult discourses. In an early attempt, Bloom et al. (1976) studied the contingent utterances of children between 21 and 36 months of age. Contingent utterances are those containing the same topic or added information to the topic identified in the preceding utterance. Bloom et al. examined the following categories of contingent discourse: social routines or formulas, yes/no responses, recoding of whole or partial repetitions, self-expansions and self-recodings, expansions that add topic information, alternatives that add information by addressing an aspect of the topic, and explanations that add topic information and introduce a related topic. Within these categories, they describe a variety of linguistic devices the children mobilized (e.g., the children could mobilize pronominal shifts in recoding). Although consideration is given to what the child knows and the information processing capacity available to him or her, Bloom et al. focused their efforts, and the whole of their taxonomy, on linguistic contingency. Thus, their coding system reflects a concern with the linguistic aspects of the child's developing system.

A somewhat different approach to child-adult discourse has been taken by Corsaro (1979). He examined discourse using 13 categories that deal with the discourse functions of initiation, topic continuation, sequencing of turns, monitoring, topic change, and discourse termination. Those categories that deal with topic continuation in Corsaro's taxonomy are topic-relevant acts and topic-relevant responses. Topic-relevant acts are turns related to the topic under discussion. If they follow other topic-relevant acts, they must elaborate or add information to the prior act. Topic-relevant responses are turns that constitute the partner's response to his or her speaker's topic-relevant act. These responses do not elaborate or add information beyond that specified in the preceding topic-relevant act. If the response does, it is double-coded a topic-relevant act and secondarily a topic-relevant response.

Corsaro (1979) coded both the children's and adults' utterances with these categories. Because adults produced the most topic-relevant acts and children produced the topic-relevant responses in his study, Corsaro chose to report the adult strategies for facilitating topic-relevant acts. Although he claims that his taxonomy is sociolinguistic in nature, his notion of topic is more semantic in nature.

***Conclusion.*** There are many ways to describe how conversational partners cooperate in the development of discourse. We have looked at some of the best known approaches in the study of language development. The orientations mobilized in these approaches are varied, and they carry different implications in clinical practice.

## Theoretical Implications

*Assessment.* The clinician who wishes to describe the child's ability to continue the topic of conversation may choose any of the methodologies described. Much like the point of our earlier discussions of assessing children's communicative intentions and revision strategies, diagnostic impressions by the clinician will be colored by the assumptions that underlie the taxonomy of choice. Thus, if Mueller's (1972) system is used, a child might be deficient both in considering the listener's perspective and in attending to nonverbal cues in the interaction. The deficits represent delays in cognitive and social skills. This is quite different from the child who, even with repetition, cannot mark a topic linguistically to continue it in conversation, as one might determine from the Keenan and Schieffelin (1976) approach. Further, if the child does not seem to be able to identify the topic, a critical consideration for both Corsaro's (1979) and Keenan and Schieffelin's (1976) approaches, the clinician is left to puzzle out the cues the child is missing. Keenan and Schieffelin's (1976) work offers a vehicle for further analyses and determination of the topic-marking devices provided by the speaker. These cues involve linguistic, paralinguistic, and nonverbal means available to speakers. The clinician has to determine the cues to which the child fails to respond.

If the clinician chooses to focus on the child's participation in contingent query sequences, the most frequently used taxonomies will again offer different characterizations of the child's performance. Bloom et al.'s (1976) approach will tend to highlight the structural linguistic aspect of the child's deficits. In a somewhat different vein, Garvey's (1979) approach will offer a coordinated assessment of linguistic and philosophical or functional abilities. The inferences drawn from these different taxonomies will differ in some obvious ways. The different underlying assumptions will influence one's clinical impression of the child.

*Intervention.* Just as differences among the underlying assumptions affect the clinician's assessment of the child, they also affect the content and form of the child's intervention program. If the clinician were to focus intervention on one of Mueller's (1972) cognitive categories, adaptation to the listener's perspective, the content of the child's intervention program might include a series of nonverbal as well as verbal interaction problems in perspective taking. Some nonverbal problems might include Piagetian perspective tasks (e.g., the view a person has of three miniature mountains or a horizontally sequenced group of different sized objects from different visual perspectives). Verbal interaction problems might include a series of screened listener situations in which the child must describe a puzzle or block to a listener sitting behind a screen who must construct a similar array. To be successful, the child must give the listener sufficient information and be sensitive to listener cues for information needed.

The content and form of intervention activities described are different from those that address the child's mobilization of linguistic forms (e.g., if one were to be concerned with linguistic strategies that map topics during successive turns). On the one hand, the clinician could simply decide to work on the development of linguistic forms on the utterance level and expect their mobilization in discourse. On the other hand, the clinician could decide to use discourse and nonverbal context to establish the conditions and cues for their use. The former intervention method is implicated most frequently in linguistically based approaches, while the latter is more frequently implicated in eclectic approaches such as those of Keenan and Schieffelin (1976) and Garvey (1979).

Thus, the character of intervention programs is affected by assumptions upon which taxonomic categories are based. Because discourse categories described here represent more than one point of view, caution must be exercised in designing the content of intervention programs. It is important to know when the child's deficits suggest that cognitive as well as linguistic activities are necessary and to know that those are the domains of interest.

## THE CURRENT DILEMMA: BAKING THE BETTER CAKE

The clinician engaged in assessment and intervention programming for pragmatic abilities in children is similar to the person who wants to bake a chocolate cake. Each will consult books for guidance. Just as the baker will find many recipes, the clinician will find a number of taxonomies of pragmatic structures, each somewhat different. Like a person choosing a recipe, a clinician can choose a taxonomy for various reasons. The taxonomy, or recipe, may be chosen because it appears quicker or easier than the others while getting the same results. Time and effort are important. Or it may be chosen because, although it may take more time and extra care than others, it promises a far superior result. Or it may be chosen because it calls for the ingredients or resources that are available. Indeed, monetary resources are a realistic consideration. Or it may be chosen because the clinician prefers or agrees with the approach. More important, it may be chosen because it is the most appropriate taxonomy for the child's needs. This last consideration is the most critical and prevalent factor in such choices. Prutting and Kirchner's (1983) taxonomy identifies the dimensions this consideration addresses and offers a clear way to progress within and across dimensions. Unfortunately, most taxonomies do not come with guidelines that identify the needs that each addresses best. The question is how the clinician decides on a taxonomy.

## Multiple Dimensions in the Context

The literature on the nature of the communication process has firmly established that it is a multidimensional phenomenon composed of social, linguistic, cognitive, and functional dimensions (Bates, 1976; Prutting & Kirchner, 1983). These dimensions are thought to interact in many ways. We do not have comprehensive information about how some dimensions take precedence over others to determine the precise choice of linguistic form that individuals make. The islands of knowledge from research indicate that no one facet or dimension has an overriding influence in all contexts. Rather, the features of some situations demand that greater emphasis be placed upon meeting the requirements of the social dimension of the interaction regardless of the linguistic form used or available for use. For example, answering the telephone demands that the individual conduct certain minimal social requirements of greeting, inquiry, and response regardless of whether a formal "Jones' residence, Arthur speaking" salutation or an ordinary "Hello" is used. Likewise, the social dimension of the situation will influence the linguistic code accessed for the message. The more formal code of greeting someone in the boardroom differs dramatically from the informal code of greeting someone on the beach or at a supermarket. By contrast, the linguistic dimension of revisions seems to overshadow the social demand by the communicative partner. Once the speaker has decided to meet his or her partner's request, the nature of the communicative choice rests on the linguistic dimensions.

It may be helpful to visualize the way these dimensions operate contextually by referring to Tversky's (1977) ideas of feature weighting. Tversky, a cognitive scientist, developed the notion that the semantic features of words or concepts may not carry equal weights in influencing an individual's interpretation of the word or concept in every situation. Rather, depending upon the situational context, one feature may be more heavily weighted than another. For example, think about the word *refrigerator*. In the context of unpacking supermarket bags filled with ice cream and other dairy products, the *functional* feature of an appliance that keeps food cold is dominant in our interpretation of the word. On the other hand, if one thinks of that same word in the context of moving one's household goods into a new home, the *perceptual* feature of size figures more heavily in our interpretation of the word.

Feature weighting can also be applied to our consideration of contextual dimensions. While all dimensions are present when the communicator begins to make pragmatic choices, some dimensions may be weighted more heavily—depending upon the context—and, therefore, may exert a greater influence on the communicative choice made. Thus, in the turn-taking situation, the linguistic dimension appears to have a more dominant influence on the communicative choices made. By contrast, the social dimension of the formality of the situation will usually dictate the linguistic code.

This suggests that clinicians should attend to the dimensions that play dominant roles in particular types of communicative interactions. The taxonomy that addresses those dimensions will be the one best suited to describe and assess the client's pragmatic performance in that area. In a sense, the taxonomy that lists or describes the necessary ingredients for your pragmatic cake is the one to be used. Baking a cake, however, is more than a list of ingredients. It is also important that the ingredients be available. Thus, it is important to know the details of the necessary ingredients or the necessary component steps or parts of the pragmatic responses as well as the child's level of skills within the dimensions of interest. One has to look within the child's own system of strengths and weaknesses.

## Individual and Dimensional Levels

The cognitive, social, functional, and linguistic dimensions are present in every communicative situation. The child has skills in these dimensions, although these skills may not seem to be at uniform levels of development. The child may be more advanced in one dimension than in another. Some children may be more advanced socially than linguistically. These children often experience greater communicative success in situations that rely less on the linguistic form of the message.

If the clinician perceives dimensions that represent the child's weaknesses, the taxonomy or approach that emphasizes the component forms or strategies within those dimensions may be the most appropriate choice. If the child has advanced social development, a taxonomy that emphasizes the social dimension is not likely to tell the clinician what the child cannot do. On the other hand, that taxonomy can be used to structure tasks to give the child optimal chances for success. Thus, the clinician's choice of taxonomy or approach should be related to the child's dimensional strengths and weaknesses. What happens when one dimension exerts an overriding influence in the child's weak dimension? Is the child doomed to communicative failure at that point?

## Interaction and Exploitation

Some youngsters, despite obvious linguistic limitations, are skilled communicators. They perform well pragmatically. As Johnston (1982) has ventured, they exploit their communicative resources. By contrast, other youngsters with far greater linguistic skills seem to misfire pragmatically at every conversational turn. What accounts for such differences?

A viable explanation for variability in pragmatic performance is provided by taking into account that (a) the dominant dimension in any one situation interacts with the child's level of skill development in that dimension, and (b) the child can exploit dimensional skills to meet the task demands.

***Dimensional Dominance and Skill Interaction.*** One dimension may be dominant in a situational context, although the others remain present and necessary. The dominant dimension plays a major part in how the situation is handled successfully. If the linguistic dimension (i.e., the linguistic form of the utterance) is crucial to the successful indirect directive, the speaker is required to produce the necessary linguistic form. Or if the cognitive dimension (e.g., the cognitive skill of being able to take on another person's perspective) is crucial to the successful message, the speaker must be at that level of cognitive development.

Children are often in possession of dimensional skills at varying stages of development. There seem to be occasions when their level of development is not sufficient to meet the demands of the situation. When this happens, they misfire or are unsuccessful at pragmatic goals. For example, if the child cannot formulate an interrogative form, it may be difficult for him or her to produce a polite request. Consequently, the child may formulate an imperative, elicit a negative response from the listener, and fail to achieve his or her pragmatic goal of obtaining a desired object. Or if the child cannot take on the listener's perspective, it may be difficult for the child to give the listener enough information to understand the child's problem or to share the funny story or experience. As a result, the child will not be able to elicit the desired empathy or response from the listener. However, some children do succeed even when they lack the dimensional resources required by the situation.

***Skill Exploitation.*** The situational context of every communicative event has many dimensions. One dimension may play a more dominant role in the event. When children lack the developmental skills necessary in the dominant dimension, they may not succeed pragmatically. When children lack the requisite skills, though, they still may be able to accomplish their pragmatic goals. As Chapman (1981) has pointed out, even a child capable of producing one word at a time can produce a polite request. "Please," with rising intonation, can meet the pragmatic demand for a polite request despite the fact that the child cannot meet the linguistic dimensional requirement of producing an interrogative sentence, preferably one containing modals. Or a child who cannot take on the listener's perspective can be pragmatically successful when he or she allows the listener to ask a series of information-gathering questions to which the child responds. Thus, children can exploit their existing dimensional skills to be successful communicators.

Whether or not they are successful, then, also depends upon whether they know how to or when to exploit their existing skills. If the baker's recipe for chocolate cake calls for a cup of sugar and the baker does not have enough, he can bake the cake if he has honey and knows how much honey to use in place of the amount of sugar listed in his recipe.

***Clinical Implications.*** In observing a child's pragmatic performance, it is important to view variability or inconsistency in performance in terms of the considerations discussed in this section. The dominant dimension should be identified, the child's dimensional levels should be ascertained, and an effort should be made to determine what is occurring in dimensional interaction and skill exploitation.

## Master Clinician

The master baker creates a masterpiece based on an understanding of what ingredients are necessary as well as the intricate proportions required for the best results. Using this knowledge, the baker can vary the products based upon the needs or desires of the patrons. The creative process of the master clinician evolves from a similar understanding. In planning pragmatic assessment and treatment, she combines her understanding of the child's cognitive, functional, linguistic, and social development with her knowledge of the dominant dimensions in the context and of the underlying assumptions of the taxonomies she uses. From this basis, she creates assessment and treatment methods that include the appropriate amount of focus in the cognitive, functional, linguistic, and social areas in the child's program. Just as each master baker expects his colleagues' recipes to work because he can identify the assumptions or principles on which they are based and knows how ingredients interact, we expect that the clinician who uses the methods and theories discussed in this chapter will experience a positive outcome in assessment and intervention.

## REFERENCES

Andersen, E. (1977). Young children's knowledge of role-related speech differences: A mommy is not a daddy is not a baby. *Papers and Reports in Child Language Development, 13,* 91–98.

Andersen, E. (1978). Will you don't snore please? Directives in young children's role play speech. *Papers and Reports in Child Language Development, 15,* 140–160.

Austin, J. R. (1962). *How to do things with words.* Cambridge: Oxford University Press.

Austin, J. L. (1970). *J. L. Austin's philosophical papers.* In J. O. Urmson & G. T. Wainock (Eds.). London: Oxford University Press.

Bates, E. (1976). *Language and context: The acquisition of pragmatics.* New York: Academic Press.

Bates, E., Benigni, L., Bretherton, I., Camaioni, L., & Volterra, V. (1979). *The emergence of symbols: Cognition and communication in infancy.* New York: Academic Press.

Bloom, L. (1973). *One word at a time: The use of single word utterances before syntax.* The Hague: Mouton.

Bloom, L., & Lahey, M. (1978). *Language development and language disorders.* New York: John Wiley.

Bloom, L., Lightbown, P., & Hood, L. (1975). Structure and variation in child language. *Society for Research in Child Development Monographs.* Chicago: University of Chicago Press.

Bloom, L., Rocissano, L., & Hood, L. (1976). Adult-child discourse: Developmental interaction between information processing and linguistic knowledge. *Cognitive Psychology, 8,* 521–552.

Brenneis, D., & Lein, L. (1977). *You fruithead!: A sociolinguistic approach to children's dispute settlement.* In S. Ervin-Tripp & C. Mitchell-Kernan (Eds.), *Child discourse.* New York: Academic Press.

Brown, R. (1973). *A first language: The early stages.* Cambridge, MA: Harvard University Press.

Chapman, R. (1981). Exploring children's communicative intents. In J. Miller (Ed.), *Assessing language production in children* (pp. 111–136). Austin, TX: PRO-ED.

Coggins, T., & Carpenter, R. (1981). The communicative intention inventory: A system for observing and coding children's early intentional communication. *Applied Psycholinguistics, 2,* 235–252. New York: Academic Press.

Corsaro, W. (1979). Sociolinguistic patterns in adult-child interaction. In E. Ochs & B. Schieffelin (Eds.), *Developmental pragmatics.* New York: Academic Press.

Dore, J. (1973). *The development of speech acts.* Doctoral dissertation, City University of New York.

Dore, J. (1975). Holophrases, speech acts and language universals. *Journal of Child Language, 2,* 21–40.

Dore, J. (1977). 'Oh them sheriff': A pragmatic analysis of children's responses to questions. In S. Ervin-Tripp & G. Mitchell-Kernan (Eds.), *Child discourse* (pp. 139–164). New York: Academic Press.

Dore, J. (1978). Variation in preschool children's conversational performances. In K. Nelson (Ed.), *Children's language* (Vol. 1). New York: Gardner Press.

Dore, J. (1979). Conversation and preschool language development. In P. Fletcher & M. Garman (Eds.), *Language acquisition* (pp. 337–361). New York: Cambridge University Press.

Ervin-Tripp, S. (1970). Discourse agreement: How children answer questions. In J. R. Hayes (Ed.), *Cognition and the development of language* (pp. 79–108). New York: John Wiley.

Ervin-Tripp, S. (1977). Wait for me roller-skate. In S. Ervin-Tripp & E. Mitchell-Kernan (Eds.), *Child discourse* (pp. 165–188) New York: Academic Press.

Gallagher, T. (1977). Revision behaviors in the speech of normal children developing language. *Journal of Speech and Hearing Research, 20,* 303–318.

Garvey, C. (1975). Requests and responses in children's speech. *Journal of Child Language, 2,* 41–63.

Garvey, C. (1977). The contingent query. In M. Lewis & L. Rosenblum (Eds.), *Interaction, conversation, and the development of language* (pp. 63–94). New York: John Wiley.

Garvey, C. (1979). Contingent queries and their relations in discourse. In E. Ochs & B. Schieffelin (Eds.), *Developmental pragmatics*. New York: Academic Press.

Glucksberg, S., & Kraus, R. M. (1967). What do people say after they have learned to talk? Studies of the development of referential communication. *Merrill-Palmer Quarterly, 13,* 309–316.

Grice, H. P. (1975). Logic and conversation. In P. Cole & J. L. Morgan (Eds.), *Syntax and semantics: Vol. 3. Speech acts*. New York: Academic Press.

Halliday, M. A. K. (1973). *Explorations in the functions of language*. London: Edward Arnold.

Halliday, M. A. K. (1975). *Learning how to mean: Explorations in the development of language*. London: Edward Arnold.

Hoar, N. (1977, October). *Paraphrase capabilities of language impaired children*. Paper presented at second annual Boston University Conference on Language Development.

Hymes, D. (1971). Competence and performance in linguistic theory. In R. Huxley & E. Ingram (Eds.), *Language acquisition: Models and methods*. New York: Academic Press.

Hymes, D. (1972). Models of the intention of language and social life. In J. J. Gumperz & D. Hymes (Eds.), *Direction in sociolinguistics: The ethnography of communications* (pp. 35–71). New York: Holt, Rinehart and Winston.

Johnston, J. (1982). *Some future directions in research in child language disorders*. Paper presented at the Symposium for Research on Child Language Disorders, University of Wisconsin, Madison.

Keenan, E. (1974). Conversational competence in children. *Journal of Child Language, 1,* 163–183.

Keenan, E. (1977). Making it last: Repetition in child discourse. In E. Ervin-Tripp & C. Mitchell-Kernan (Eds.), *Child discourse* (pp. 125–138). New York: Academic Press.

Keenan, E., & Schieffelin, B. (1976). Topic as a discourse notion: A study of topic in the conversations of children and adults. In C. Li (Ed.), *Subject and topic* (pp. 336–384). New York: Academic Press.

Kraus, R. M., & Glucksberg, S. (1967). The development of communication competence as a function of age. *Child Development, 4* , 225–260.

Leonard, L., Wilcox, J., Fulmer, K., & Davis, G. (1978). Understanding indirect requests: An investigation of children's comprehension of pragmatic meanings. *Journal of Speech and Hearing Research, 21*, 528–537.

Levinson, S. (1983). *Pragmatics.* New York: Cambridge University Press.

Meline, T. (1978). *Referential communication by normal and deficient language children.* Paper presented to the American Speech and Hearing Association, San Francisco.

Mitchell-Kernan, C., & Kernan, K. (1977). Pragmatics of directive choice among children. In S. Ervin-Tripp & C. Mitchell-Kernan (Eds.), *Child discourse.* (pp. 189–210) New York: Academic Press.

Mueller, E. (1972). The maintenance of verbal exchanges between young children. *Child Development, 43*, 930–938.

Nippold, M., Leonard, L., & Anastopoulas, A. (1982). Development in the use and understanding of polite forms in children. *Journal of Speech and Hearing Research, 25*, 193–202.

Parisi, D., & Antinucci, F. (1978). *Essentials of grammar* (Elizabeth Bates, Trans.). New York: Academic Press.

Piaget, J. (1963). *The origins of intelligence.* New York: Norton.

Prutting, C., & Kirchner, D. (1983). Applied pragmatics. In T. Gallagher & C. Prutting (Eds.), *Pragmatic assessment and intervention issues in language* (pp. 29–64) San Diego: College-Hill Press.

Rees, N. (1978). Pragmatics of language: Applications to normal and disordered language development. In R. Schiefelbusch (Ed.), *Bases of language intervention.* Baltimore: University Park Press.

Schegloff, E. (1971). Notes on a conversational practice: Formulating places. In D. Sudnow (Ed.), *Studies in social interaction* (pp. 95–135). New York: Free Press.

Schegloff, E. (1972). Sequencing in conversational openings. In Gunperz & Hymes (Eds.), *Directions in sociolinguistics* (pp. 346–380). New York: Holt, Rinehart and Winston.

Schegloff, E., Jefferson, G. & Sacks, H. (1977). The preference for self-correction in the organization of repair in conversation. *Language, 53*, 361–382.

Searle, J. (1969. What is a speech act? In M. Black (Ed.), *Philosophy in America.* Ithaca, NY: Cornell University Press.

Searle, J. (1969). *Speech acts.* Cambridge, MA: Cambridge University Press.

Simon, C. (1984). Functional-pragmatic evaluation of communication skills in school-aged children. *Language, Speech and Hearing Services in the School, 15*, 83–97.

Tough, J. (1977). *The development of meaning.* New York: Halsted Press.

Tversky, A. (1977). Features of similarity. *Psychological Review, 84*, 327–352.

Tyack, D., & Ingram, D. (1977). Children's production and comprehension of questions. *Journal of Child Language, 4*, 211–224.

Wiig, E. H. (1982). *Let's talk: Developing prosocial communication skills.* Columbus, OH: Charles E. Merrill.

Wiig, E., & Semel, E. (1984). *Language assessment and intervention for the learning disabled.* Columbus, OH: Charles E. Merrill.

Wood, B. S., & Gardner, R. (1980). How children "get their way": Directives in communication. *Communication Education, 29*, 264–272.

# 9

# *Pragmatic Deficits in Emotionally Disturbed Children and Adolescents*

CHRISTIANE A. M. BALTAXE AND
JAMES Q. SIMMONS III

"I AM SURE I DIDN'T MEAN—" ALICE WAS BEGINNING, BUT THE RED QUEEN INTERRUPTED HER IMPATIENTLY.

"THAT'S JUST WHAT I COMPLAIN OF: YOU SHOULD HAVE MEANT! WHAT DO YOU SUPPOSE IS THE USE OF A CHILD WITHOUT ANY MEANING? EVEN A JOKE SHOULD HAVE A MEANING—AND A CHILD IS MORE IMPORTANT THAN A JOKE, I HOPE. YOU COULDN'T DENY THAT, EVEN IF YOU TRIED WITH BOTH HANDS."

"I DON'T DENY THINGS WITH MY HANDS," ALICE OBJECTED.

"NOBODY SAID YOU DID," SAID THE RED QUEEN. "I SAID YOU COULDN'T IF YOU TRIED."

"SHE IS IN THAT STATE OF MIND," SAID THE WHITE QUEEN, "THAT SHE WANTS TO DENY SOMETHING—ONLY SHE DOESN'T KNOW WHAT TO DENY!"

"A NASTY, VICIOUS TEMPER," THE RED QUEEN REMARKED; AND THEN THERE WAS AN UNCOMFORTABLE SILENCE FOR A MINUTE OR TWO.

**LEWIS CARROLL**—*Through the Looking Glass*

In the above fairy tale Lewis Carroll charms his readers with this dialogue between Alice and the Red and White Queens. A similar dialogue encountered in a clinical setting would

Preparation of this chapter was supported by research grants DD (59P-45192-13), MCH (MCT-0927-13), and Share. Appreciation is extended to the language fellows of the University Affiliated Training Program, University of California at Los Angeles, who in the context of clinical work and discussions contributed to the elaboration of pragmatic parameters in some of the individual case studies.

probably evoke the strong suspicion of disordered communication. Through grammatically correct, the language in the interaction itself does not follow the expected pattern of language use in a social context. A mental health professional who frequently makes a diagnosis of psychotic or emotional disorder based on verbal and nonverbal interaction might consider such a dialogue as *concrete*, *illogical*, and as evidence of *loose associations*, at least on the part of one of the interlocutors. Despite the absence of more specific grammatical deficits in the preceding dialogue, a communication specialist today would identify such a dialogue as communicatively disordered and focus on the pragmatic aspects of the interchange.

Pragmatics is defined as the use of language in a social context and has been characterized as the "soft underbelly" of formal linguistic theory and as "a border area within which the correct use of language required knowledge about the speaker, the listener, and the social and physical setting of an ongoing discourse" (Bates, 1976, p. xi). This area has only recently become a serious focus of investigation in normal and deviant child language development. Studies in pragmatics have included both verbal and nonverbal behaviors relevant to communication, and such studies carried out to date have covered a considerable range of topics. Fey and Leonard (1983) classified these topics as those related to conversational participation, discourse, regulation, referential skills, code switching, and speech acts. Others have used more specific taxonomic classifications (Chapman, 1981; Damico & Braziel, 1981; Dore, 1975; Gallagher & Prutting, 1983; Halliday, 1975; Halliday & Hasan, 1976; Rees & Wollner, 1981). These taxonomies covering specific areas of language use in context have been applied, modified, and enlarged in various studies with normal and language disordered children (Bloom, Rocissano, & Hood, 1976; Boskey & Nelson, 1980; Johnston, 1982; Keenan, 1974; Leonard, 1984; Leonard, Camarata, Rowen, & Chapman, 1982; McLean & Snyder-McLean, 1978; McShane, 1980; Miller, 1981; Prizant & Duchan, 1981; Prutting & Kirchner, 1983; Schank & Abelson, 1977; Snyder, 1975; Teas, 1983; and others).

The importance of studies relating to interactional patterns in the framework of normal and deviant child development and in language acquisition has now been clearly recognized. The available data on children suffering from a variety of communication deficits and/or cognitive delays or disorders indicate that such populations frequently are delayed in pragmatic development as well. While most of such studies suggest that language disordered children exhibit the same range of pragmatic strategies as normal children at a comparable level of language development (Bricker & Carlson, 1980; Fey, Leonard, & Wilcox, 1981; Gallagher & Darnton, 1978; Shatz, Shulman, & Bernstein, 1980; Skarakis & Greenfield, 1983; Snyder, 1975; Van Kleeck & Frankel, 1981), there is also some evidence that the extent to which such children use these strategies leads to unique as well as qualitatively distinct profiles. Thus, various authors suggest in this context that it may be erroneous to think that language disordered children are merely delayed when compared to normal children (Prutting & Kirchner, 1983; Teas, 1983). One might also add that the actual presence of such deficits may go unrecognized and distinctions from normal children may be missed unless procedures are employed that allow for the discovery of potential deficits in the interactional corpus of language disordered children instead of applying preexisting taxonomies (Baltaxe, Roblee, & Guthrie, 1984). Considerable work remains to be done to identify and establish communicatively relevant pragmatic parameters and behaviors in normal as well as language deficient children.

While pragmatic studies with language disordered children still present a confusing picture, even less information is available when it comes to children with emotional disturbances. Three principal aspects of development—linguistic, cognitive, and social—have been identified as interfacing and providing the basis for pragmatic development (Bates, 1976; Dore, 1975; Halliday, 1975) One may thus assume that delays and/or deficits in any of these areas are also reflected in pragmatic abilities.

Another dimension, which may not have been sufficiently differentiated from social development, is the development of affect, emotions, or feelings. Development along this dimension appears to be highly significant in the acquisition of pragmatic competence. In trying to understand affect, its development, and its influence on the pragmatics of language, it might be useful to utilize a framework provided by Lewis and Rosenblum's (1978) description of four essential components. These components include (a) the appearance of or the alteration in an internal physiological state or a change in the cognitive set in the individual; (b) a concomitant change in the overt or surface expression of the individual; (c) the individual's perception of the pattern of such changes; and (d) the individual's personal experience or interpretation of these perceived changes in himself or herself as well as in others.

In considering the relationship of affect to pragmatics, all four of these components appear relevant and are generally signaled verbally or nonverbally in a communication interchange. The first component may translate into different feeling states such as happiness, anger, sadness, shyness, fear, or enthusiasm. It may also produce a general attitude affecting the interactional process. As for the second component, concomitant external changes may include facial expression as well as body positioning and movement. This second component may also relate to the vocal characteristics of the speaker and to more specific formal linguistic aspects of the interchange. In addition, it may include metalinguistic features such as hesitations and pausing, distinct prosodic patterns, an emphasis on the connotative meaning of words, the choice of specific syntactic patterns, and other types of verbal and nonverbal behaviors. The last two components may translate into the speaker's awareness and monitoring of these emotional states—their changes and external expression in the speaker as well as in the speaker's ongoing interpretation of, and reaction to, the expression of these feeling states on the part of the listener.

Pragmatically, it may not matter what the underlying physiological mechanism of an affective state is in the individual. What seems important are the learned and unlearned responses to affect in both the speaker and the listener. In the case of learned behaviors, there may be specific social and/or linguistic conventions that lend themselves more readily to interactional interpretation. In either case, however. the learned as well as unlearned signals associated with specific emotional states and their changes will affect the interactional process. Such signals include a myriad of general as well as specific characteristics. These constitute an integral part of what might be called the pragmatics of language. The expression or external manifestation of an affective state, its change and interpretation, thus plays an important role in the speaker-hearer role relationship in a communicative context.

When pragmatic development is viewed as the interface of four, rather than three, principal developmental dimensions (i.e., linguistic, social, cognitive, and affective), it may also be argued that children who suffer from lags, deficits, or disorders in emotional development may be at risk for pragmatic deficits. Furthermore, the kind of emotional lag, deficit, or disorder may be predictive of the type of pragmatic deficit seen. The relationship among these four dimensions is complex, however. Deficits along any of these dimensions are not mutually exclusive, and cause-and-effect relationships are poorly understood. Thus, children impaired in their emotional development may also suffer from cognitive, linguistic, and social impairment. Similarly, children with impairments or delays in these areas may also suffer from emotional disorders.

This chapter focuses on what we currently know about pragmatic deficits in children and adolescents who are also considered emotionally disordered. They may have additional linguistic, cognitive, and social deficits, and no claim is made with respect to the primary role of any one of these. The term *emotional disorder* is a loosely used, broad categorization for psychiatric disorders that encompasses more than a specific developmental lag or disorder of emotion, affect, or feeling. The term in its broader sense coexists and overlaps extensively, however, with its more narrow meaning of primary disorder of affect, feeling, or emotion. In the present context, the broader meaning of the term is retained. The following areas are addressed: (a) definition and scope of emotional disturbances of childhood and adolescence; (b) pragmatic deficits in emotionally disturbed children and adolescents inferred from the behavioral descriptions of these populations; (c) pragmatic deficits inferred from the criteria used for the diagnosis of emotional disorders; and (d) studies by various researchers that focus more specifically on pragmatic deficits in the emotionally disturbed and clinical case studies carried out in our own laboratory.

## DEFINITION AND SCOPE OF EMOTIONAL DISORDERS

In examining the concept of emotional disorders in childhood and adolescence, one is faced with a lack of uniform and clear-cut definitions as well as with a diversity of interpretation, depending on background and expertise, as to the scope of such disorders. Thus, for the lay person, "emotional disorder" may encompass almost any psychiatric disturbance. For the communication specialist, emotional disorder may be closely linked with children diagnosed as autistic, those who have behavioral problems, and children who attend special classes for the seriously emotionally handicapped in the public school system. Emotional disorders may also be cited as a secondary characteristic to a more basic speech and language deficit.

A more specific meaning of emotional disorder has evolved in the educational system as a result of Public Law 94-142 with its more stringent requirements for appropriate school placement. However, Forness, Sinclair, and Russell (1984) point out that "notions of appropriate definition and classification of these children are not fully worked out" (p. 22). Although the designation *emotional disorder* in the educational literature has been largely replaced by the term *behavioral disorder* (Rutherford & Pietro, 1978–1983; Forness et al., 1984), emotional disorder or disturbance remains at the base of the educational classification system. For example, the concept of *seriously emotionally disturbed* (SED) derives from the Right to Education for All Handicapped Act, which "forces the schools to document an *intrapsychic* problem in order to serve a child with behavior disorders" (Forness et al., 1984, p. 23). The emphasis is thus on an underlying emotional disorder rather than on the specific behaviors of a particular child. It is interesting to note, as these authors state, that the emphasis on "intrapsychic" problems has led parents of autistic children to lobby the U.S. Department of Education for changes in federal regulations. This has resulted in the removal of *autism* from the category of *seriously emotionally disturbed* and placed it into the legal category of *other health impaired*. Nevertheless, the communication specialist continues to adhere to the concept that autistic children are emotionally disturbed.

The definition of *seriously emotionally disturbed* under the Right to Education for All Handicapped Act is that of a condition exhibiting one or more of several characteristics present over a long period of time and to a marked degree, which adversely affects educational performance. These characteristics are (a) an inability to learn that cannot be explained by intellectual, sensory, or health factors; (b) an inability to build or maintain satisfactory interpersonal relationships with peers and teachers; (c) inappropriate types of behavior or feelings under normal circumstances; (d) a general pervasive mood of unhappiness or depression; or (e) a tendency to develop physical symptoms or fears associated with personal or school problems. The term does not include children who are "socially maladjusted" or "behavior disordered" unless it is determined that they also show one or more of the specific characteristics described above (Forness, personal communication, August 1985). According to a 1982 U.S. Department of Education report, nearly 350,000 children and adolescents enrolled in the public school system are identified as severely emotionally disturbed. This population thus represents the fourth largest group of handicapped individuals served by that system (Forness et al., 1984).

In contrast to the educational system, the mental health professions generally identify emotional disorder more clearly with the term *mental disorder*. The *Diagnostic and Statistical Manual for Mental Disorders* (DSM-III) provides the current framework for diagnosis and treatment of such disorders. DSM-III defines a mental disorder as a "clinically significant behavioral or psychological syndrome or pattern that occurs in an individual and that is typically associated with either a painful symptom (distress) or impairment in one or more important areas of functioning (disability)" (p. 6). The diagnosis of a mental disorder also carries with it the inference that "there is a behavioral, psychological, or biological dysfunction" (DSM-III, p. 6). Since for most such disorders, etiology or pathophysiological processes are unknown, the approach to these disorders is descriptive. DSM-III provides a multiaxial system to assist in diagnosis, treatment, and prognosis. It identifies clinical syndromes and lists the essential features that need to be present to make a diagnosis, associated features that are often, but not invariably, present, age of onset, course, impairment, complications, predisposing factors, prevalence, sex ratio, familial pattern, and differential diagnosis. DSM-III thus provides a broader framework than that used in the public school system, and the two systems are not directly interchangeable. DSM-III also includes such disorders as mental retardation, autism, stereotyped movement disorders, specific developmental disorders such as severe developmental language disability, dyslexia, agraphia, and other disorders with physical manifestations which will be excluded from this text unless also specified for a more specific psychiatric disorder. In this context it is also of interest to note that mentally retarded children have a prevalence rate for psychiatric disorders six times that of the general population, while brain-damaged children have five times the rate, and physically handicapped children without direct central nervous system involvement have twice the rate of the general population (Rutter, Graham, & Yule, 1970; Rutter, Tizard, & Whitmore, 1970). In addition to emotional, behavioral, or mental disorders, the terms *psychiatric disorder* and *psychopathology* are also frequently used in the literature. For purposes of this text, where our own studies are concerned, the DSM-III system of diagnosis is adhered to. When reference is made to other studies, the descriptive terminology used in these studies is followed.

## PRAGMATIC DEFICITS INFERRED FROM BEHAVIORAL DESCRIPTIONS

Not surprisingly, our review of the literature on pragmatics and emotional disorders revealed only a very small number of studies that addressed the area of pragmatics specifically. These are discussed further in the following paragraphs. Based on the premise that pragmatic deficits represent a subset of communication handicaps, we assumed that studies of children with disorders in communication would also include pragmatic studies. Our search of the literature on communication handicaps and emotional disturbances again proved of low yield with respect to pragmatic studies or details. Our review did show, however, that it is possible to infer pragmatic deficits from the behavioral descriptions that accompanied most of these studies as well as from the type of emotional disorder implicated. We will therefore provide a review of studies on communication deficits and emotional disorders and identify those behaviors from accompanying descriptions that we consider pragmatically weighted. Two approaches are used in this review. In the first, the communication handicap is treated as the index problem, and the emotional disorder is considered a secondary or concomitant characteristic. In the second approach, the emotional disorder is treated as the index problem, and the communication handicap is considered concomitant or secondary. The term *emotional disorder* is being used here in the broad sense described previously and includes psychiatric disorder, behavioral disorder, mental disorder, and psychopathology as they identify the population in the studies reviewed below.

Studies that treat the communication handicap as the index problem are extensive in number, while those that treat the emotional disorder as the index are more limited in scope. In the first group of studies, emphasis has been placed on the central role of language in cognitive, emotional, and social development as well as in the development of self-image and in educational advancement. In the second group, psychopathology received major attention and assumed a central role. It is of interest that in both groups impairment in peer relationships was cited as a major characteristic. These studies, although interesting and provocative, need to be viewed with some degree of caution. In a review of the literature, Cantwell and Baker (1977) and Baker and Cantwell (1982) noted that most studies suffered from significant methodological limitations. These limitations involved problems in the definition of the psychiatric (emotional) disorder, the precise delineation of the type of communication handicap seen, reliability and validity of techniques used to assess both the presence of a communication handicap and the presence of psychopathology, sampling bias, inadequate sample size, and failure to consider other associated factors such as mental retardation and brain damage. The above methodological criticisms must also be considered in assessing the pragmatic interpretations offered on the basis of the behavioral descriptions accompanying these studies.

Tables 9.1 and 9.2 provide a summary of individual studies including the authors, details relating to sample size, communication handicap, emotional disorder, and associated behaviors reported in the individual studies. Behaviors that appear as pragmatically weighted are italicized. Unmarked behaviors are interpreted as being neutral with respect to pragmatics. Studies in which the communication handicap serves as the index are listed in Table 9.1; studies in which the emotional disorder is the index are in Table 9.2.

In inferring pragmatic deficits from these behaviors, the specifics of such deficits will have to await the actual analysis of interactional patterns in such children. However, from the description of these behaviors one may surmise far-reaching involvement, ranging from various violations of the Gricean conversational postulates to impairment in turn-taking ability, initiation of conversation, conversational repair, code switching, referencing and sequencing ability in discourse, differentiation of old and new information, establishment of topic-comment schemata, pragmatic use of prosody, and various other aspects of speaker-hearer role relationships. With the information currently available, it is probably useless to speculate on whether the inferred deficits are due to the emotional disorder, the communication handicap, or to the co-occurrence of both. The point of interest is the fact that the deficits can co-occur.

## PRAGMATIC DEFICITS INFERRED FROM CRITERIA USED FOR THE DIAGNOSIS OF EMOTIONAL DISORDERS

As noted earlier, pragmatic deficits can also be inferred from the criteria used for the diagnosis of emotional disorders. Some of these deficits, such as autism and childhood onset pervasive developmental disorder, co-occur with other communication handicaps. In contrast, children and adolescents who suffer from schizophrenia and various types of major affective disorders such as depression or mania have more adequate linguistic skills in syntax and phonology. Pragmatic deficits in this population may constitute the sole communication handicap and present an essential diagnostic characteristic of the emotional disorder itself. To date, little formal research has been carried out with respect to these populations. The exception is studies of autistic children (Baltaxe, 1977, 1984; Duchan, 1983; Duchan & Palermo, 1982; Prizant, 1978, 1983; Prizant & Duchan, 1981; Tager-Flusberg, 1981), which have been carefully reviewed by Duchan (1984). We will therefore refrain from duplicating such a review in the present context.

A more formal pragmatic analysis of the discourse and interactional patterns of children and adolescents who suffer from schizophrenia and major affective disorders may also present a viable, more formalized alternative to current impressionistic practices of diagnosing a thought disorder. The critical issue here is the relationship between language and thought, since such children suffer from what has been called disorganized thinking or a "thought disorder" (Andreason, 1979a, 1979b; American Psychiatric Association, 1980).

The complex relationship between language and thought has been a serious topic in many disciplines. In psychiatry, which has been no exception, the distinction among thought, language, and speech is frequently poorly delineated, and changes in speech production and communication are also taken as evidence of disordered thinking or of a thought disorder. Such changes are most easily translated into problems in pragmatics. Although somewhat indirectly, these essential diagnostic characteristics are actually described in pragmatic terms in the psychiatric literature (American Psychiatric Association, 1980; Andreason 1979a, 1979b). The issue of what constitutes a thought disorder is therefore also relevant in the present discussion.

Two types of thought disorder are sometimes differentiated, one relating to *content of thought*, the other to what is called a *formal thought disorder*. A disorder of content of thought involves delusional thinking, which may consist of delusions of persecution and delusions of reference in which events, objects, or other people are given particular and unusual significance, usually of a negative or pejorative nature. Although a disorder of content of thought may involve false speaker-hearer presuppositions and imply deficits in language usage (e.g., restricted topic formation, inappropriate use of prosody, and frequent self-reference, to name a few), impairments in interactional behavior are more specifically identified in the description of a formal thought disorder. An example of this is *loosening of associations*, in which "ideas shift from one subject to another

TABLE 9.1

## Studies of Communication Disorders

| Authors | Communication Handicap | Psychiatric/Behavioral Emotional Disorders | Associated Behaviors |
|---|---|---|---|
| Orton (1937) | communication handicap | secondary social behavior problems | |
| Chess (1944) | 7 cases, language handicapped children | personality distortion, behavior problems | 'extra wild', stubborn, temper tantrums, refuses explanations, expectations of failure, difficulties adapting to group, difficulties understanding directions |
| Carrell & Bangs (1957) | language deficit in children | significant alteration in child's behavior | |
| Fitzsimmons (1958) | 70 articulation disordered, 70 normals, 1st grade | articulation disordered significantly more behavior problems | destructiveness, eating problems, fears, jealousies nervousness, shyness, refusal to obey, temper tantrums, thumbsucking |
| Ingram (1959) | 80 communication handicapped children | 10 with psychiatric problems | withdrawal, immaturity, thumbsucking, temper tantrums, enuresis, excitability, nightmares, inability to form normal relationships with peers and caretakers, comprehension problem |
| Trapp & Evan (1960) | normal children, children with articulation disorders | anxiety significantly greater with articulation disorders | sleep disturbances, fears, anxieties, tensions, poor peer relationships, poorer adjustment |
| Solomon (1961) | 40 articulation disordered, 40 normal controls | significantly more (psychiatric) disturbances in articulation disordered | orality: thumbsucking, crying; passivity: shyness, eagerness to please; internalizing: restlessness, worrying; externalizing: destructiveness, cruelty |

**TABLE 9.1.** Continued

| Authors | Communication Handicap | Psychiatric/Behavioral Emotional Disorders | Associated Behaviors |
|---|---|---|---|
| Butler, Peckham, & Sheridan (1973) | 7-year-olds with speech difficulties | 50% maladjusted | |
| Chess & Rosenberg (1974) | 139 children | 99 behavior disorders, reactive disorder, neurotic thought disorder | listener strain, deviation of defensive behaviors, teasing by other children, tantrums, extreme sullenness, frustration, angry, withdrawn, hyperactivity, adaptive difficulties, disorganized thinking, poor peer relationships, separation anxiety, withdrawal, distinguished from normals by inappropriate gestures and facial expressions, abnormal anticipations, abnormal attention span, problems of hand/eye coordination |
| Affolder, Brubaker, & Bischofberger (1974) | 30 language deficient children (3 to 10 years) | | |
| DeAjuriaguerra, Jaeggi, Guignard, Kocher, Maquard, Roth, & Smid (1976) | follow-up 17 dysphasic children | 7 developmental disequilibrium with anxiety, preneurotic state, 5 serious personality disorders | difficulties in social behaviors |
| Cantwell & Baker (1977) | speech and language disordered children as a group | probability of increased prevalence of psychiatric disorder | |
| Stevenson & Richmond (1978) | 22 language delayed children | 59% psychiatric problems, 14% in random sample of 705 children | |

**TABLE 9.1.** Continued

| Authors | Communication Handicap | Psychiatric/Behavioral Emotional Disorders | Associated Behaviors |
|---|---|---|---|
| Cantwell, Baker, & Mattison (1980) | 100 communication handicapped (mean age 5½ years) | 53% psychiatric diagnosis of these 19 attention deficit disorder, 13 oppositional disorder, 12 anxiety disorder | both groups: frustration, feelings of easily being hurt, disobedience, shyness, irritability, eating problems |
| Baker, Cantwell, & Mattison (1980) | 99 children communication handicapped (46 speech disorders, 53 speech and language disorders), mean age 5 to 8 years | speech and language more severe and frequent behavioral abnormalities, both groups: conduct disorder, emotional problems, poor peer relationships | speech and language group: immaturity, restlessness, short attention span, excitability, tantrums, solitary behaviors—speech only: stomach aches, nightmares, fights with siblings |
| Baker & Cantwell (1982) | 200 children with communication handicap (1.9–14.3 years) | 53% psychiatric diagnosis (107 subjects), major categories: 28 attention deficit disorder[1], 15 shyness-anxiety disorder[2], 14 oppositional disorder[3], 10 adjustment disorder[4], 8 unspecified mental disorder<br>*Total psychiatric categories*: 28 | [1]often does not seem to listen, short attention span, inability to concentrate, difficulty completing task, misinterpretation of tasks, does not seem to listen to instructions, excess motor restlessness, frequent interruptions, difficulty waiting turn, poor frustration tolerance, frequent talking out of turn in class, often fails to finish things started<br><br>[2]excessive shrinking from contacts with strangers, interference with peer functioning, extreme distress in separating from parents, home, or familiar surroundings, clinging behavior, morbid fears and preoccupations, excessive worry and fearful behavior, somatic complaints |

**TABLE 9.1.** Continued

| Authors | Communication Handicap | Psychiatric/Behavioral Emotional Disorders | Associated Behaviors |
|---|---|---|---|
| | | | [3]opposition to all authority, 'no' sayers, negativistic, provocative, refusal to comply, argumentativeness, interference of behavior with productive activity and relationships, temper tantrums, stubbornness, violation of minor rules |
| | | | [4]impairment in social functioning, maladaptive behaviors to identification of events, including recklessness, depression, anxiousness, anger, ambivalence |

TABLE 9.2

## Studies of Emotional Disorders

| Authors | Communication Handicap | Psychiatric/Behavioral Emotional Disorders | Associated Behaviors |
|---|---|---|---|
| Wylie, Feranchak, & McWilliams (1965) | 15% communication handicap | 292 cases; no commonly recognizable clinical syndromes | headbanging, hyperactivity, involuntary movements, rocking, compulsions, rituals, soiling, thumbsucking, wetting, firesetting, poor regard for personal safety, shyness, friendlessness, feeling inferior, sensitive to criticism, fighting with parents, difficulty sleeping |
| Chess & Rosenberg (1974) | 139—some kind of language difficulty | 593 cases of psychiatric referrals | |
| Friedlander, Wetstone, & McPeek (1974) | receptive difficulties | children with emotional disturbances | |
| Grinnell, Scott-Hartnett, & Larson-Glasier (1983) | 64 communication handicap | 80 nonhearing impaired children preadolescent and adolescent psychiatric patients | |
| Gualtieri, Koriath, van Bourgondien, & Saleeby (1983) | 50% language problems | 40 psychiatric cases (4.1–13.4 years) including attention deficit disorder, adjustment reaction conduct disorder[1], schizoid disorder[2], schizophrenia[3] | Severe behavior problems<br>[1]repetitive and persistent pattern of aggressive behavior toward others, +/- failure to establish normal degree of affection, empathy, or bond with others, lying<br>[2]no close friends, no interest in making friends, no pleasure from peer interactions, general avoidance of nonfamilial social contacts, especially peers, no interest in activities involving other children<br>[3]content of language disturbed, incoherence, loosening of associations, illogical thinking, poverty of content delusions, social isolation, digressive, vague, overelaborate, circumstantial, metaphorical speech, odd or bizarre ideation, magical thinking |

completely unrelated or only obliquely related without the subject speaker showing any awareness that the topics are unconnected. Statements that lack a meaningful relationship may be juxtaposed, or the individual may shift idiosyncratically from one topic to another." Another example is *poverty of content of speech*, in which "speech is adequate in amount but conveys little information because it is vague, overly abstract, overly concrete, repetitive or stereotyped," thus violating the Gricean principle of relevance. "The listener can recognize this disturbance by noting that little, if any information has been conveyed, although the individual has spoken at some length" (American Psychiatric Association, 1980, p. 182).

Traditionally, the presence of a formal thought disorder is diagnosed on the basis of impressions collected in an interview situation and, until recently, without even a consistent framework and a specific methodology. Moreover, there had been no experimental studies that examined the possible presence of such characteristics in contrast groups. Subjectively applied categories used without concise definitions included loosening of associations, word salad, incoherence, loss of goal, and so forth. In an attempt to formalize the assessment process, Andreason (1979a, 1979b) developed a rating scale that lists 20 separate categories of linguistic behaviors: laconic speech or poverty of speech, poverty of content of speech, pressure of speech, distractible speech, tangentiality, derailment, incoherence, illogicality, clanging, neologisms, word approximations, circumstantiality, loss of goal, perseveration, echolalia, blocking, stilted speech, and self-reference. Using this scale to examine the interactional patterns of the patient, the psychiatrist rates a 50-minute doctor-patient interview for the presence of these behaviors from mild to severe. Andreason considers each of these characteristics a separate thought disorder. She calls her scale a Thought-Language-Communication Scale, thus recognizing the difficulties with diagnosing a thought disorder and with distinguishing among thought, language, and communication. Despite an apparent contradiction in terms, Andreason divides her 20 separate "thought disorders" into those she considers more specifically *communication disorders*, because

> most of the time, language behavior involves a dyadic interaction between a speaker and a listener, and the disorder occurs because the speaker fails to follow a set of rules which are conventionally used to make it easier for listeners to understand. When the speaker fails to take the various needs of the listener into account, the result is usually a *communication disorder*. (Andreason, 1978, p. 2)

From the above definition of communication disorder (which includes Andreason's categories of poverty of content of speech, pressure of speech, distractible speech, tangentiality, derailment, stilted speech, echolalia, self-reference, circumstantiality, loss of goal, perseveration, and blocking), it is clear that the thought disorders in this group are in effect pragmatic deficits. The term *language disorder* is used for yet another set of thought disorders within Andreason's 20 categories. Included in this set are those categories in which the speaker violates the syntactic and semantic conventions that govern the use of language (i.e., the categories of incoherence, clanging, neologisms, and word approximations). The concept of thought disorder is used to identify a third group of characteristics "in which thinking alone seems to be aberrant" (p. 2). This group of thought disorders includes poverty of speech and "aberrant inferential process," which is characterized by a pattern of speech in which "conclusions are reached which do not follow logically" and in which a "logical inference is made between two clauses which is unwarranted or illogical."

It is clear that the various ways in which the term *thought disorder* is used in the above framework are confusing. Yet all of these are viable characteristics in the diagnosis of a thought disorder. The significant fact for us to consider is that linguistic interaction and its analysis are brought explicitly into the arena of emotional disorders and their diagnosis.

Although Andreason's scale presents a significant step forward in articulating pragmatic deficits in the emotionally disturbed, it can be criticized for being impressionistic and subjective and for relying on rater recall without the benefit of transcribed records. In addition, the definitions provided for each of these categories are still somewhat inadequate or overlapping, and reasonable interrater reliability can be achieved only after considerable practice and experience. Also, although the focus is clearly on communicative interaction, the method used is not very illuminating linguistically. It does not tell us much about the specific parameters of pragmatics that appear deficient. Thus, although the scale may be useful for diagnostic purposes, its implications for therapeutic intervention are difficult to translate into actual treatment programs. An inspection of the 20 language behaviors rated will also quickly reveal that such behaviors cannot be considered unique to a schizophrenic thought disorder, for example. Individual behaviors or combinations thereof can be found in normal speakers, where they may be related to speech errors (Fromkin, 1975), states of fatigue or stress (Stengel, 1947), and where they may also be exploited as literary devices as in the quote from *Through the Looking Glass* at the beginning of this chapter. Significantly, some of these behaviors may also be found in affective disorders (Andreason, 1979a, 1979b; Durbin & Marshall, 1977), in cases of organic brain dysfunction (Shaffer, 1973), and in the adult aphasias (Gerson, Benson, & Frazier, 1977). Nonetheless, it is the *pattern* in which various of these thought disorders appear in combination that is diagnostically significant for the schizophrenic population.

Another problematic issue that requires further exploration is whether such a scale can be reliably applied to children and adolescents. While current DSM-III criteria for adult and childhood schizophrenia are the same, children's language behaviors may be further confounded by developmental linguistic, cognitive, and experiential issues. Nevertheless, the scale is currently being applied to this younger population as well.

## STUDIES OF EMOTIONALLY DISTURBED CHILDREN AND ADOLESCENTS IN A PRAGMATIC FRAMEWORK

The problem of thought disorder has been approached from a different perspective by another group of investigators (Rochester & Martin, 1979; Rochester, Martin, & Thurston, 1977). They focused more specifically on the apparent parallels between a thought disorder and pragmatic deficits. They observed that thought-disordered speakers present two pragmatic difficulties to the listener. First, they alert the listener to search for information that is either never given or that is given in an ambiguous form. Second, thought-disordered speakers use limited (linguistic) bonds to tie their discourse together in a cohesive fashion. The speaker thus "puts the listener on hold as he (the listener) searches for the anticipated information." Thus, "the listener clearly has to work harder to understand the speaker" (Rochester, Martin, & Thurston, 1977, p. 111). Broadly stated, the thought-disordered speaker fails to take the point of view of the listener, a prerequisite of effective communication.

### Halliday and Hasan Model of Discourse Analysis

The same group of investigators approached the study of a thought disorder more formally, using the Halliday and Hasan (1976) model of discourse analysis based on coherence of discourse. This model elaborates on the concept that, for the speaker and the listener to communicate, their speech productions have to be coherent and their discourse has to adequately establish connections between the various elements of discourse. These connections are linguistically marked and are discoverable through linguistic analysis. Halliday and Hasan (1976) define coherence or cohesion of discourse as follows.

> Cohesion occurs where the interpretation of some element in the discourse analysis is dependent on that of another. The one presupposes the other, in the sense that it cannot be effectively decoded except by recourse to it. When

> this happens, a relation of cohesion is set up and the two elements, the presupposing and the presupposed, are thereby at least potentially integrated in the text. (Halliday & Hasan, 1976, p. 4)

Major categories of cohesion within this model include a category of reference, which can be pronominal, demonstrative, or comparative in nature; substitution and ellipsis, which can be nominal, verbal, or clausal; and conjunction, which can be additive, adversative, causal, temporal, or continual. Finally, there is a lexical category, which includes same root, synonym, superordinate, and a general item. Based on this model and categorization, Rochester and Martin (1979) were able to show that the speech productions of thought-disordered and nonthought-disordered schizophrenics (thought-disordered here refers to formal thought disorder; nonthought-disordered refers to content of thought) and normal subjects could be clearly differentiated. They had used three contexts on which they based their analysis: an interview situation, the description and interpretation of cartoons, and the retelling of a narrative. Their subjects consisted of 10 of each group, with a mean age for the thought-disordered of 23.3, for the nonthought-disordered of 25.8, and for the normal of 31.0. The productions of the thought-disordered subjects were characterized by a low amount of cohesion and the use of inferior cohesive strategies. They were deviant in reference patterns, provided fewer links between clauses, and used less informative types of cohesive reference. Also, reference to nonexistent objects as well as ambiguous reference was frequent. In addition, the majority of reference clues provided the listener were situational rather than retrievable from the text itself. The major difference from the normal subjects was that the thought-disordered subjects were less cohesive and also differed in the type of cohesive strategies used.

## Application to Children

Again, the application of this type of analysis to the speech productions of similar contrast groups in children, where developmental factors may result in an unpredictable effect, must be questioned.

Two studies are of interest here. Leaper (1981), of our own UCLA study group, used the Halliday and Hasan (1976) analysis with two children diagnosed as schizophrenic and having a formal thought disorder, based on the Andreason scale and psychiatric assessment. The subjects, aged 6 and 9, were matched by age with two normal children. The language samples used in the analysis included those collected in a structured interview, description of Thematic Apperception Test (TAT) cards, and a story retelling paradigm using the "Three Little Bears."

Results showed that the discourse of the two thought-disordered children had a strikingly similar pattern to that seen in the thought-disordered adults of the Rochester and Martin (1979) study. Two prevalent patterns were the excessive use of lexical cohesion, including repetitions of the same root, the use of synonyms, or the use of a superordinate or a specified (general) vocabulary item to refer to an element previously mentioned. The second pattern consisted of reliance on situational rather than contextual verbal reference. As with adults, the thought-disordered children differed significantly from the normal subjects.

More recently, Harvey, Weintraub, and Neale (1982) used the Halliday and Hasan approach to analyze the speech productions of 153 children and adolescents between the ages of 7 and 18 who were the offspring of schizophrenic individuals (N = 23) and adults suffering from unipolar (N = 43) and bipolar (N = 38) affective disorders as well as the offspring of normal individuals (N = 53). The study was based on the premise that the offspring of disturbed individuals are at risk for similar disorders. These authors limited their language sampling to descriptions of five TAT cards and their analysis to examining reference, conjunction, and lexical cohesion. Their results showed that the offspring of all the psychopathology groups could be differentiated from each other and from the offspring of the schizophrenic individuals as well as from those of the normal individuals. The offspring of the schizophrenic group showed the most deviant performance across all dependent measures. They were less verbally productive and had poorer patterns of cohesion among ideas than did children of normal individuals. They also produced more unclear and ambiguous reference than did the other groups. In agreement with the earlier Leaper (1981) study, the authors' general finding was that the patterns of deficit produced by the children at risk for schizophrenia were similar to those found in the speech performance of adult thought-disordered schizophrenics. They showed a high degree of undesirable lexical cohesion, situational rather than verbal contextual reference, and a high degree of nonproductive addition. The schizophrenic offspring group was maximally differentiated from children with normal parents. However, deviant discourse patterns were also identified for the offspring of all psychopathological groups, with offspring of individuals suffering from a unipolar affective disorder being more deviant than offspring of manic individuals and nearly as deviant as those of schizophrenic individuals. A combination of environmental and genetic factors is proposed in accounting for their findings, and the term *cognitive slippage* instead of *thought disorder* is suggested to describe the results for this population. The results and possible clinical significance of the above findings are further supported by a prospective longitudinal study, using a nonpragmatic approach, of children of severely schizophrenic mothers (Parnas, Schulsinger, Schulsinger, Mednick, & Teasdale, 1982).

## Case Studies

In yet another set of nine individual case studies of children and adolescents diagnosed as having emotional disturbances (Baltaxe, in preparation), language samples were collected in a structured interview situation and based on a story retelling paradigm. The samples were transcribed and analyzed for pragmatic characteristics based on naturalistic methods of data analysis, with earlier work in pragmatics serving as a guideline. The subjects of these case studies ranged in age between 6 and 15 years. Six were male and three were female. Socioeconomic class ranged from lower class to upper middle class. Six subjects were identified as having or suspected of having a formal thought disorder. Three suffered from depression, one was diagnosed as having elective mutism, and one as having a gender identify disorder. At least two of the subjects showed a significant difference between performance and verbal IQ, another two had a history of language delay, and for one of these children there also was substantial evidence of organicity, which included a seizure disorder and a moderate hearing loss. All but three of the subjects had an IQ, as measured by formal IQ tests, that was in the normal or superior range, two were borderline, and one was mentally retarded. Significantly, none showed serious deficits in syntax and phonology, although language skills were not necessarily age appropriate. Individual pragmatic profiles are shown in Table 9.3.

As Table 9.3 shows, all of the subjects were observably deficient in pragmatic functioning. In the broadest sense, all of the deficits identified presented violations of speaker-hearer presuppositions and a failure to take the listener's perspective. These deficits related to conversational participation, discourse regulation, referential skills, code switching, and speech acts.

Although the group of subjects is too small to provide even a reasonable hypothesis as to the effect on pragmatics of such variables as type of diagnosis, IQ, and socioeconomic class, it is of interest that those subjects suspected of or having a thought disorder had reasonably similar patterns of pragmatic deficits, and these differentiated them from the other subjects, although individual deficits showed an overlap.

## A VIEW TOWARD THE FUTURE

The review and report on our own work in progress discussed in the preceding paragraphs underscores the fact that the domain of emotional disorders has only begun to be explored with respect to identifying pragmatic behaviors. Apart from problems of nosology, definitions, the scope of emotional disorders, and the identification of specific subject groups for study, pragmatic data obtained on emotionally disturbed children and adolescents must be interpreted with special care. As discussed previously, emotional disorders occur at a much higher rate in association with other cognitive, mental, linguistic, and physical handicaps than in the normal population. Unless these variables are carefully controlled for, pragmatic characteristics may also reflect such impairments and may not be due solely to the emotional disorder. There is no doubt, however, that the domain of emotional disturbances provides a rich and exciting new frontier in the exploration of pragmatics. We believe that the identification and interpretation of behavioral descriptions of children and adolescents with emotional disorders offered in the study in progress present reasonable first steps, as does the careful scrutiny of the diagnostic criteria necessary for the identification of specific subgroups of emotional disturbances. Together, they provide useful guidelines as to the types of pragmatic characteristics that might be predicted and the kinds of hypotheses that might be formulated. Diagnostic approaches, as exemplified by the Andreason (1979a, 1979b) scale, strongly point to the common interest of the psychiatrist and the communication specialist in an area that links speech, language, and thought and that is not immune to theoretical as well as practical difficulties. The application of formalized taxonomies to research on language in context is well demonstrated by the Halliday and Hasan (1976) approach, which identifies specific parameters of deficits in these populations and provides a useful basis for comparison between normal and emotionally disturbed subjects. Naturalistic methods, applied to individual case studies and used in combination with past findings in pragmatic studies, guard against some of the limitations inherent in the use of preexisting scales alone. The rich texture of language use in context gone awry in children and adolescents with emotional disturbances thus provides a promising interdisciplinary arena where professionals from the mental health fields and communication can collaborate and benefit from one another's contributions.

TABLE 9.3

## Clinical Case Studies for Pragmatic Deficits

| IQ | Language: Phonology | Language: Syntax | Psychiatric Diagnosis | Pragmatic Deficits |
|---|---|---|---|---|
| **Case I:** 6 years of age, female | | | | |
| low normal | low normal | low normal | schizophrenia, thought disorder<br><br>*Complicating factors*:<br>history of early language delay, history of possible sexual abuse | *Specific focus*: Application of Gricean model to clinical sample<br>Violation of Gricean conversational postulates (Grice, 1975)<br><br>*be polite*—violated by:<br>• refusal to cooperate<br>• use of words belonging to child's repertoire of offensive language<br><br>*be relevant*—avoid obscurity or ambiguity, violated by:<br>• obscure topic change within turn<br>• obscure topic change between turns so that response is unrelated to question<br>• volunteering irrelevant information<br>• providing incomprehensible information by the use of neologisms<br><br>*be informative*—violated by:<br>• giving insufficient, irrelevant, or no information<br>• being perseverative<br>• using routines with little information content<br><br>*be truthful*—violation of truth value of speaker-hearer presuppositions by:<br>• providing counterfactual responses<br>• use of counterfactual routines<br>• exploitation of the maxim of truthfulness through the use of metaphors with sexual reference<br><br>(*Other*: deficits occurred only with male interlocutors) |

**TABLE 9.3.** Continued

| IQ | Language: Phonology | Language: Syntax | Psychiatric Diagnosis | Pragmatic Deficits |
|---|---|---|---|---|
| **Case II:** 7 years of age, male | | | | |
| normal range | normal range | normal range | gender identity confusion, "bizarre behavior," emotional disturbances | *Specific focus*: interactional differences contingent on hearer differences<br><br>*Speaker—mother*<br>questions: 43% of discourse with mother<br>• overuse of rhetorical questions<br>• preponderance of questions of apparent immediate concern relating to gender identity and personal appearance<br>• overuse of requests with apparent intent to change behavior of conversational partner<br>• creation of interactional ambiguity by mother's responses (hedged responses) by listener<br>• hedged responses, empty (filler) responses<br>• repetition of speaker's requests<br>• provision of conflicting information to interlocutor |
| **Case III:** 10 years of age, male | | | | |
| full scale IQ, superior range | no obvious difficulties | | behavior problems, depression<br><br>*Complicating factors:* 58 points difference between verbal, performance IQ, bilingual (English-French) | *Specific focus*: Speaker's knowledge of speaker-hearer presupposition relevant to discourse<br>• failure to orient listener by establishing relevant background information for discourse<br>• difficulties in establishing topic<br>• difficulties in establishing reference for the listener<br>• use of noncontextual situational rather than verbal reference<br>• failure to differentiate old and new information<br>• use of personal, demonstratives, deictic pronouns when information was used for the first time<br>• lack of providing background information for proper nouns in discourse<br>• lack of appropriate turn-taking behavior<br>• inappropriate topic switch within and between utterances as well as between turns<br>• failure to clarify questions of immediate concern<br>• failure to relate coherent narrative<br>• difficulties in describing and sequencing events in time |

TABLE 9.3. Continued

| IQ | Language: Phonology | Language: Syntax | Psychiatric Diagnosis | Pragmatic Deficits |
|---|---|---|---|---|
| | | | | • paucity of speech<br>• lack of initiation of speech<br>• lack of attention to speaker<br>• difficulties in describing and sequencing events in time |
| **Case IV:** 12 years of age, female | | | | |
| borderline | commensurate with intellect, functioning; word-finding difficulties | | schizophrenic, possible thought disorder<br><br>*Complicating factors*: history of early language delay, seizure disorders, history of physical and sexual abuse, moderate hearing loss, use of hearing aid | *Specific focus*:<br>• failure to orient listener by establishing relevant background information for discourse<br>• inappropriate between and within turn reference switch<br>• use of conversational routines<br>• manipulation of conversation through use of rhetorical expression (rhetorical gambit)<br>• perseveration on limited set of conversational routines<br>• inappropriate use of rhetorical questions as greeting<br>• inappropriate topic switch through use of rhetorical questions<br>• inappropriate use of ellipsis<br>• inappropriate topic switch to self<br>• use of deviant prosodic patterns |
| **Case V:** 13 years of age, male | | | | |
| gifted range | normal range | normal range | depression, possible thought disorder | *Specific focus*: Gricean conversational postulates (Grice, 1975) *violation*: relevancy, informativeness principle<br><br>*Specific focus*: speaker's knowledge of speaker-hearer presuppositions<br>• failure to orient listener by establishing background information relevant to discourse<br>• use of noncontextual situational reference acting as if listener knows situational reference<br>• failure to differentiate between new and old information by not:<br>—providing referent noun phrases for personal, demonstrative, deictic pronouns or for general lexical items<br>—not establishing background information for proper nouns |

TABLE 9.3. Continued

| IQ | Language: Phonology | Language: Syntax | Psychiatric Diagnosis | Pragmatic Deficits |
|---|---|---|---|---|
| | | | | • improper use of pronouns, definite articles, and demonstrative noun phrases to mark new information<br>• inappropriate topic switch where the topic was semantically related but irrelevant to present discourse<br>• inappropriate topic expansion between sentences where the topic was related grammatically but irrelevant to discourse<br>• inappropriate reference switch singular to plural<br>• inappropriate reference switch to self |
| **Case VI:** 13 years of age, male | | | | |
| normal | normal range | normal range | schizophrenic, thought disorder<br>*Complicating factors*: head injury at 4 years of age | *Specific focus*: speaker's knowledge of speaker-hearer presuppositions, pragmatic abilities in story telling<br>• failure to orient the listener by establishing background information relevant for discourse<br>• difficulties in establishing topic of discourse<br>• failure to differentiate new and old information<br>• use of definite articles and pronouns for new information<br>• difficulties in establishing reference for personal, demonstrative, deictic pronouns used in discourse<br>• inappropriate use of rhetorical questions to induce contingent queries on the part of the listener<br>• difficulties in describing events in time<br>• difficulties in logically sequencing utterances within discourse |
| **Case VII:** 9 years of age, male | | | | |
| borderline | no obvious deficit | | bizarre behavior and ideation, possible thought disorder, schizotypal | *Specific focus*: speaker's knowledge of speaker-hearer presuppositions relevant to discourse<br>• failure to orient listener by establishing relevant background information for discourse<br>• difficulties in establishing topic<br>• difficulties in establishing reference for the listener<br>• failure to relate coherent narrative and difficulties in describing and sequencing events in time |

TABLE 9.3. Continued

| IQ | Language Phonology Syntax | Psychiatric Diagnosis | Pragmatic Deficits |
|---|---|---|---|
| | | | • use of noncontextual situational rather than verbal reference<br>• failure to differentiate old and new information<br>• use of personal, demonstrative, deictic pronouns when information is used for the first time<br>• lack of providing background information for proper nouns in discourse<br>• lack of appropriate turn-taking behavior<br>• inappropriate topic switch within and between utterances as well as between turns<br>• failure to clarify questions of immediate concern |
| **Case VIII:** 13 years of age, male | | | |
| borderline line | commensurate with intellectual function, no obvious difficulties | schizophrenia, thought disorder | • failure to orient listener by establishing background information relevant for discourse<br>• difficulties in establishing reference for the listener<br>• failure to differentiate old and new information<br>• use of personal, demonstrative, diectic pronouns when information used for the first time<br>• lack of appropriate turn-taking behavior<br>• inappropriate topic switch within and between utterances and between turns<br>• use of noncontextual situational reference<br>• lack of providing background information for proper nouns for listener |

**TABLE 9.3.** Continued

| IQ | Language: Phonology | Language: Syntax | Psychiatric Diagnosis | Pragmatic Deficits |
|---|---|---|---|---|
| **Case IX:** 15 years of age, female | | | | |
| MR | no obvious difficulty | grammatically acceptable, but minimal, rp complex utterances | elective mutism<br><br>*Complicating factor*: early history of language delay | *Specific focus*: language in different context, self, mother, and others<br><br>*Self-conversations*<br>• increase in linguistic complexity<br>• whispered voice<br>• perseveration on topic<br>• spontaneous initiation of speech<br><br>*Conversations with mother*<br>• clear articulation and appropriate loudness of voice<br>• ritual play with conversational routines by both speaker and hearer<br>• overuse of solicited and unsolicited contingent queries<br>• rhetorical use of solicited and unsolicited contingent queries<br>• ritual play consisting of assertion/counter assertion games<br><br>*Others*<br>• lack of initiation of speech<br>• paucity of speech<br>• low voice pitch<br>• monotonous intonation |

## REFERENCES

Affolder, F., Brubaker, R., & Bischofberger, W. (1974). Comparative studies between normal and language disturbed children based on performance profiles. *Acta Otolaryngol, Supplement 323*, 1–32.

American Psychiatric Association. (1980). *Diagnostic and statistical manual for mental disorders* (3rd ed.). Washington, DC: Author.

Andreason, N. (1978). *Scale for the Assessment of Thought, Language, and Communication* (memeograph).

Andreason, N. (1979a). The clinical assessment of thought, language, and communication disorders: The definition of terms and of their reliability. *Archives of General Psychiatry, 36*, 1315–1321.

Andreason, N. (1979b). Thought, language, and communication disorders II: Diagnostic significance. *Archives of General Psychiatry, 36*, 1325–1330.

Baker, L., & Cantwell, D. (1982). Language acquisition, cognitive development and emotional disorder in childhood. In K. E. Nelson (Ed.), *Children's language* (Vol. 3., pp. 286–321). Hillsdale, NJ: Lawrence Erlbaum.

Baltaxe, C. (1977). Pragmatic deficits in the language of autistic adolescents. *Journal of Pediatric Psychology*, 2(4), 176–180.

Baltaxe, C., (1984). The use of contrastive stress in normal, aphasic, and autistic children. *Journal of Speech and Hearing Research, 27*, 97–105.

Baltaxe, C., Roblee, M., & Guthrie, D. (1984). A comparison of two approaches used to identify communicative behaviors. *Proceedings, Symposium on Research in Child Language Disorders*, Madison, WI: University of Wisconsin Press.

Baltaxe, C., & Simmons, J. Q. (1985). *Pragmatic behaviors in emotionally disturbed children and adolescents*. Paper presented at the annual meeting of ASHA. Washington, DC.

Bates, E. (1976). *Language in context*. New York: Academic Press.

Bloom, L., Rocissano, I., & Hood, L. (1976). Adult-child discourse: Developmental interaction between information processing and linguistic knowledge. *Cognitive Psychology, 8*, 521–552.

Boskey, M., & Nelson, K. (1980). *Answering unanswerable questions: The role of imitation*. Paper presented at the Boston Conference on Language Development, Boston.

Bricker, D., & Carlson, L. (1980). *The relationship of object and prelinguistic social-communicative schemes to the acquisition of early linguistic skills in developmentally delayed infants*. Paper presented at the Conference on Handicapped and At-Risk Infants: Research and Application, Asilomar, CA.

Butler, N., Peckham, C, & Sheridan, M. (1973). Speech defects in children aged 7 years: A national study. *British Medical Journal, 1*, 253–257.

Cantwell, D., & Baker, L. (1977). Psychiatric disorder in children with speech and language retardation: A critical review. *Archives of General Psychiatry, 34*. 583–591.

Carrell, J., & Bangs, J. (1957). Disorders of comprehension associated with idiopathic language retardation. *Nervous Child, 9*, 64–76.

Chapman, R. (1981). Exploring communicative intents. In J. Miller (Ed.), *Assessing language production in children* (pp. 111–136). Austin, TX: PRO-ED

Chess, S. (1944). Developmental language disability as a factor in personality distortion in childhood. *American Journal of Orthopsychiatry, 14,* 483–493.

Chess, S., & Rosenberg, M. (1974). Clinical differentiation among children with initial language complaints. *Journal of Autism and Childhood Schizophrenia, 4,* 99–109.

Damico, J., & Braziel, K. (1981). *Systematic observation of communicative interaction: A naturalistic language assessment technique*. Paper presented at the American Speech-Language Hearing Association, Los Angeles.

De Ajuriaguerra, J., Jaeggi, A., Guignard, F., Kocher, F., Maquard, M., Roth, S, & Schmid, E. (1976). The development and prognosis of aphasia in children. In D. Morehead & A. Morehead (Eds.), *Normal and deficient child language* (pp. 345–385). Austin, TX: PRO-ED.

Dore, J. (1975). Hollow phrases, speech acts, and language universals. *Journal of Child Language, 2,* 21–40.

Duchan, J. (1983). Autistic children are non-interactive or so we say. *Seminars in Speech and Language,* 53–61.

Duchan, J. (1984). Clinical interactions with autistic children. *Topics in Language Disorders,* 4(4), 62–71.

Duchan, J., & Palermo, J. (1982). How autistic children view the world. *Topics in Language Disorders,* 2(1), 10–15.

Durbin, M., & Marshall, R. (1977). Speech in mania: Syntactic aspects. *Brain and Language, 4,* 208–218.

Fey, L., & Leonard, L. (1983). Pragmatic skills in children with specific language impairment. In T. Gallagher & C. Prutting (Eds.), *Pragmatic assessment and intervention issues in language* (pp. 65–82). San Diego: College-Hill Press.

Fey, M., Leonard, L., & Wilcox, K. (1981). Speech style modifications of language impaired children. *Journal of Speech and Hearing Disorders, 46,* 91–97.

Fitzsimmons, R. (1958). Development, psychosocial and educational factors in children with non-organic articulation problems. *Child Development, 29,* 481–489.

Forness, S., Sinclair, E, & Russell, A. (1984). Serving children with emotional or behavior disorders: Implications for educational policy. *American Journal of Orthopsychiatry, 54*(1), 22–32.

Friedlander, B., Wetstone, H., & McPeek, D. (1974). Systematic assessment of selective language listening deficits in emotional disturbed children. *Journal of Child Psychology and Psychiatry, 15,* 1–12.

Fromkin, V. (1975). A linguist looks at 'schizophrenic language.' *Brain and Language,* 2(4), 498–503.

Gallagher, T., & Darnton, B. (1978). Conversational aspects of the speech of language disordered children: Revision behaviors. *Journal of Speech and Hearing Research, 21,* 118–135.

Gallagher, T., & Prutting, C. (Eds.). (1983). *Pragmatic assessment and intervention issues in language*. San Diego: College-Hill Press.

Gerson, S., Benson, D. F., & Frazier, S. (1977). Schizophrenia versus posterior aphasia. *American Journal of Psychiatry, 134,* 906–969.

Grice, H. (1975). Logic and conversation. In P. Cole & L. H. Mortan (Eds.), *Syntax and semantics, Vol. 3: Speech Acts* (pp. 41–58). New York: Academic Press.

Grinnell, S., Scott-Hartnett, D., & Larson-Glasier, M. (1983). Language disorders in the Napa State Hospital Children's Program [Letter to the editor]. *Journal of the American Academy of Child Psychiatry, 22,* 580–581.

Halliday, M. (1975). *Learning how to mean.* London: Edward Arnold.

Halliday, M., & Hasan, R. (1976). *Cohesion in English.* London: Longmans.

Harvey, P., Weintraub, S., & Neale, J. (1982). Speech competence in children vulnerable to psychopathology. *Journal of Abnormal Child Psychology, 10*(3) 373ka-2-388.

Ingram, T. T. S. (1959). Specific development disorders of speech in childhood. *Brain, 82,* 450–467.

Johnston, J. (1982). The language disordered child. In N. Lass, L. McReynolds, J. Northern, & D. Yoder (Eds.), *Speech, language and hearing* (Vol. 2). Philadelphia: W. B. Saunders.

Keenan, E. (1974). Conversational competence in children. *Journal of Child Language, 1,* 163–184.

Leaper, C. (1981). *The discourse of schizophrenic children.* Paper presented at the Sixth Annual Boston Child Language Conference, Boston.

Leonard, L. (1984). Normal language acquisition: Some recent findings and clinical implications. In A. Holland (Ed.), *Language disorders in children* (pp. 1–36). San Diego: College-Hill Press.

Leonard, L., Camarata, S., Rowen, L., & Chapman, R. (1982). The communicative functions of lexical usage by language impaired children. *Applied Psycholinguistics, 3,* 109–116.

Leonard, L., & Wilcox, M. (1984). Developmental language disorders: Preschoolers. In A. Holland (Ed.), *Language disorders in children* (pp. 100–128). San Diego: College-Hill Press.

Lewis, M., & Rosenblum, L. (1978). Introduction: Issues in affect development. In M. Lewis & L. Rosenblum (Eds.), *The development of affect* (pp. 1–10). New York: Plenum Press.

McLean, J., & Snyder-McLean, L. (1978). *A transactional approach to early language training.* Columbus, OH: Charles E. Merrill.

McShane, J. (1980). *Learning to talk.* Cambridge: Cambridge University Press.

Miller, J. (1981). *Assessing language production in children,* Austin, TX: PRO-ED.

Orton, S. (1937). *Reading, writing, and speech problems in children.* New York: W. W. Norton.

Parnas, J., Schulsinger, M., Schulsinger, H., Mednick, S., & Teasdale, T. (1982). Behavioral precursors of schizophrenia spectrum. *Archives of General Psychiatry, 39,* 658–665.

Prizant, B. (1978). *An analysis of the function of immediate echolalia in autistic children.* Doctoral dissertation, State University of New York, Albany.

Prizant, B. (1983). Echolalia in autism: Assessment and intervention. *Seminars in Speech and Language, 4,* 63–77.

Prizant, B., & Duchan, J. (1981). The function of immediate echolalia in autistic children. *Journal of Speech and Hearing Disorders, 46,* 241–249.

Prutting, C., & Kirchner, D. (1983). Applied pragmatics. In T. Gallagher & C. Prutting (Eds.), *Pragmatic assessment and intervention issues in language* (pp. 29–64). San Diego: College Hill Press.

Rees, N., & Wollner, S. (1981). *A taxonomy of pragmatic abilities: The use of language in conversation*. Paper presented at the Annual Convention of the American Speech-Language-Hearing Association, Los Angeles.

Rochester, S., & Martin, J. (1979). *Crazy talk: A study of the discourse of schizophrenic speakers*. New York: Plenum.

Rochester, S., Martin, J., & Thurston, S. (1977). Thought process disorder in schizophrenia: The listener's task. *Brain and Language, 4*, 95–114.

Rutherford, R., & Pietro, A. (Eds.). (1978–1983). *Severe behavior problems of children and youth* (Vol. 1–6). Reston, VA: Council for Children with Behavior Problems.

Rutter, M., Graham, P., & Yule, W. (1970). *A neuropsychiatric study of childhood*. Lavenham, Suffolk, England: Lavenham Press.

Rutter, M., Tizard, J., & Whitmore, K. (Eds.). (1970). *Education, health and behavior*. London: Longmans Green.

Schank, R., & Abelson, R. (1977). *Scripts, plans, goals, and understanding*. Hillsdale, NJ: Lawrence Erlbaum.

Shaffer, D. (1973). Psychiatric aspects of brain injury in childhood: A review. *Developmental Medicine and Child Neurology, 15*, 211–220.

Shatz, M., Bernstein, D., & Shulman, M. (1980). The responsiveness of language disordered children to indirect directiveness in varying contexts. *Applied Psycholinguistics, 1*, 295–306.

Skarakis, E., & Greenfield, P. (1983). *The role of new and old in the verbal expression of language disabled children*. Paper presented at the Fourth Annual Boston Conference on Language Development, Boston.

Snyder, L. (1975). *Pragmatics in language disabled children: Their prelinguistic and early verbal performatives and suppositions*. Unpublished doctoral dissertation, University of Colorado.

Soloman, A. (1961). Personality and behavior patterns of children with functional defects of articulation. *Child Development, 32*, 731–737.

Stengel, E. (1947). A clinical and psychological study of echo reaction. *Journal of Mental Science, 93*, 598–612.

Tager-Flusberg, H. (1981). *Pragmatic development and its implication for social interaction in autistic children*. Paper presented at the International Symposium on Autism Research, Boston.

Teas, E. (1983). *Discourse of preschool children: A contextual analysis*. Doctoral dissertation, University of Colorado, Boulder.

Trapp, E., & Evan, J. (1960). Functional articulatory defect and performance on a non-verbal task. *Journal of Speech and Hearing Disorders, 25*, 176–180.

Van Kleeck, A., & Frankel, T. (1981). Discourse devices used by language disordered children: A preliminary investigation. *Journal of Speech and Hearing Disorders, 46*, 250–257.

Wylie, H., Feranchak, P., & McWilliams, B. (1965). Characteristics of children with speech disorders seen in a child guidance center. *Perceptual Motor Skills, 20*, 1101–1107.

# 10

# *Application of Pragmatics to Severely Mentally Retarded Children and Youth*

JAMES E. MCLEAN AND
LEE SNYDER-MCLEAN

An important trend can be observed in the intensive study of human language that has held forth for the past 25 years. Gradually, the dominant theoretical models of human language have shifted from idealized models of the language system per se to models that focus on the relationship between language and the human being who creates and uses it. For example, models of phonology have shifted away from those focused on the distinctive features of the phonological system (e.g., Jakobson, Fant, & Halle, 1963) to process models that consider the effects of selective pressures of the human auditory system and articulatory mechanisms on the production of speech sounds (Ingram, 1976). Similarly, the dominant model of semantics is no longer the idealized feature model described by Katz and Fodor (1963), but rather one that views semantic notions and relationships as the encoding of a speaker's internalized knowledge (e.g., Bloom, 1970; Bowerman, 1973; Leonard, 1976; Rosch, 1973; Slobin, 1973). Even syntax has undergone a similar shift, as the abstract model of generative grammar offered by Chomsky (1957) has been resynthesized in case-grammar systems (e.g., Fillmore, 1968) that consider syntactic structures in relationship to the propositional content they encode. When viewed from this perspective, pragmatics can be seen simply as a more inclusive master-model for this general trend aimed at returning language to its users.

---

The work reported in this chapter was supported in part by NICHD grants HD 18955 and HD 02528 to the University of Kansas, Bureau of Child Research

Such a trend is enormously attractive to those interested in individuals who manifest severe language deficiencies. Paradoxically, in all the efforts of the past two and a half decades to better describe and thus better understand human language, we actually have learned very little about people who have such deficiencies. Certainly, we have documented and quantifed the severity of their deficiencies by comparing their language output with idealized models of our language systems. However, we have not generally described the communicative behaviors and systems such individuals do have. And, while we have designed intensive procedures aimed at training idealized language forms, we have concentrated primarily on input variables and rarely on the client's needs for and role in acquiring communication and language.

There is no small irony in this fact that, while we have learned much about language systems, we have learned little about the people who have severe language deficiencies—knowledge that might help us better understand human language and human language acquisition. Such a lack of productivity in describing and evaluating the communicative status of people with severe language deficiencies points to limitations that are inherent in the idealized and reductionistic theoretical models of the past, with their exclusive focus on linguistics and "verbal behavior." This relative lack of productivity with severely language deficient clients in some way accounts for the rapid and enthusiastic acceptance of pragmatics in the clinical sector. Hope is strong among clinical language workers that a return to a psychological model of language, as opposed to linguistic models focused on language form or behavioral models focused on extreme empiricist descriptions (Skinner, 1957), will allow a better understanding of language in human terms. Implicit in this view is the belief that such an understanding can be applied to language deficient individuals and populations, and that such applications will provide new information that is productive in both the assessment and treatment of such people.

## ORGANIZING PERSPECTIVES ON PRAGMATICS

Overall, the pragmatics model is a psychological model of human language. At a *macro* level, it focuses on human language as a specialized system of interactive behaviors used by people to create, coordinate, and maintain social environments that are cooperative and productive (DeLaguna, 1963). At a *micro* level, however, a pragmatics view considers that the forms of language people create and use are heavily influenced by multiple psychological factors such as speakers' intents in interacting with others (Austin, 1962; Searle, 1969); speakers' histories and relationships with their receivers (Andersen, 1977); and a culture's rules for use of such behaviors (Grice, 1975). Such perspectives provide important supplements to the idealized and reductionistic models of language as either linguistic structure controlled by innate predispositions to acquire syntax (Chomsky, 1965) or as verbal behavior acquired through a process of imitation and controlled by objective antecedent and consequent stimuli (Skinner, 1957). These perspectives of the psychological bases and social functions of language clearly have been underrepresented in the treatment processes offered over the past two decades.

The question now is, how appropriate and productive can we make the pragmatics model for human populations that manifest severe deficiencies in language? Clearly, the data are not all in at this time. However, the anecdotal reports and preliminary data available appear to be quite positive. First, the pragmatics model provides an excellent framework for better describing the communicative and language repertoires of severely language deficient people. These richer descriptions, in turn, provide an important base for revising our assessment procedures for such clients. Second, the pragmatics model is useful in the prescription of some initial treatment goals that are significantly different from goals of the past and that seem both appropriate and productive for such clients. Third, the pragmatics model is productive in guiding the development of new and quite different procedures and contexts for communicative training. For example, a recent report (McLean & Snyder-McLean, 1984a) of various strategies used for facilitating language acquisition among handicapped children by a number of clinical researchers reflects a strong disposition to apply a pragmatics model.

In this chapter we report specifically on the efforts and results of applications of various elements of pragmatics to a population of severely mentally retarded children and youth who demonstrate severe language deficiencies. While these efforts must be clearly marked as exploratory and their results seen as preliminary rather than definitive, we think they indicate clear potential for the clinical productivity of the pragmatic or communicative perspective for severely mentally retarded clients. In addition, there are indications that the data emanating from such applications may eventually make important contributions to our understanding of human language and the products and processes of its acquisition.

We begin with a brief discussion of the characteristics of the topic population of severely language deficient persons who suffer severe mental retardation. Next, we identify specific elements subsumed in the overall pragmatics model that appear to be most pertinent to this population. Finally, we discuss the operationalization of these elements of pragmatics as taxonomies of behaviors that can be observed and, thus, objectively applied in the clinical processes of assessment and treatment.

In this context we present some preliminary findings from our own applications of these taxonomies to samples of severely retarded clients.

## CHARACTERISTICS OF THE TOPIC POPULATION

Representative definitions rather consistently identify four critical features of *mental retardation* (cf. McLean & Snyder-McLean, 1980). First, the problem is deemed to be *developmental* in that it is not the result of any immediate trauma and is manifest throughout the human developmental period (up to 18 years of age). Second, the problem is considered to be *mental* in that it reflects impairment in general intellectual or cognitive functioning. Third, mental retardation is considered to be *pervasive* in that it affects the individual's ability to function in all activity spheres, as opposed to a more specific learning disability whose effects might be manifested in only one sphere. Fourth, mental retardation is fully defined only by inclusions of measures of the relative abilities of people to adapt themselves to a *normal environment*. Such adaptive abilities include, among others, domains such as independent functioning (e.g., toileting and other self-care behaviors); language development; self-direction; and socialization. Adaptive functioning can be further evaluated by considering any actual *maladaptive* behaviors that might be demonstrated. Thus, persons with stereotypic behaviors; destructive or violent behaviors; and/or self-injurious behaviors, among others, would be judged to be lower on overall adaptive behavior scales (cf. Nihira, Foster, Shellhaas, & Leland, *AAMD Adaptive Behavior Scale*, 1969).

Our focus in this chapter is on persons classified as *severely* mentally retarded. This means that our topic population includes individuals whose IQs fall in the range between 20/25 and 35/40, based upon a measure of general intellectual functioning, and who have been judged to demonstrate concomitantly low levels of adaptive behaviors (Grossman, 1983). It also means that individual members of the topic population are either nonverbal or exhibit oral or manually signed language repertoires generally well below those of a normally developing 3-year-old. Clearly, this is a population with severe and pervasive impairments. Experience suggests, however, that it is also a heterogeneous population in terms of the levels of adaptive and communicative behaviors of its members. Definition of the differences that exist in the communicative behaviors among members of this population is critical to any truly individualized treatment efforts. In addition, better definition of communicative differences among such clients could prove to be important to the overall knowledge base in child language. It is to the better description and analysis of these differences that we have begun to apply the elements of a pragmatics perspective.

The substance of this chapter reflects much information provided by others working in both child language and mental retardation. In addition, much of it is based on the authors' own relatively intensive experience in experimental treatment and laboratory research contexts with two sample groups of this overall population of severely mentally retarded children. It is important to note that these sample groups may not be representative of the total population of severely mentally retarded children and youth. There may be other subsets of this population that would provide patterns of behavior and abilities different from those we describe in this chapter. The population from which our samples were drawn and upon which we base our observations is that of mentally retarded youngsters and adolescents who are, in varying degrees, ambulatory, toilet-trained, and largely self-sufficient in feeding and other self-help skills. All persons in our current samples reside in the custodial-care environment of a state institution for mentally retarded persons. All persons in our samples have had several years of behavioral training in both educational and speech and language programs.

Members of our sample groups move about the grounds of the institution with minimal constraints but under constant supervision. These individuals have many contacts with both peers and adult authority figures. However, these children and youths live in environments that are essentially devoid of the natural interactional opportunities and consequences that characterize mainstream human social environments. That is, their environments are highly structured and offer few opportunities for self-determined schedules and activities. Although intensive efforts to change these conditions are ongoing, the institutional environment most often offers minimal representation of the responsiveness and cooperation that characterize normal environments in Western cultures. As a result, it is possible that the population sample we are considering may exhibit communicative deficiencies that are the result of environmental processes that have primary effects on communicative performance; and that the performances we describe may not be accurate reflections of client communicative competence (Hymes, 1971). In most cases, however, we judge that the communicative deficits we are describing are rooted in serious depressions of communicative competence that have been exacerbated by concomitant depressions of the communicative environment.

Although in this work we focus on the benefits that this population may derive from applications of the elements of pragmatics, we further suggest that this population may produce perspectives and data that are useful in the analysis of some current issues in the field of pragmatics. Since the elements of pragmatics have been identified on the basis of data collected from competent speakers, it is interesting to investigate their relative representation among speakers who appear to be less than competent. The pragmatic elements represented in the communicative behaviors of severely language deficient clients may be considered to be more generic to communication than to language, and a further investigation of the relationship between the two domains in a nonnormal population is important. This suggests the need for studies of the basic elements of pragmatics and the order of their emergence among populations who manifest significantly atypical development in many behavioral domains, including communication. Such data would appear to have important potential for contributing to a better understanding of the relationships that exist between various human social and cognitive attainments and communication and language performance, including the relative continuity or discontinuity of preverbal and linguistic communicative behaviors (cf. Bloom, 1983).

## SELECTING PRAGMATIC ELEMENTS FOR APPLICATION

The field of pragmatics is a broad and complex collection of philosophical, theoretical, and empirical elements rooted strongly in analyses of normal language usage and normal language acquisition processes. Its most recent representations in the child language literature have ranged from the classical, philosophical expositions of Bates (1976) to eclectic approaches designed to parse and operationalize its many elements for both clinical and research applications (cf. Baltaxe & Simmons, Chapter 9 of this volume; Bates, Camaioni, & Volterra, 1975; Craig, 1983; Duchan, 1984; Kaiser & Warren, Chapter 16 of this volume; McLean & Snyder-McLean, 1984b; Prutting, 1982; Rees, 1978; Snyder & Silverstein, Chapter 8 of this volume). Whatever the final orientation and applications may be, any discussion of pragmatics must begin with the awareness that it is concerned with the relationships between language and its human users. In her philosophical orientation, Bates (1976) notes that Peirce (1932) introduced the term *pragmatics* as a branch of the study of *semiotics* (signs) and that Morris (1946) differentiated it as the branch of linguistics concerned with the relationships of signs to their users, as compared to *semantics*, the branch concerned with the relationship of signs to their referents, and *syntactics*, the branch concerned with the relationship of signs to each other. Such definitions are critical in setting up the boundaries and logical place of pragmatics in the overall linguistic hierarchy; but such definitions are somewhat abstract for those needing to operationalize pragmatics for clinical use. The more eclectic expositions of the various elements of pragmatics and their taxonomies have contributed toward this needed operationalization of pragmatics. Pragmatics is a curious area, however; although its elements are related at a single and basic philosophical level, its scope is so broad and its elements so disparate that they do not lend themselves to neat, systematic expositions. Duchan's (1984) excellent analysis of the historical bases of pragmatics and its applications indicates that the prevalent method of organizing and synthesizing pragmatics for clinical and research purposes has been simply to develop checklists of the elements that are of interest or appear to have special utility for the problem or population of interest. While such approaches are somewhat unsatisfying because of their relative fragmentation, they seem to be the only feasible way of managing the complexity of this particular body of theory and knowledge.

In developing our checklist of pragmatics elements for application to severely language deficient clients, we have chosen to consider three aspects of pragmatics: (a) speech acts and performatives; (b) products and processes involved in speech act acquisition; and (c) discourse skills and their prelinguistic forms. The substance and data basic to these three topics allow us to identify the questions and taxonomies that we apply to the communicative behaviors of severely language deficient clients suffering severe mental retardation.

## Speech Acts and Performatives

The most basic elements of a pragmatics perspective are rooted in a view of language utterances as *acts* (Bates, 1976). Austin's (1962) discussion of *speech acts* offers a view of language utterances as social acts and suggests that, like all acts, speech acts reflect some aspect of the intent or the state of their emitter (illocutions). Like all acts, they have some effects upon their receivers (perlocutions). Like all acts, they have some specific form or topography (locutions). Because competent language users are intuitively aware of all of these dimensions of their speech acts, their utterances are influenced by each of them. Speakers, therefore, construct utterances that are designed to maximize the probability that their intended effects will be attained. This means, then, that the grammar of these speech acts will be appropriate to their audience; their propositions and semantic content will be cast in ways that will be understood and considered appropriately respectful and polite by their audiences; and, to the degree that politeness allows, their utterances will be constructed to be efficient and ever-mindful of information that can be presupposed because of past history, current context, and previous utterances shared with any particular audience (Austin, 1962; Bates, 1976; Searle, 1969).

The overall notion of speech acts that carry speaker intentions and have effects on receivers begs a further question about the specific uses or functions of speech acts in a social milieu. Considerations of such functions lead to taxonomies of early speech act intentions (Dore, 1975) and effects (Halliday, 1975) drawn from observational data on young children.

The taxonomy of intents by Dore, for example, listed the following: requesting action, calling, protesting, greeting, labeling, requesting answer, repeating, answering, and practicing. Practicing, of course, can be considered a speech act but not a socially communicative function.

The pertinence of such empirically identified speech act functions for severely language deficient clients is that they provide a basis for revising the taxonomies of arbitrary language functions that have become prominent in many of the behavioral language treatment programs. Arbitrarily selected functions appear to have concentrated on labeling both actions and objects, and requesting both objects and actions. Often, both the labeling and requesting functions were evoked in an answer context, for example, "What this?" (label given) or "What want?" (label given). Thus, such programs have tended to slight many of the functions required in natural social discourse contexts. In other cases, speech act functions carried in treatment programs for severely language deficient children and youth suffering mental retardation have been derived from linguistic form classes in a function-follows-form paradigm, rather than the pragmatic paradigm of form following needed functions (e.g., Ruder & Smith, 1974; Waryas & Stremel-Campbell, 1978). In summary, the pragmatically oriented research that identified functions of speech acts or *performatives* (Austin, 1962) has brought a new perspective to the assessment and training of "functional" language repertoires in severely language deficient clients. This research shifts the focus of treatment goals to social communication as opposed to linguistic form and thus alters completely the matrices applied in determining desired treatment outcomes. Such a move to a communicative perspective suggests the need for complete revision of the goals, procedures, and contexts of behavioral treatment programs that were designed to bring linguistic forms under the control of objective stimuli like pictures and objects. In considering such revisions, the data and perspectives provided by studies of the acquisition of communication and speech acts among normally developing children have been highly productive.

## Products and Processes of Speech Act Acquisition

Consideration of the products and processes of speech act acquisition among normally developing infants and young children is a hybrid operation that cannot be contained within the framework of pragmatics. It has become a standard component of pragmatic applications, however, because the view of language and communication as social behavior carrying speaker intentions demands the ability to document the presence of such intentions, both in the observable behaviors of speakers and in the responses to such perceived intents among receivers. Such documentation is straightforwardly accomplished among mature language users. However, the documentation of the relative place of such intents and effects in the behaviors of infants and young children who are just acquiring communicative behaviors is not as easily available. Thus, researchers began to concentrate on describing the psychosocial aspects of early infant behaviors; their course of development and refinement; and their possible relationships to later linguistic forms and speech act performatives. As evidenced in a burgeoning literature regarding communicative development, this research has been both successful and prolific. As we discuss later in this chapter, behaviors that seem to reflect communicative intent can be reliably observed even in the nonlinguistic behaviors of young babies. The emergence of such intent and the expansion and refinement of its topographical forms appear to follow an orderly and relatively standard course of development. The effects that such intentional communicative behaviors have on receivers also have been documented in studies of the responses of caregivers in interactions with young children. We shall describe the data from observational research carried out with normally developing infants and young children later. First, we would like to briefly discuss an issue related to the use of these data in applications to the population being considered in this chapter.

Some professionals object to the application of so-called *developmental* data to children and youth suffering mental retardation. While we understand the concerns that underlie these objections, we have come to believe that it is more valid to use empirically derived descriptions of the products and processes of language acquisition by real children than to create arbitrary representations of these through extrapolations from either linguistic or behavioral descriptions of idealized adult language. For this reason, we, and many others, have looked carefully at the data on the acquisition of language repertoires to identify those aspects of language acquisition by normally developing children that might be considered as *generic* (characteristic and constant) to language acquisition by anyone. It has not seemed logical to us that severely mentally retarded children would acquire language repertoires in ways that were totally unique or variant from the ways that other humans acquire them. While we do not assume total isomorphism between retarded and normal learners, neither do we expect the relative heteromorphism that is implied in the arbitrary products and processes contained in many of the early behavioral programs (e.g., Gray & Ryan, 1973; Guess, Sailor, & Baer, 1974; Kent, 1974). Thus, we believe that the data that track the acquisition of language among normally developing children are worthy of careful examination and analysis through applications to severely language deficient children and youth.

Prominent in the results of the analyses of normal development are four basic findings about the acquisition of communicative repertoires. First, the data show that infants' earliest reflexive or procedural motor acts have *effects* on their social environment, even though the infant has no apparent intent to have such effects; and that clearly identifiable intentional communicative acts emerge between 8 and 12 months of age in normally developing infants (Bates et al., 1975; Carpenter, Mastergeorge, & Coggins, 1983; Harding, 1983; Sugarman-Bell, 1978). Second, the developmental data show that the behavioral forms of intentional communicative acts reflect a cumulative evolutionary process in which motor acts become more and more specialized and *conventionalized* for communicative functions (e.g., gestures for *requesting*, *showing*, *giving*, and *indicating* develop) and then are supplemented by linguistic forms (Bates et al., 1975; Carpenter et al., 1983; Harding, 1983; Sugarman, 1984). Third, the developmental data indicate that even the earliest intentional communicative acts reflect multiple performatives (or proto-performatives), including functions such as protests, requests for actions and objects, directing attention, comments on actions and objects, and answering (Bates, 1976; Carpenter et al., 1983; Harding, 1983). Fourth, these data also indicate that the communicative acts of young children gradually reflect an increasing *decontextualization* from their referents (Bates, 1979; Moerk, 1977; Werner & Kaplan, 1963). For example, an early gesture might involve the holding out of a cup to request "more juice." A later gesture would omit the cup and simply involve pointing directly toward the juice container, perhaps accompanied by an intonated vocalization signaling some urgency. Such a process of decontextualization is considered to indicate progress along a continuum of symbolic ability.

The data bases underlying each of these four observations provide important quantifications of products and processes observed in the acquisition of communication and language repertoires. Researchers like Bloom (1983) and Sugarman (1984) correctly point out that one cannot assume that continuity exists between the nonlinguistic and linguistic communicative repertoires observed in the normal developmental process. However, this caution does not alter the fact that the pattern of communication and language acquisition includes the following characteristics: (a) the emergence of communicative intentions; (b) the movement of communicative signals from primitive motor acts to specialized and conventionalized motor acts; (c) the presence of multiple functions for communicative acts at the earliest levels of communicative intentions; and (d) the gradual distancing or decontextualization of communicative signals from their referents. Later, we will look for representations of each of those seemingly generic products and processes in the communicative repertoires of severely language deficient children and youth classified as severely mentally retarded.

## Discourse Skills and Their Nonlinguistic Forms

Basic to, but separate from, speech acts per se are the rules for their use in interactive episodes with other people. Such discourse or conversational performances subsume all of the elements of pragmatics that we have discussed to this point and, in addition, offer other elements unique to the discourse level itself. While many of the elements of pragmatics that assure effectiveness, efficiency, and appropriateness of utterances exist at the utterance level, many elements come into play only in discourse and conversations. These elements are reflected in Grice's (1975) notion that conversation or discourse between people is based on an initial assumption that such exchanges will be cooperative and, thus, will be truthful, sincere, and relevant to the purpose of the discourse. Violations of these assumptions occur, of course, and such violations provide the bases for humor, for politeness, and for marking a speaker's assumption of social subordinance to a receiver (Andersen, 1977; Bates, 1976). In addition to these subtle, but powerful, effects on the structure and content of utterances, the cooperative principles outlined by Grice (1975) also extend to the patterns of discourse. Thus, speakers allow receivers their turns in the conversation and, in reciprocation, fill their own turns when they come around again. They also maintain the topic of the conversation or note their changes of topics with elaborate conventions.

When we first began to review the literature emanating from pragmatics, we saw little immediate application for the rules related to discourse or conversation to our severely language deficient population. Such skills were so far beyond the language levels of the clients for whom we were seeking help that we simply passed over discourse on our way to more study of the speech act–based taxonomies. However, as we reviewed the elements of discourse skills (e.g., topic, topic maintenance, and adjacency) simultaneously with Bruner's (1975) discussions of mother-child interaction patterns (including joint focus, joint actions, and turn taking), we saw the potential of yet another continuum relationship existing between nonverbal interaction patterns and the verbal interaction patterns of conversation. In fact, we were quite late in seeing this potential, because it had already been noted by several others including Bateson (1971), who applied the term *proto-conversations* to the vocal interactions between mothers and children; Bruner (1975), who discussed the young child's "routines for assuring joint reference"; and Kendon (1967), who applied the term *dialogic exchange* to the interactional gaze patterns of the caregiver-infant dyad.

In our applications of pragmatics to severely language deficient clients, then, we have incorporated both the data that characterize the nonverbal "dyadic interaction" patterns (Moerk, 1977) carried out between young children and their caregivers and those data that quantify later patterns of discourse or conversation. We have found that these data yield additional taxonomies for designing both assessment and treatment targets for severely language deficient clients. Both nonverbal dyadic interaction skills and discourse skills reflect a competence for social exchange and interaction that is critical to communication and language acquisition. In a sense, such dyadic patterns provide the envelope within which both communicative and speech acts are issued and their effects realized. The discourse rules that govern linguistic exchanges make demands that are not placed on nonlinguistic exchanges. Thus, the argument against nonlinguistic to linguistic continuity may obtain in this domain as well as in speech acts. It should be noted, however, that nonlinguistic communicative acts and dyadic interaction patterns may well create the interactive envelopes that are critical to the acquisition of both linguistic responses and eventual specific conversational devices (Bruner, 1975; Ratner & Bruner, 1978). Without such an envelope, social acts are out of context and, in fact, are difficult to construct. It is important, then, to observe the performance of severely mentally retarded clients in their interactions and to attempt to ascertain their competence to create and maintain these patterns of social interaction by either verbal and/or nonverbal means. The details and applications of these taxonomies to severely mentally retarded clients will also be considered in a later section of this chapter.

## Summary of Potentially Applicable Pragmatic Elements

All of the foregoing discussion has been intended to highlight those aspects of the broad and complex field of pragmatics that have appeared pertinent and functional in designing both descriptive and prescriptive assessment and treatment for severely language deficient children and youth. The application of these assessments has provided us with the potential for obtaining much richer data regarding both the communicative performance and the competence of our mentally retarded clients. We would like, now, to share the results of some beginning applications of these elements. In doing so, we should note these applications are just beginning—not only in our own work but in the work of many others. As a result, many of the findings that we will be discussing are unpublished, and many of our speculations at this point are only that—speculations. We think, however, that it is important to begin to share such clinical experience and its implications for this population of severely communicatively handicapped children and youth. We find many past descriptions of the communicative behaviors of severely mentally retarded persons to be both narrowly focused on linguistic forms and overgeneralized across varying levels of mental retardation. Thus, there is much that we might learn about people suffering mental retardation and about communication if we were to apply the pragmatic perspectives and elements that we have highlighted in the preceding sections of this chapter.

## APPLICATIONS TO ASSESSMENT AND TREATMENT

As we have noted previously, a model of human language that includes pragmatics stands in contrast to previous idealized and reductionistic models which described language only in terms of its form and the relationship of that form to certain objective stimuli. A model that includes the pragmatics of language would at least recognize the psychological states and processes that must underlie the production of specific speech acts. The treatment generated by such a model would be two-dimensional, with one dimension focused on the appropriate cognitive and/or psychological underpinnings of sociocommunicative acts per se and the other dimension focused directly on the psychological processes required for acquisition of the appropriate highly specialized linguistic forms of such acts. Since initial communicative forms could be prelinguistic, a relatively robust communicative system might be attained long before clients attained linguistically appropriate forms.

The possibility of being able to attain a nonlinguistic, but socially effective, communicative repertoire with severely language deficient clients has important clinical implications for such clients. In addition to the opportunity to exploit the immediate social utility of such a repertoire, there is the added potential that such a repertoire might enhance the possibilities that a higher level linguistic repertoire might also be attained. The semantic revolution fueled by Bloom (1970), Bowerman (1973), and Slobin (1973) emphasized a process of linguistic form "mapping onto" already existing child knowledge. It seems at least a possibility that higher level linguistic speech acts might also map onto previously existing nonlinguistic communicative acts. This mapping possibility does not require one to assume that nonlinguistic forms and linguistic forms reflect continuity in their development. Even though one might consider that linguistic learning is different from nonlinguistic learning, the presence of an already established competence in social communication might still be viewed as having potential positive effects in facilitating the acquisition of linguistic response forms to carry out such established functions. In fact, such a facilitating function is implicit in the developmental data that document a steady process of conventionalization and escalation of communicative form to encode a rather consistent repertoire of social functions among normally developing children (Bates, 1976; Bates et al., 1975; Sugarman, 1984; Sugarman-Bell, 1978).

As we have also noted previously, such implications seem to be far-reaching and deserving of rigorous empirical testing, especially among populations of severely language deficient children and youth. The task at hand, then, is to begin to test the validity of pragmatic elements in terms of their specific productivity when applied to the assessment and treatment of severely language deficient clients. This task requires three distinct operations: (a) The elements of pragmatics that have been identified as being potentially clinically useful need to be operationalized in behavioral taxonomies that can be objectively measured; (b) behaviors included in these taxonomies need to be sampled in the topic population; and (c) the results of these samples need to be analyzed and interpreted in terms of what they might indicate about a client's competence to act communicatively. The products of these operations could, in turn, guide the identification of both general and specific treatment goals, treatment procedures, and treatment contexts. We begin this process in the remaining sections of this chapter.

The three major dimensions of pragmatics discussed previously are productive of many elements for application to our topic population. These elements are not mutually exclusive and, in application, are observed to be interactive in many ways. Thus, the elements of pragmatics that we apply come from all three of the dimensions already identified; namely, speech act theory and performatives; products and processes of speech act acquisition; and discourse skills.

Those researchers studying child language from a pragmatics perspective have tended to specify the behaviors that constitute speech acts and discourse devices and to sample their occurrence in the repertoires of various subjects. When such behaviors have been consistently observed across many subjects, these researchers have assumed that the psychological bases for such behaviors are indeed extant and can be inferred from the observed behaviors. Bruner (1983) takes such a psychological model position and suggests that observed pragmatic competence in a speaker reflects the speaker's "orientation to social reality" in communicative contexts. Thus, the speaker's communicative behaviors are in resonance with the communicative rules for his or her culture. Ideally, such a view would suggest that by sampling and analyzing the communicative behaviors of severely language deficient clients suffering mental retardation, we might draw some conclusions about their knowledge of sociocommunicative reality and, thus, the communicative conventions of society, including the specialized behavioral forms used in carrying out these conventions. Even further, it seems reasonable to assume that some conclusions about what such clients know about the communicative process might be highly prescriptive in the selection of treatment goals and the design of procedures for attaining those goals.

From this perspective, there are four initial questions about their knowledge base for communication and language that are both important and possible to "ask" severely mentally retarded clients, many of whom may be nonverbal. We offer these questions below with each identified initially by the element of pragmatics from which it has been derived, and then we discuss each of the questions in terms of the taxonomies available for asking them. These four questions are:

1. *Communicative Intentions*: Do such clients' current communicative behaviors demonstrate that they understand their ability to have effects on other people?
2. *Signal Level of Intentional Speech Acts*: If intentional, do such clients understand that there are several types of specific and specialized behavioral forms that can be used to have these effects?
3. *Performatives*: Do such clients' intentional communicative repertoires demonstrate that they understand that there are several different types of effects that they can have on other people around them?
4. *Dyadic Interactions and Discourse*: Do the behaviors of such clients demonstrate that they understand that social interactions in general, and communicative behaviors in particular, follow a pattern of reciprocal, turn-taking responses around a referent or topic that is jointly shared with a receiver and, additionally, that this referent or topic is routinely maintained for several turns in the interaction?

We have begun to ask these questions of severely language deficient clients who are classified as severely mentally retarded. In the following sections, we identify the taxonomies from pragmatics theory and data that serve in asking the questions. We also discuss some of the preliminary data that have come from these applications in our research setting.

## Communicative Intentionality

In assessing communicative intentions, we have found the three-level taxonomy offered by Bates et al. (1975) to be directly applicable. As noted previously, Bates and her colleagues have used terminology from Austin's (1962) speech act theory to classify three stages in the emergence of intentional communicative responses among normally developing infants. The first of these is the *perlocutionary* stage, in which adults assign communicative intent to infant behaviors that carry no apparent intent on the part of the child. Thus, adult caregivers assign intent to generalized behavioral states such as fussing, hand sucking, smiling, or excitation and respond in accordance with the intents that they have thus assigned. Later, as both Bates et al. (1975) and Sugarman-Bell (1978) report, children begin to direct their action behaviors to adults and often alternate their attention and actions between their adult receivers and some referent object or event. Such coordinated attentions between referents and receivers allow communicative intentions on the part of the child to be reliably observed at this point. Bates et al. refer to this stage, in which communicative intentions can be reliably judged, as the *illocutionary* stage. A final stage, in which specific linguistic response forms emerge and are used to carry the intent of a child's act, is labeled the *locutionary* stage.

In our applications we have maintained this specialized terminology for classifying levels of communicative intentionality among language deficient subjects, because it functions to emphasize that we are classifying only *communicative* behaviors. This terminology thus reduces the potential for confusing intentional communication behaviors with other purposeful (but noncommunicative) motor acts. Table 10.1 shows this taxonomy and the behavioral criteria that we use to determine which stage best characterizes a client's communicative acts.

In working with nonverbal clients, we find it useful to describe and classify those behaviors that can be reliably observed as being directed toward, and intended to have effects on, other people. It seems logical to assume that a client who does not emit some behaviors that appear to

**TABLE 10.1**

**Emergence of Communicative Intentionality**

| Stage/Level | Child Behavior | Adult Behavior |
|---|---|---|
| *Perlocutionary* | Single focus on object or person; no communicative intent apparent | Assigns "intent" to behaviors observed |
| *Illocutionary* | Alternating or dual focus on referent object and adult; behavior directed at receiver; behavior persistent | "Reads" intent and responds in kind |
| *Locutionary* | Specialized communicative form (e.g., linguistic) | Decodes message and responds |

Adapted from Austin (1962); Bates, Camaioni, & Volterra, (1975); Bates, (1976)

"map" communicative intentions has little basis for specific linguistic training. This view is disputed by the behaviorists' "remedial logic" model (e.g., Guess, Sailor, & Baer, 1977), which denies the possibility of being able to identify preverbal prerequisites to speech and/or linguistic responses and, therefore, suggests that only the end behaviors of language (i.e., linguistic utterances) be targeted in treatment programs.

Another criticism of attempts to assess the presence of communicative intentionality also comes generally from behaviorists. Specifically, some behaviorists may challenge the assumption that one can observe or assess an "inside" event like communicative intentions. The data offered by Bates et al. (1975), Carpenter et al. (1983), and Sugarman-Bell (1978) appear to be reliable in identifying responses that at least can be consistently labeled by mature speakers as intentional communicative acts among normally developing children. Our own experience, and that of colleagues like Cirrin and Rowland (1985), indicates that communicative intentions can also be reliably judged among severely language deficient, nonverbal clients. To attain this interjudge reliability, we have used the coordinated attention between a referent and a receiver as a primary criterion for assigning intentionality to a response. In addition, we apply secondary, corroborating criteria such as proximity, receiver directionality, persistence in a behavior, and cessation of the behavior upon the meeting of the assumed intent. In making such judgments, the topography of the intentional communicative signal is also considered. The factor of signal level has implications beyond just the issue of identification of intentional communicative responses, however, and it will be discussed in more depth in the following section.

Clearly, the key judgment at this initial level of testing with severely language deficient, nonverbal clients is between *perlocutionary* levels of behavior, which have no apparent speaker intentions underlying them, and *illocutionary* levels, in which speaker intentions can be reliably classified. By applying the classifications and general criteria shown in Table 10.1, we are effectively asking clients about their understanding of their ability to have effects on others.

The methods used in investigations of intentionality with severely language deficient subjects generally follow procedures patterned after those used by Snyder (1975) in her research with normal and language delayed children. A situation is baited with a collection of objects and a person carrying out various routines with the objects. The objects and the routines carried out with them are designed to be both appealing and inviting to the subjects. In the interactive situation, there are critical breaks in the routines which both invite and allow subjects to issue some communicative act. Any such communicative acts by subjects are counted and described. Later, the acts are analyzed from videotapes and classified as to their performative class at the speech act level and the discourse level (Chapman, 1981).

Investigations in our setting have provided data that suggest high variability in such intentional communicative act behaviors among populations of severely language deficient adolescents suffering severe mental retardation. For example, we studied one sample of 15 such subjects, originally selected because they were never observed to use any spoken or signed words in spontaneous communication and therefore could be classified as nonverbal. Following a classroom intervention phase, in which teaching staff were instructed to increase both opportunities for and responsiveness to communicative acts, we observed these subjects in two baited interactive sessions. Our data indicated that all subjects issued some behaviors that could be reliably classified as *illocutionary* using one or more of the criteria identified above but specifically including coordinated attention to both an object or action-event and a receiver (Cirrin & Rowland, 1985; McLean, Snyder-McLean, & Cirrin, 1981). Some of these intentional repertoires were extremely fragile and in some instances consisted of only five such responses in two 20-minute sessions. In other instances, however, the intentional repertoires were extremely robust, with one subject issuing 209 such communicative acts in the two sessions in the baited context.

The presence of such intentional or illocutionary communicative acts among severely handicapped, nonverbal clients indicates that they may have at least some minimal understanding of their ability to have effects on other people. The availability of such an understanding could provide the keystone to treatment aimed at making this response class of intentional acts directed toward other people more robust among some clients and at escalating the level of specialized communicative responses among other of these clients. We discuss both the elements and the direction of such treatment in the next section as we look at the signal levels represented among the members of this population.

## Signal Level of Intentional Communicative Acts

Our second question related to whether or not severely language deficient clients indicate that they understand that many special behaviors are available for encoding intentional communicative acts. The data obtained in our setting (Cirrin & Rowland, 1985; McLean et al., 1981) revealed that these 15 subjects exhibited a wide range of signal behaviors. The nature of these varying signal levels appears to be significant from both a theoretical and a treatment perspective.

Specifically, these data indicated that our 15 subjects could be classified into three distinctly different groups in terms of the level of their intentional communicative signal behaviors (McLean et al., 1981). First, 7 of the 15 subjects emitted signals that consisted primarily of simple action schemata directed toward both people and objects. These schemata included actions such as reaching toward a desired object; a pulling-away motion from people or objects; contact gestures in which the object was used in a gesture (e.g., proffering a cup); and actions on people such as tugging at them or placing another person's hand on an object.

A second level of nonverbal action schemata was observed among 6 subjects in this sample of 15. This second level of signal consisted of subject repertoires that, in addition to the primitive action schemata and contact gestures described above, also contained gestures that were "decontextualized" in that they did not include specific contact with an object or person. In many cases these gestures were accompanied by intonated vocalizations. The distal point was a highly significant gesture, because it was the presence of this gesture that most clearly identified those subjects whose signal levels had moved away from the more primitive action schemata and into fuller repertoires of more conventionalized and specialized communicative signal levels. In addition, some subjects that we included in this level produced a few (less than 5) highly ritualized and stimulus-bound words or proto-words. These generally took the form of food-related manual signs (e.g., *eat* and *drink*) that were produced only in the presence of some food or drink and that generally had long histories of conditioning in previous training programs.

Still a third level of signal was emitted by 2 of the 15 subjects included in the study. At this third level, communicative repertoires included more than 5 standard manual signs, which were used in spontaneous and nonritualized communication, as well as many decontextualized conventional gestures. Further, and significantly we think, these subjects showed extremely low rates of the primitive action repertoires observed in other subjects in the sample. The quantitative differences of the communicative repertoires of subjects at these three levels appeared to be quite clear-cut, and they served to "trichotomize" our subject sample. We have chosen to classify these three levels of subjects for further research and clinical use. The behavioral criteria for these three levels of communicative signals are shown in Table 10.2. We have classified these three differential levels as *primitive, conventionalized,* and *referential*.

The taxonomy presented in Table 10.2 specifies these three levels and describes the criterion behaviors that we have been applying for placing clients in each level. By describing and clustering the types of behaviors that our clients use in their encoding of intentional communicative acts, we hope, eventually, to be able to draw some conclusions about the processes that are functioning for them in their acquisition of an effective repertoire of sociocommunicative behaviors. Interestingly, it appears that this taxonomy will direct us to more questions about symbolic processes than strictly social ones.

TABLE 10.2

**Three Intentional Communicative Signal Levels Observed In Severely Retarded Subjects**

| Primitive Act | Conventionalized Act | Referential |
|---|---|---|
| Gestures with object (e.g., proffers cup to request more) | Request gesture (open palm without object in hand) | Single word utterances (5 or more; accurate phonological/manual form, single word responses used in spontaneous, nonritualized interactions) |
| Acts on object (e.g., tries to unscrew lid on jar with alternating attention to adult) | Show gesture (offers object but does not give it up) | Multi-word utterances (word forms co-occur) |
| Acts on adult (e.g., takes adult's hand and places on jar lid) | Give gesture (offers object and allows taking) | Grammatical utterances word order; grammatical) |
| Pulls away (to signal "no" or to protest) | Point gesture (extends finger—no contact with object) | |
| Vocalizations | Wave gesture (bye-bye or hello) | |
| | Nodding or No gesture | |
| | Intonated vocalizations (with or without other actions/ gestures) | |
| | Proto-words (e.g., consistent phonological form or gesture, single word responses [fewer than 5] in repertoire) | |

The data from investigations in our setting to this point indicate that the topographies of the communicative acts of three distinctly differing types of severely language deficient children and youth are still of the same genre as those reported in the descriptions of emerging communicative acts among normally developing infants and young children reported by such investigators as Bates et al. (1975) and Bates (1976). That is, the communicative responses of a population of adolescents suffering severe mental retardation include primitive actions; refined action schemes; standard gestural repertoires; and, finally, nonverbal equivalents of words (manual signs and proto-words). In addition to demonstrating signal types similar to those observed in normally developing children, these severely retarded subjects also demonstrated hierarchical clustering reminiscent of the normal developmental processes of decontextualization and coventionalization. Thus, the levels characterized as primitive, conventional, and referential appear to be ordinal in that subjects classified as *conventional* might occasionally use some primitive signals (though they rarely did so); whereas the reverse pattern was never observed.

Because these signal-type clusters were relatively exclusive, and because each succeeding cluster was a progression on the preceding one, it seems reasonable to consider that the same processes that appear to operate in the acquisition of communicative signals among normally developing young children may also obtain in a population of severely handicapped clients. That is, the differences among the three classes of signals exhibited by members of our sample reflect a process of both *conventionalization* (i.e., a move from primitive actions to conventional gestures and thence to true signs) and *decontextualization* (i.e., a move from actions with objects and people to actions/gestures distanced from objects and people). Clearly, more research is needed in this general area. This finding does suggest, however, that some aspects of a pragmatic model lead directly to speculations about the role of cognition in these apparent processes among severely retarded individuals, parallel to such speculations in considerations of pragmatics and language development among normally developing children (e.g., Bates, 1976, 1979). These perspectives on the differential functioning of the conventionalization and decontextualization processes among severely mentally retarded subjects also lead directly to the questions being raised by investigators of normal language acquisition about whether there is continuity among nonlinguistic communicative behaviors and linguistic forms (Bloom, 1983; Shatz, 1983; Sugarman, 1984).

When the data on both intentionality and signal levels are integrated, the result is a taxonomy that provides a dual matrix for classifying the basic communicative status of severely language deficient clients. This matrix allows the three-level classification of communicative acts to be expanded to six sublevels which reflect important quantitative as well as qualitative differences. Table 10.3 shows this summary taxonomy, which we have found to be helpful in describing the differential levels exhibited in our population of clients suffering severe mental retardation. Similar matrices have been suggested by others working with both developmentally young children and other severely language delayed populations (e.g., Prutting, 1979; Seibert & Hogan, 1982).

Apparently, the taxonomies derived from the developmental literature that describe and classify both the products and processes observed in the emergence of intentionality and communicative forms among normally developing children can be productively applied to highly atypical populations. Such applications suggest, for example, that severely language deficient clients do not demonstrate communicative

**TABLE 10.3**

**Dual Matrix for Classifying Clients: Levels of Communicative Intentionality and Conventionality of Signals**

| Stage/Level | Behavior | Adult-Assigned Meaning |
|---|---|---|
| *Perlocutionary* | | |
| Reactive | "Fussing" vocalization or excitation | What's wrong? What can I do for you? |
| | Regards/attends to entity or event of interest | What do you see? I see the bus, too. See the people in it? |
| | Laughs aloud in response to playful action with adult | Do you like that? Want more? I'll do it again. |
| Proactive | Tries to get food by reaching response | You're hungry! Well, let's eat. Here's your sandwich. |
| *Illocutionary* | | |
| Primitive | Holds up object and extends it toward adult | What do you have there—a new radio? Shall we turn it on? |
| | Alternates visual regard from adult to desired puzzle | Do you want that puzzle? Okay, I'll get it for you. |
| | Pulls person to desired activity | Do you want me to come? Okay, let's go. |
| Conventional | Hands cup to adult, points to refrigerator, vocalizes with inflection | More juice? You want more. More juice, okay. Here's more juice. |
| *Locutionary* | | |
| Emerging | Says, "Help"; Holds up gloves | Want me to help? Okay. I'll help put the gloves on. |
| Conventional | Says, "Help me with my gloves." | OK, I'll help you. Can you say please? |

Adapted from Austin (1962); Bates, Camaioni, & Volterra (1975); McLean, Snyder-McLean, & Sack (1982) forms that are deviant from those observed at various points along the developmental continuum followed by normal children. The data, at this point at least, also indicate that the general sequence of signal form development observed in normal development obtains in cases of severe language deficiency. While there are obvious quantitative differences in the behaviors of normally developing children and severely language deficient subjects at these various levels, such general concordance in acquisition products and processes suggests that it might prove feasible to design treatment approaches that follow the patterns demonstrated by normally developing children rather than to create arbitrary sequences for application to severely language deficient clients. Certainly, such a hypothesis deserves a rigorous empirical testing effort.

## Communicative Effects and Functions

Our third question in the application of the pragmatics model relates to the understanding severely language deficient clients have about the functions or performative classes that are characteristic of human communicative systems. The functions that are routinely carried out through speech acts in Western cultures have been classified in several taxonomies. Most notable among these have been those offered by Chapman (1981), Dore (1975), Searle (1969), and Halliday (1975). Probably the most important attribute of human language functions offered by these researchers is that they specify the social aspects of speech acts and thus remove them from the limited perspective of their relationship to archetypical referents. Notions of language functions rendered almost exclusively in terms of their referent relationships have limited the teaching of language to endless lists of object names, verbs, and color names. The need to assess the functions of speech acts at multiple levels, including the functions that are specific to discourse, is basic to a pragmatics approach to language assessment (Chapman, 1981). In this context, then, Table 10.4 offers a simple taxonomy of language functions that we have used in investigations with severely language deficient children and youth suffering severe mental retardation. It is important to observe the communicative functions reflected in the communicative acts of such clients and to determine whether or not their repertoires reflect the range and types of functions that are characteristic of normal speakers and, thus, are adequate for normal social environments or contexts.

Again, investigations in our setting have provided interesting preliminary data regarding the performatives that are reflected in the communicative responses of our original population of 15 severely mentally retarded, nonverbal subjects as well as a more recent sample of 18 similar subjects. These data on performatives again reflect quantitative and

**TABLE 10.4**

**Categories of Communicative Functions Used in Research with Severely Retarded Subjects**

*Request Object*: Seeks the receipt of a specific object from the listener where the child awaits a response.The object may be out of reach due to some physical barrier.

*Request Action*: Seeks the performance of an action by the listener where the child awaits a response. The child may specify the action (e.g., "sit"), or the child's immediately preceding behavior gives evidence that he or she realizes that some action is a necessary step to obtaining some object (e.g., signaling "help" to open a jar).

*Protest*: An indication that the speaker opposes or disapproves of the listener's behavior or action.

*Direct Attention to Self*: Direction of listener's attention to the child himself or herself as a general attention-getter for some unspecified social purpose.

*Direct Attention for Communication*: Direction of listener's attention to self as a preface to another communicative behavior that follows immediately.

*Direct Attention to Object*: Direction of listener's attention to an external, observable referent or some object identified by the child. This includes the speaker taking notice of an object or labeling an object in absence of a request.

*Direct Attention to Action*: Direction of listener's attention to an ongoing action or event in the environment. The focus may be the movement or action of an object rather than the object itself. A "comment" on some ongoing activity.

*Answer*: A communicative response from a child to a request for information from the adult listener. This typically takes the form of indicating a choice or answering a question.

*Request Other*: Seeks information, approval, or permission from the listener where the child awaits a response. This includes directing the listener to provide specific information about an object, action, or location.

Adapted from "Communicative Assessment of Nonverbal Youths with Severe, Profound Mental Retardation" by F. M. Cirrin & C. M. Rowland, 1985, *Mental Retardation*, *23*, 52-62.

qualitative differences among the repertoires of different members of this subject sample. Again, these differences appear to cluster subjects. In fact, when we consider both the number of function types and the frequency of use by various subjects, these data cluster subjects into the identical groups created by the signal level data. Thus, there are clear differences in the number, types, and frequency of various performative classes among subjects classified *primitive*, conventional, or referential in accordance with their signal levels. It is important to note, however, that the major differences in this domain were evidenced in the comparison of the *primitive* group with both the *conventional* and the *referential* groups.

The predominant functions carried in the communicative acts of the group classified as *primitive* were requests for objects, requests for actions, and protests. When we move to the group classified as *conventional* and *referential* in their communicative forms, we found that directing attention to objects was a more frequent function than requests for objects or actions. The overall pattern of subjects classified as *referential* was basically the same as that demonstrated by those subjects classified as *conventional*. Figure 10.1 shows the relative frequencies for all functions for all three groups. This general pattern of differential proportions of communicative functions was replicated in a sequel study that we have recently completed (details are available from the authors), which involved a greater number of *referential* and *conventional* subjects in slightly more structured communication assessment sessions.

Because of space limitations in this reporting format, we will not discuss these data in any detail. We simply note what we consider an important difference between the *primitive* group and the other two groups; namely, that the *primitive* group's performatives were dominated by imperatives, while the other two groups showed a robust repertoire of declarative-type functions (i.e., directing attention of others as opposed to requesting objects and actions). In fact, no subject classified in the *primitive* group in our original study displayed a purely declarative function that we could identify with certainty. However, the *primitive* subjects' lack of a conventionalized point gesture need not preclude the expression of a declarative. After all, very young, normally developing children express declaratives by their gaze behaviors and their contact gestures with objects. Our current conclusions from these findings are that, while children at a *primitive illocutionary* level do understand their ability to affect other people, they do not reflect the full range of communicative functions generic to truly social exchanges which involve other people in ongoing interaction episodes. As is demonstrated in the succeeding section, such a speculation would be borne out by the general dyadic interaction patterns that characterize subjects in the *primitive* group.

In summary, we can see again that severely language deficient clients classified as severely mentally retarded demonstrate considerable heterogeneity in their apparent understanding of the functions of communicative acts. Both the *conventional* and the *referential* groups showed a relatively full range of functions. The group of subjects classified as *primitive* in their communicative forms, however, showed severe constraints in their representations of the functions that are characteristic of human communication repertoires. As we make this point, we must avoid

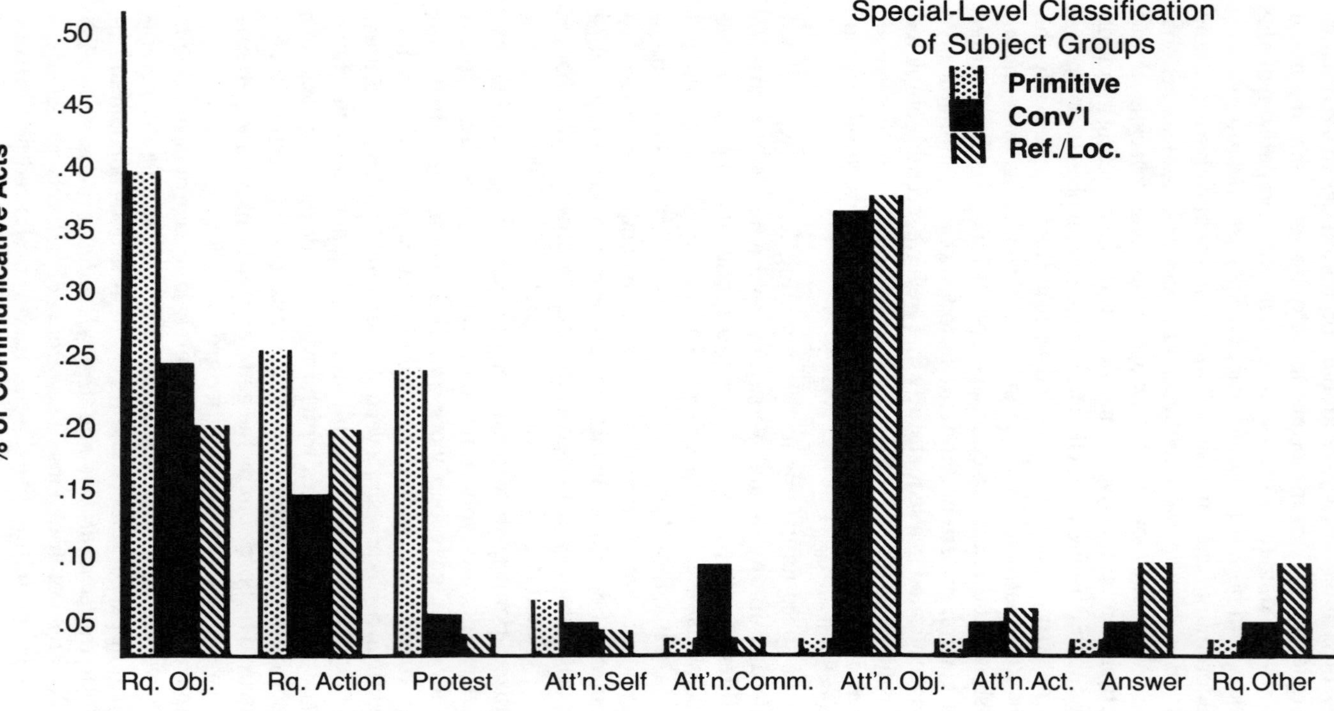

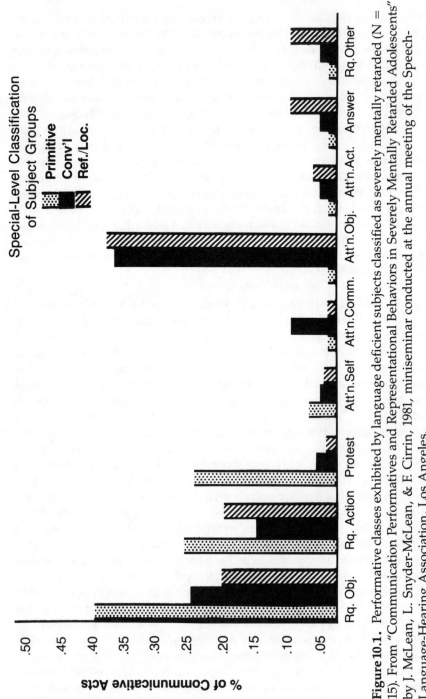

**Figure 10.1.** Performative classes exhibited by language deficient subjects classified as severely mentally retarded (N = 15). From "Communication Performatives and Representational Behaviors in Severely Mentally Retarded Adolescents" by J. McLean, L. Snyder-McLean, & F. Cirrin, 1981, miniseminar conducted at the annual meeting of the Speech-Language-Hearing Association, Los Angeles.

giving the counterimpression that our higher communicative groups were fully competent communicative agents; they were not. Their overall realization forms were limited; their grammar-form levels were extremely low or nonexistent; and their general patterns of interaction were still highly atypical. However, they did indicate that they understood that their specialized communicative behaviors could function in many ways and that many of these ways were specific to the human penchant for social interaction.

The obvious treatment implications of these findings would be reflected in attempts to increase the numbers and types of performatives expressed by severely language deficient clients. A successful demonstration of just such an attempt has been reported by Reichle, Rogers, and Barrett (1984), who trained the discriminative production of a *request*, a *rejection*, and a *comment* with a severely mentally retarded adolescent girl.

## Dyadic Interaction Patterns

Our fourth and final question for guiding pragmatic applications with severely language deficient clients pertains to the investigation of such clients' understanding of the general reciprocal and cooperative patterns that characterize human social and communicative interactions. As we noted previously, our interest in general human interaction patterns extends from Grice's (1975) "conversational maxims" to Moerk's (1977) nonverbal "dyadic interaction" patterns. The taxonomy that we have derived for clinical application in this domain is shown in Table 10.5. The elements of interaction listed in this taxonomy are observed early in the social and communicative development of normal children and are still present in the patterns of linguistic discourse among mature language users. This, then, is another area in which development occurs along a continuum from nonlinguistic to linguistic behaviors and which, therefore, has important potential for applications to our topic population.

Although we do not have formal data and analyses of these dyadic behaviors from the investigations that we have been describing, we do have some distinct impressions and general descriptions from this experience that we shall discuss. As the reader might anticipate, we did observe quantitative and qualitative differences in the dyadic interaction patterns of subjects classified as *primitive* when compared to those subjects classified in either the *conventional* group or the *referential* group. Among members of the group classified as *primitive*, we generally observed low representation of these interaction patterns. Most often, joint focus was fleeting, and turn-taking and turn-filling patterns were quite short-lived or nonexistent. In interacting with subjects in the *primitive* group, we had the overwhelming impression that these individuals were not robustly

**TABLE 10.5**

**Dyadic Interaction Skills**

*Preverbal*
- Attend to other person
- Attend to/maintain joint focus of interaction
- Fill turn (adjacency)
- Fill turn with relevant response (contextually contingent)
- Initiate interaction/evoke attention of other
- Establish joint focus/direct other's attention to entity or event

*Early Discourse Skills*
- Adjacency (fill your turn and wait your turn)
- Contextual/linguistic contingency (talk about joint topic)
- Contextual presuppositions (don't talk about obvious)

Reprinted with permission from *A transactional approach to early language training: A mediated program for inservice professionals* by J. E. McLean, L. Snyder-McLean, & S. Sack (1982). Columbus, OH: Charles Merrill.

"social." Such an impression is consistent with all of the other pragmatic elements that we have examined with these subjects. The reader will recall that subjects in this group had primarily imperative communicative functions.

In contrast, subjects classified as either *conventional* or *referential* appeared to be more "socialized." Generally, individuals in these two groups shared a focus; took and filled turns; initiated new shared focuses; and maintained a ritualized interactive pattern for some period of time. Interestingly, however, in our experience with these subjects, it was only the subjects classified as *referential*, and who thus had symbolic communicative forms, who provided the highest levels of socialization in that their behavior episodes reflected humor and high levels of playfulness. These observations that subjects who demonstrate higher symbolic levels in their communicative signals also demonstrate higher levels in their dyadic interaction patterns again suggest that the social aspects of human interaction and communication must be viewed as critically linked with certain elements of the cognitive processes.

The treatment implications in the dyadic interaction area are straightforward and are beginning to be represented in a number of clinical programs. The first such implication is that the elements of dyadic interaction should be targeted in all social contexts. The establishment and maintenance of common focuses for interactions can be targeted in any and every interaction routine—verbal or nonverbal. Maintenance of focus appears also to be generic and thus productive at any interactive or communicative level, as are turn taking and turn filling. All such skills will help a handicapped client function more appropriately in social contexts. Any of these skills acquired in nonverbal social routines can be extended to any later verbal repertoires that might be attained.

The second major implication of work in the area of dyadic interaction skills is reflected in the strong move toward training communicative repertoires in social contexts. This trend has multiple roots ranging from Bruner's (1975) look at the social ontogenesis of language to philosophical bases established in Wittgenstein's (1958) notions of the "language game" as playable only in context. This in situ training trend is obvious in the work of language treatment specialists of all schools of thought from psycholinguists like Snow (1984) to behaviorists like Kaiser and Warren (Chapter 16 of this volume), Halle (1984), and Hart (1981) and eclectic speech pathologists and special educators like Creaghead (1984), Culatta (1984), and McLean and Snyder-McLean (1984a, 1984b). All such social training contexts teach communication within "routines" that model and reinforce the patterns of interaction that characterize both discourse and nonverbal exchanges (e.g., Snyder-McLean, Solomonson, McLean, & Sack, 1984). The data on such approaches are now beginning to appear, and the results to date are highly encouraging.

## SUMMARY AND CONCLUSIONS

We began this chapter with an observation that language is being returned to its users, and we identified the psychological model of pragmatics as a master-model for such a perspective. In the remainder of the chapter, we identified and operationalized those elements of the overall pragmatics model that have high potential for being productive in the assessment and treatment of severely language deficient clients classified as severely mentally retarded. In reviewing the preliminary data obtained in applications of the various taxonomies available in pragmatics to a small sample of such a population, we have shown that such applications are both appropriate and productive.

We can (and have) learned much about the communicative systems of seriously handicapped persons through the applications of this model. We have seen evidence that suggests that severely language deficient clients can have reliably identifiable communicative intentions and that these intentions are encoded in a wide range of signal behaviors that are not atypical of those signal behaviors observed among individuals who acquire language normally. We have seen that certain of our subjects demonstrated extremely constrained communicative functions and that others of them displayed a near normal range of such communicative functions. We also described our impressions of the general interactive, social-skill patterns observed among our topic population. We stated that we found many such handicapped children to be sorely lacking in appropriate interactive skill patterns and others to be at least minimally competent at nonverbal or emerging verbal levels.

We should emphasize here that, despite all these generally positive descriptive data from our severely handicapped subjects, none of these subjects provided communicative repertoires and patterns that would qualify them as even approaching competence as mature human communicators. Even our *referential* clients, who showed relatively full repertoires of communicative functions and symbolic level signals, did not come near the communicative competence of a normal 3-year-old child. The critical question for us, then, is whether we can discover the means to effectively raise the overall competence of clients like those we have been discussing by focusing more on communication and language in their relationships to their human users. And, in better describing the seriously deficient levels of communicative competence that exist among certain of our fellows, can we learn more about this behavior that builds and maintains our social systems and allows us to have effects on the conditions of our existence?

## REFERENCES

Andersen, E. S. (1977). *Learning to speak with style: A study of the sociolinguistic skills of children*. Unpublished doctoral dissertation, Stanford University, Stanford, CA.

Austin, J. L. (1962). *How to do things with words*. London: Oxford University Press.

Bates, E. (1976). *Language and context*. New York: Academic Press.

Bates, E. (1979). *The emergence of symbols: Cognition and communication in infancy*. New York: Academic Press.

Bates, E., Camaioni, L., Volterra, V. (1975). The acquisition of performatives prior to speech. *Merrill-Palmer Quarterly, 21*, 205– 226.

Bateson, M. C. (1971, January). *The interpersonal context of infant vocalizations*. Quarterly Progress Report, Research Laboratory of Electronics, Massachusetts Institute of Technology, No. 100, 170–176.

Bloom, L. (1970). *Language development: Form and function in emerging grammars*. Cambridge, MA: MIT Press.

Bloom, L., (1983). Discussion of continuity and discontinuity, and the magic of language development. In R. M. Golinkoff (Ed.), *The transition from prelinguistic to linguistic communication* (pp. 79–92). Hillsdale, NJ: Lawrence Erlbaum.

Bowerman, M. F. (1973). *Learning to talk: A cross-linguistic comparison of early syntactic development, with special reference to Finnish*. London: Cambridge University Press.

Bruner, J. S. (1975). The ontogenesis of speech acts. *Journal of Child Language, 2*, 1–19.

Bruner, J. (1983). The acquisition of pragmatic commitments. In R. M. Golinkoff (Ed.), *The transition from prelinguistic to linguistic communication* (pp. 27–42). Hillsdale, NJ: Lawrence Erlbaum.

Carpenter, R. L., Mastergeorge, A. M., & Coggins, T. E. (1983). The acquisition of communicative intentions in infants eight to fifteen months of age. *Language and Speech, 26*, Part 2, 101–116.

Chapman, R. S. (1981). Exploring children's communicative intents. In J. F. Miller, *Assessing language production in children: Experimental procedures* (pp. 111–136). Austin, TX: PRO-ED.

Chomsky, N. (1957). *Syntactic structures*. The Hague: Mouton.

Chomsky, N. A. (1965). *Aspects of the theory of syntax*. Cambridge, MA: MIT Press.

Cirrin, F. M., & Rowland, C. M. (1985). Communicative assessment of nonverbal youths with severe, profound mental retardation. *Mental Retardation, 23*, 52–62.

Craig, H. (1983). Application of pragmatic language models for intervention. In J. Gallagher & C. Prutting (Eds.), *Pragmatic assessment and intervention issues* (pp. 101–127). San Diego: College-Hill Press.

Creaghead, N. A. (1984). Strategies for evaluating and targeting pragmatic behaviors in young children. *Seminars in Speech and Language, 5*(3), 241–252

Culatta, B. (1984). A discourse-based approach to training grammatical rules. *Seminars in Speech and Language, 5*(3), 253–263.

DeLaguna, G. A. (1963). *Speech: Its function and development*. Bloomington, IN: University Press. (First published 1927)

Dore, J. (1975). Holophrases, speech acts and language universals. *Journal of Child Language, 2*, 21–40.

Duchan, J. F. (1984). Language assessment: The pragmatics revolution. In R. C. Naremore (Ed.), *Language science* (pp. 147–180). San Diego: College-Hill Press.

Fillmore, C. (1968). The case for case. In E. Bach & R. T. Harms (Eds.), *Universals in linguistic theory* (pp. 1–88). New York: Holt, Rinehart and Winston.

Gray, B., & Ryan, B. (1973). *A language program for the nonlanguage child*. Champaign, IL: Research Press.

Grice, H. P. (1975). Logic and conversation. In P. Cole & J. L. Morgan (Eds.), *Syntax and semantics: Vol. 3. Speech acts*. New York: Academic Press.

Grossman, H. J. (1983). *Classification in mental retardation*. Washington, DC: American Association on Mental Deficiency.

Guess, D., Sailor, W., & Baer, D. (1974). To teach language to retarded children. In R. L. Schiefelbusch & L. L. Lloyd (Eds.), *Language perspectives—Acquisition, retardation, and intervention* (pp. 529–563). Austin, TX: PRO-ED.

Guess, D., Sailor, W., & Baer, D. (1977). A behavioral-remedial approach to language training for the severely handicapped. In E. Sontag (Ed.), *Educational programming for the severely and profoundly handicapped* (pp. 360–377). Reston, VA: The Council for Exceptional Children.

Halle, J. W. (1984). Arranging the natural environment to occasion language: Giving severely language-delayed children reasons to communicate. *Seminars in Speech and Language, 5*(3), 185–198.

Halliday, M. (1975). Learning how to mean. In E. Lenneberg & E. Lenneberg (Eds.), *Foundations of language development: A multi-disciplinary approach* (Vol. I, pp. 239–265). New York: Academic Press.

Harding, C. G. (1983). Setting the stage for language acquisition: Communication development in the first year. In R. M. Golinkoff (Ed.), *The transition from prelinguistic to linguistic communication* (pp. 93–113). Hillsdale, NJ: Lawrence Erlbaum.

Hart, B. (1981). Pragmatics: How language is used. *Analysis and Intervention in Developmental Disabilities, 1*, 299–313.

Hymes, D. (1971). Competence and performance in linguistic theory. In R. Huxley & E. Ingram (Eds.), *Language acquisition: Models and methods* (pp. 3–23). London: Academic Press.

Ingram, D. (1976). *Phonological disabilities in children*. New York: Elsevier.

Jakobson, R., Fant, C. G. M., & Halle, M. (1963). *Preliminaries to speech analysis: The distinctive features and their correlates* (2nd ed.). Cambridge, MA: MIT Press.

Katz, J. J., & Fodor, J. A. (1963). The structure of a semantic theory. *Language, 39*, 170–210.

Kendon, A. (1967). Some functions of gaze-direction in social interaction. *Acta Psychologica, 26*, 22–63.

Kent, L. R. (1974). *Language acquisition program for the severely retarded*. Champaign, IL: Research Press.

Leonard, L. (1976). *Meaning in child language*. New York: Grune & Stratton.

McLean, J., & Snyder-McLean, L. (1980). Communication disorders associated with mental and behavioral deviations. In R. J. VanHattum (Ed.), *Communication disorders: An introduction* (pp. 463ka-2-508). New York: Macmillan.

McLean, J., & Snyder-McLean, L. (Eds.). (1984a). Strategies of facilitating language development in clinics, schools and homes. *Seminars in Speech and Language, 5*(3), 213–228.

McLean, J., & Snyder-McLean, L. (1984b). Recent developments in pragmatics: Remedial implications. In D. J. Muller (Ed.), *Remediating children's language* (pp. 55–82). San Diego: College-Hill Press.

McLean, J., Snyder-McLean, L., & Cirrin, F. (1981). *Communication performatives and representational behaviors in severely mentally retarded adolescents*. Miniseminar conducted at the annual meeting of the Speech-Language-Hearing Association, Los Angeles.

McLean, J., Snyder-McLean, L., & Sack, S. (1982). *A transactional approach to early language training: A mediated program for inservice professionals*. Columbus, OH: Charles E. Merrill.

Moerk, E. L. (1977). *Pragmatic and semantic aspects of early language development*. Austin, TX: PRO-ED.

Morris, C. (1946). *Signs, language and behavior*. Englewood Cliffs, NJ: Prentice-Hall.

Nihara, K., Foster, R., Shellhaas, M., & Leland, H. (1969). *AAMD Adaptive Behavior Scale: Manual*. Washington, DC: American Association on Mental Deficiency.

Peirce, C. (1932). *Collected papers*. C. Jartshorne & P. Weiss (Eds.). Cambridge, MA: Harvard University Press.

Prutting, C. (1979). Process/prä/ses/n: The action of moving forward progressively from one point to another on the way to completion. *Journal of Speech and Hearing Disorders, 44*, 3–30.

Prutting, C. (1982). Pragmatics as social competence. *Journal of Speech and Hearing Disorders, 47*, 123–133.

Ratner, N., & Bruner, J. (1978). Games, social exchange and the acquisition of language. *Journal of Child Language, 5*, 391–401.

Rees, N. S. (1978). Pragmatics of language. In R. L. Schiefelbusch (Ed.), *Bases of language intervention* (pp. 191–268). Austin, TX: PRO-ED.

Reichle, J., Rogers, N., & Barrett, H. C. (1984). Establishing pragmatic discrimination among the communicative functions of requesting, rejecting, and commenting in an adolescent. *The Journal of the Association for Persons with Severe Handicaps, 9*(1), 31–36.

Rosch, E. H. (1973). On the internal structure of perceptual and semantic categories. In T. E. Moore (Ed.), *Cognitive development and the acquisition of language* (pp. 111–144). New York: Academic Press.

Ruder, K. F., & Smith, M. D. (1974). Issues in language training. In R. L. Schiefelbusch & L. L. Lloyd (Eds.), *Language perspectives—acquisition, retardation, and intervention* (pp. 565–605). Austin, TX: PRO-ED.

Searle, J. R. (1969). *Speech acts: An essay in the philosophy of language*. London: Cambridge University Press.

Seibert, J. M., & Hogan, A. E. (1982). A model for assessing social and object skills and planning intervention. In D. P. McClowry, A. M. Guilford, & S. O. Richardson (Eds.), *Infant communication: Development, assessment, and intervention* (pp. 21–54). New York: Grune & Stratton.

Shatz, M. (1983). On transition, continuity and coupling: An alternative approach to communicative development. In R. M. Golinkoff (Ed.), *Transition for prelinguistic to linguistic communication* (pp. 43–55). Hillsdale, NJ: Lawrence Erlbaum.

Skinner, B. F. (1957). *Verbal behavior*. New York: Appleton-Century-Crofts.

Slobin, D. I. (1973). Cognitive prerequisites for the development of grammar. In D. I. Slobin & C. Ferguson (Eds.), *Studies of child language development* (pp. 175–208). New York: Holt, Rinehart and Winston.

Snow, C. E. (1984). Parent-child interaction and the development of communicative ability. In R. L. Schiefelbusch & J. Pickar (Eds.), *The acquisition of communicative competence* (pp. 69–108). Austin, TX: PRO-ED.

Snyder, L. S. (1975). *Pragmatics in language disabled children: Their prelinguistic and early verbal performatives and presuppositions.* Unpublished doctoral dissertation, University of Colorado.

Snyder-McLean, L., Solomonson, B., McLean, J., & Sack, S. (1984). Structuring joint action routines: A strategy for facilitating communication and language development in the classroom. *Seminars in Speech and Language, 5*(3), 213–228.

Sugarman, S. (1984). The development of preverbal communication: Its contribution and limits in promoting the development of language. In R. L. Schiefelbusch & J. Pickar (Eds.), *The acquisition of communicative competence* (pp. 23–68). Austin, TX: PRO-ED.

Sugarman-Bell, S. (1978). Some organizational aspects or pre-verbal communication. In I. Markova (Ed.), *The social context of language* (pp. 49–66). New York: John Wiley.

Waryas, C., & Stremel-Campbell, K. (1978). Grammatical training for the language delayed child. In R. L. Schiefelbusch (Ed.), *Language intervention strategies* (pp. 145–192). Austin, TX: PRO-ED.
Werner, H., & Kaplan, B. (1963). *Symbol formation*. New York: John Wiley.
Wittgenstein, L. (1958). *Philosophical investigations*. Oxford: Basil, Blackwell & Mott.

SECTION V

# *Assessment*

GERALD M. SIEGEL, EDITOR

# 11

# *Issues in Language Assessment*

GERALD M. SIEGEL

Assessment is at the heart of informed remediation and teaching and provides the basis for determining which aspects of a therapy program are working well, which need revisions, and which may be totally inappropriate. The creative application of assessment methods yields information that is of immediate use to the clinician and client, and also information that adds to the inventory of knowledge the clinician can call on when assisting a new client. At its best, assessment helps the clinician learn about basic principles in the organization of skills and behaviors, as well as guiding the course of instruction for an individual client.

## A CHANGING VIEW OF ASSESSMENT

Numerous issues in assessment remain unresolved and continue to preoccupy teachers, clinicians, and researchers. As concepts concerning the nature of language change, the available instruments must also be changed or redefined to reflect the newer concepts. Commercial testing instruments are not easily altered, especially if they have been carefully standardized to provide a normative basis for comparisons. Informal methods are more readily modified, but these approaches typically don't come with the rich reservoir of normative data that make the standardized tests appealing for some applications. The clinician will also be divided between the need to use new tests that reflect current orientations to language and the desire to retain methods that have proven useful in the past. Language research and theory are currently in flux, and those of us in applied fields cannot help feel a sense of alarm as familiar ground gives way to new theories and models of language. It is not only the process whereby children acquire language that is being scrutinized but the very nature of language itself.

The original *Language Perspectives* volume included topics ranging from speech perception of normal infants to language intervention for the mentally retarded, but it did not contain a section dedicated to assessment. Perhaps that omission reflected the view that all of the topics considered in that volume had implications for assessment in that they raised issues involving measurement, description, and evaluation of some aspect of the data of child language. The clinical practice of speech and language therapy is intertwined with basic developments in theory and research. A future archeologist, digging through the remains of twentieth century special classrooms and speech and hearing clinics, would undoubtedly posit the existence of Chomsky, though he might not be sure whether Chomsky was one person or an entire cult. In either case, the shift from atheoretical, descriptive measures to tests based on a theory of linguistic knowledge would be evident. It would also be evident that the Chomsky edifice was soon altered, and that on these stones there grew new structures of semantics, pragmatics, cognition. The evidence would be there in the heaps of language tests, kits, programs, manuals, and the proliferation of textbooks in education, linguistics, and cognitive psychology, with perhaps some sprinkling of artifacts reflecting primitive applications of computer technology to language testing and remediation.

The measurement chapters in the current book reveal a changing concept of assessment. As Broen points out (Chapter 12 of this volume), assessment is not synonymous with testing but is rather a broader concept that incorporates testing as one form of gathering knowledge about a client's status and needs.

> In an assessment, an attempt is made to understand the performance of an individual in the environment in which that individual functions. It is an evaluative and interpretive appraisal of performance. Information from a variety of sources can be used in an assessment. Some of that information may come from informal, norm-referenced tests, some may come from informational observation; some of the information may be gathered directly by the clinician, and some may come from other individuals; some of the information may be quantitative, and some may be qualitative. An assessment will draw from all available and appropriate sources including parents, teachers, and other professionals and will interpret information relative to the particular questions that are being asked and the particular situation in which the child is found. (Broen, Chap. 12 of this volume)

## COORDINATING ASSESSMENT THEORY AND PRACTICE

It is not enough to use a test battery to rank a child relative to his or her peers. Assessment must be keyed to the clinician's model or theory of language. This implies that the clinician should be able to articulate such a model and to recognize where available commercial tests do or do not fit this model. This view of assessment liberates the clinician from absolute dependence on the test maker's concept of language, but it also imposes an obligation on the clinician to have an alternative concept. Within this framework, it is not only the child's score, but, more important, the content of the child's performance, that concerns the clinician. Assessment becomes integrated with intervention because both proceed from the same underlying model of the nature of language and communication and because the purpose of assessment is not to label or describe the child so much as to describe his or her knowledge, skills, and performance.

Chomsky's views of language have also created some problems for the clinic. His preoccupation with competence, almost to the exclusion of performance, does not square entirely with the clinician's concern for improving the client's communication. Communication involves performance, both in listening and speaking. In an earlier era, when clinicians characterized their work as *articulation* therapy, problems in "carry-over" (generalization) were bemoaned but not unexpected. Now that articulation disorders have become *phonological* disorders, it is harder to understand why the child who has mastered the phonological rules in one setting (e.g., the clinic) should not incorporate those same rules in all settings. The view of misarticulation as representing a failure in underlying knowledge has the effect of characterizing articulatory performance in static forms, since the knowledge is not viewed as fleeting or unstable. Clinicians and teachers have had to step back from unequivocally embracing a knowledge-based approach to language so that the performance components can be kept in view. Even though children have acquired the relevant phonological rules, their articulation will continue to reflect the habitual ways of responding that they have practiced during their tenure as speakers. Though performance may reflect competence, other factors also influence performance, and these will not automatically fall into place once competence has been achieved.

For assessment, these observations indicate that when the child has demonstrated the appropriate linguistic rule in some setting, it is still necessary to examine performance across a variety of situations. An adequate assessment must be sensitive to the role of contextual or situational variables in determining behavior. Assessment should not cease at the boundaries of the clinic, and it is not only children's speech that must be evaluated but also the reactions of the significant persons in their environment. I recall an instance when the mother of a child with whom we were working was convinced that the lisp we were attempting to eradicate was preferable to the new sound we were trying to teach ("It sounds so shrill"). Unfortunately, it took many therapy sessions before we discovered these discrepant preferences and learned that the mother's discomfort was precisely with the skill we were attempting to teach her child.

Reichle and Karlan's chapter in this section (Chapter 13) reveals still another application of assessment in plotting a course of therapy, in this instance for children with limited vocal skills. The decision to teach a child a nonspeech form of communication carries significant implications for the child and the family, and yet, as Reichle and Karlan note, "Decisions regarding the use of augmentative communication systems are seldom empirically motivated." The decision rules that Reichle and Karlan review emanate from a set of systematic observations of the child and his or her circumstances—that is, they are based on assessments. Indeed, the rules that have been used to determine whether to use augmentative communication are similar to the kinds of information that might routinely be collected as part of a speech and language assessment: status of the speech production mechanism; information about the cause of the problem; previous response to instruction; the extent of language development in comprehension and production; the level of cognitive and pragmatic development; evidence of emotional problems; and, finally, an item that should be included in any evaluation, the reactions of the child's family and other environmental sources to the child's problem and to the remediation procedures being planned.

Though the decision rules are arrived at through assessment procedures, the selection and weighting of the information that is collected reflect the point of view of the examiner. Assessment provides information that is then filtered through the examiner's theoretical framework. The assessment procedure will not determine whether a certain level of cognitive attainment is necessary before the child can be taught sign language. That decision comes from the current theory about the relationship between cognition and linguistic acquisition and the supportive evidence and interpretations that have been placed on the evidence. In this instance, as in the language assessment procedures discussed by Broen, assessment is guided by theory and research. The choice of certain decision rules and not others reflects the clinician's implicit view of the factors that underlie successful acquisition of a communication system, whether vocal or nonvocal.

## USE OF NONVOCAL COMMUNICATION SYSTEMS

The recognition that vocal communication is not the most efficient method for all children has led to the development of the augmentative or nonvocal systems described in this text and has provided new opportunities for children who would otherwise be communicatively mute. It has also, however, introduced new problems because the decision to elect the nonvocal mode is not an easy one to make. The use of a communication board, or even of sign, intrinsically limits the range of situations in which communication can occur or the partners who can be engaged.

In the past it has seemed that the decision to use an augmentative system was irrevocable; when all else has failed, we must be willing to consign the child to the extraordinary world of nonspeech communicators. Reichle and Karlan raise the prospect that the decision need not be so portentous, that nonvocal communication may actually foster speech development, and that the choice of a particular augmentative system is not irrevocable. It may even be profitable to mix systems. The key to success in these various combinations, however, is continuing assessment. Reichle and Karlan refer to modality sampling as the basis for making choices, an approach that is entirely consistent with the view of testing as the systematic sampling of behavior. The use of decision rules to select the appropriate method of communication for a severely handicapped child points out the need to apply a systematic chain of logic in arriving at such decisions. It also highlights the fact that there are many assumptions that enter into the logical chain, assumptions that must ultimately be checked by empirical research, and that the application of the rules to a particular child requires careful ongoing assessment.

## OTHER ASSESSMENT ISSUES

There are other issues in assessment that are not considered in this section because of limits of space but that represent important insights into the role of assessment in the entire remediation process. For example, maintenance, transfer, and generalization of skills taught in the clinic to other settings and environments have long been of concern. Procedurally, the question is how such generalization can be accomplished. Linked to that concern is the question of how we can tell whether generalization has occurred. This is an assessment issue. What is the proper method to monitor the performance of our clients in other environments? What value can we place on self-report or on the reports of others? To what extent is it feasible or even ethical to monitor surreptitiously in nonclinical situations? What relationship should we establish between the formal measures used to monitor progress in the clinic and information obtained in other situations? If we use test data in the clinic and language samples outside, are the comparisons meaningful? Ingham and Costello (1984) have raised questions with respect to stuttering that apply to all facets of speech and language. Though problems in generalization have long been recognized, it is only recently that such problems have invited the development of specific behavioral technology (e.g., Siegel & Spradlin, 1978; Stokes & Baer, 1977) and concern for assessment as part of that technology.

There is an issue, too, in deciding when it is time to end therapy. Often the decision is made by factors outside of the clinician's control: The client moves, transfers, or graduates. Behavioral objectives are often established at the beginning of a program, but they are likely to need revision as the therapy progresses. The more specific the initial goals, the less likely they are to seem appropriate as therapy proceeds. Once a severely handicapped child has learned to communicate some very particular needs, we immediately want to broaden his or her communicative skills. Part of the issue is, again, a question of generalization.

Manning and Ortman (1980) and Manning, Keappock, and Stick (1976) have demonstrated that some proportion of children who appear to be ready for dismissal from therapy on the basis of ordinary articulation test scores perform much more poorly when tested in the presence of background noise and, further, that performance under the noise is a good prognostic indicator of whether the children will maintain their recently learned articulation skills outside of the clinic. In the attempt to interpret these results, Manning and his colleagues have speculated that some children remain inappropriately dependent on auditory feedback to produce error-free speech, and that loss or interference with that feedback causes them to revert to patterns of misarticulation. One implication of this view is that articulation therapy ought to incorporate procedures to ensure that children shift from auditory to other forms of feedback monitoring until they eventually become fully automatic in the production of the new sounds.

While there has been some disagreement with Manning's interpretation of these data (Yanez, Siegel, Garber, & Wellen, 1982), it is important to note that an in-depth assessment provides information that predicts whether additional therapy will be needed and that the standard assessment methods used to monitor progress during therapy—the articulation test as ordinarily administered—may not be sensitive enough to provide these predictive indications. Articulation tests are usually administered in such a way as to give the child every advantage. The stimuli are selected to display the sounds under question; the environment is usually quiet and free from distraction; only the child is speaking; there is no competition for the floor; the turn-taking routines are clearly established. These conditions are appropriate for obtaining indications of the child's best performance, but they may not be closely related to ordinary performance in less ideal communication contexts.

Manning's findings demonstrate the potential interaction of research, practice, and theory. The research emanates from a theory about the role of feedback in acquiring articulation skill. To test the theory, research was conducted that has important implications for identifying which children have stabilized their articulation gains. Confirmation of the theory leads to further hypotheses and to suggestions concerning the use of feedback during initial therapy. Clearly, assessment has been an integral part of this movement from theory to practice and back to theory.

## SUMMARY

This section on assessment focused particularly on the contribution of assessment to planning and monitoring a course of remedial instruction and the contribution of assessment to the decision rules that are applied in deciding whether a child should be engaged in augmentative or alternative communicative modes. In discussing these topics other issues were raised, at least partly because assessment is so embedded in all phases of teaching. The perspectives on assessment depart from conventional approaches in that assessment was located throughout the therapy process rather than solely at the beginning and was shown to be intimately involved in decisions concerning generalization, therapy outcome, and changes that occur in the ongoing process of providing help to handicapped children. Assessment is not only what the clinician does at the start of therapy to describe and plot a course. The course is constantly changing, and assessment must make continuing contributions as new courses are prepared.

## REFERENCES


Ingham, R. J., & Costello, J. M. (1984). Stuttering treatment outcome evaluation. In J. Costello (Ed.), *Speech disorders in children* (pp. 313–346). San Diego: College-Hill Press.

Manning, W. H., Keappock, N. E., & Stick, S. L. (1976). The use of auditory masking to estimate automatization of correct articulatory production. *Journal of Speech and Hearing Disorders, 41*, 143–149.

Manning, W. H., & Ortman, K. J. (1980). Use of auditory masking to estimate automatization of correct articulation in children. *Folia Phoniatrika, 32*, 29–38.

Siegel, G. M., & Spradlin, J. E. (1978). Programming for language and communication therapy. In R. L. Schiefelbusch (Ed.), *Language intervention strategies.* (pp. 357–398). Austin, TX: PRO-ED.

Stokes, T. F., & Baer, D. M. (1977). An implicit technology of generalization. *Journal of Applied Behavior Analysis, 10*, 349–367.

Yanez, E. A., Siegel, G. M., Garber, S. R., & Wellen, C. J. (1982). The effects of different masking noises on children with /s/ or /r/ errors. *Journal of Speech and Hearing Disorders*, *47*, 150–153.

# 12

# *Plotting a Course: The Ongoing Assessment of Language*

PATRICIA A. BROEN

Discussions of the assessment of language disorders in children usually focus on two outcomes: the identification of the child with a language disorder and the differential diagnosis of disorders that affect various components of language. Assessment procedures may evaluate the child's ability to comprehend language or to produce language; they may evaluate syntactic, semantic, pragmatic, or phonological components of language. Such an assessment usually involves the use of standardized, norm-referenced tests as well as informal observation and some analysis of a language sample. When a good language assessment has been completed, the clinician will be able to describe the child's language skills relative to those of other children of the same age or cognitive ability and will be able to describe the relative strengths and weaknesses of the child's performance on tests of the various components of language. Procedures for this kind of assessment have been described in a number of places (Darley & Spriestersbach, 1978; Emerick & Hatten, 1979; Lund & Duchan, 1983; McCormick & Schiefelbusch, 1984; Miller, 1981; Newhoff & Leonard, 1983). The end result of such an assessment should be the starting place for therapy. This chapter begins at that point. It is assumed that the clinician has a model of language and a procedure for evaluating language within that model. It is assumed that the child with a language disorder has been identified and that the specific language areas that are in need of remediation have been determined. The problems of monitoring progress in therapy and of determining when the goals of therapy have been met are considered.

The tests that were used originally in the identification of a child as language delayed or language disordered are usually inappropriate for monitoring progress. The scope of the test is frequently too broad. For example, an initial assessment of syntactic skills surveys or samples from a wide range of syntactic structures, while a teaching program may only teach the distinction between present progressive and past progressive verbs or the production of singular and plural nouns; an assessment of phonological skills may sample all of the phonemes in the language in several phonetic contexts, but a remedial program may only teach /t/ or initial voiceless stops.

An initial assessment typically does not test a specific language skill in enough depth. There may be only one or two test items in the area of interest rather than a comprehensive or exhaustive set of items. In most cases, tests are not designed to allow interpretation of performance on individual items, though such interpretation has sometimes been proposed (Owens, Haney, Giesow, Dooley, & Kelly 1983). Both Muma (1978) and Lund and Duchan (1983) provide a good discussion of these problems. What is needed to monitor ongoing therapy is a test or assessment procedure that samples repeatedly and in a comprehensive way the language skill that is being taught. For example, if the remedial goal is the productive use of plurals, the assessment could include several examples of the [s], [z], and [ə] plural allomorphs and a sample of various irregular plural forms including those where no change occurs (*soap, sheep*), those that change the vowel (*man, foot*), and those forms like *leaf* and *loaf* that are regular except that voicing of the final consonant changes in the plural form. Such an assessment would provide a broad sample of plural production and would provide enough items so that change during the course of an intervention program could be observed. Like a criterion-referenced test, this procedure would test knowledge of a particular content area: plural noun production. The clinician would have to decide how to interpret performance on such a measure.

Interpretation would reflect the goals of the teaching program and expectation for generalization. For example, teaching a child a *rule* for the production of regular plural forms should result in the correct production of regular plurals on the ongoing assessment measure; one might also expect the child to generalize the plural rule to the irregular plurals, producing "soaps," "sheeps," and "foots." If teaching focused on the plural *rule*, these overgeneralizations would be counted as correct because they provide additional evidence that the child has the rule. Later, if a set of irregular plurals were being taught, overgeneralization of the regular plural rule would be considered incorrect. In this way, interpretation of a child's performance on such an assessment would be tied directly to the goals of teaching and the language model used in teaching.

In the example above, when the plural rule was being taught, the assessment might not include the specific words that were used in teaching because the rule would be expected to generalize to novel or new nouns. However, if the child is being taught irregular plural forms, either they are by definition not rule governed, or the rules are too obscure to be used, in which case the assessment tool should include the *words* that are being taught or that will eventually be taught. No generalization beyond that set would be expected.

Unfortunately, language tests or assessment procedures to monitor ongoing therapy are not generally available. However, assessment tools and procedures can be designed by the clinician (Lund & Duchan, 1983); they can be borrowed from research studies (Miller, 1981); or they can be adapted from commercially available materials. All three of these alternatives are considered later in this chapter.

## DEFINITIONS

First, here are definitions of some words that are used in several ways in the speech pathology literature resulting in some confusion. A common understanding of these terms is basic to an understanding of the assessment process. The definitions were derived primarily from Salvia and Ysseldyke (1981) and from Anastasi (1968) and should help to clarify some of the issues in this area.

### Assessment

In an assessment, an attempt is made to understand the performance of an individual in the environment in which that individual functions. It is an evaluative and interpretive appraisal of performance. Information from a variety of sources can be used in an assessment. Some of that information may come from formal, norm-referenced tests, and some may come from informal observation; some of the information may be gathered directly by the clinician, and some may come from other individuals; some of the information may be quantitative, and some may be qualitative. An assessment will draw from all available and appropriate sources including parents, teachers, and other professionals and will interpret information relative to the particular questions that are being asked and the particular situation in which the child is found. An assessment can be used to make a number of decisions including identification, placement, and planning.

## Test

A test is "an objective and standardized measure of a sample of behavior" (Anastasi, 1968, p. 21). A joint committee including members of the American Psychological Association, the American Educational Research Association, and the National Council on Measurement in Education has defined a test as "a set of tasks or questions intended to elicit particular types of behaviors when presented under standardized conditions to yield scores that have desirable psychometric properties" (1974, p. 2). As Salvia and Ysseldyke (1981) point out, testing and assessment are not synonymous. The outcome of a test is a score that can be interpreted. While testing may be a part of the process of assessment, assessment can include much more than testing.

## Norm-Referenced Test

A norm-referenced test compares the performance of a child to that of other children of the same age. It allows the examiner to place the child on some continuum relative to other children. Norm-referenced tests are particularly useful in the identification of children who are significantly different from the average child.

***Developmental Scores.*** Performance on a norm-referenced test may be described in terms of either developmental scores or scores that reflect relative standing. In the language area, developmental scores are typically age-equivalent scores. For example, if a 5-year-old child has a Mean Length of Utterance (MLU) of 4.4, she would be said to be performing at the 4-year level, because the average MLU for 4-year-olds is 4.4 (Miller & Chapman, 1981).

Developmental scores should be interpreted with caution, because they do not take into account the variability that may occur within a particular age group. The 5-year-old with an MLU of 4.4 will be said to be one-year delayed in expressive language. Such a description implies that the child has a significant problem. However, by definition, half of the children tested will score below the mean and, therefore, below age level. We want to know if a child is different enough to warrant treatment. The mean alone provides no information about the distribution of scores at a particular age. In the example cited above, the mean for 5-year-old children is 5.6. If the standard deviation at 5 years were .5, this child would score more than two standard deviations below the mean for her age or in the bottom 3% of the population of 5-year-old children (assuming a normal distribution). In this case we would still interpret this child's performance as indicating a rather significant delay. However, if, as is the case, the standard deviation at 5 years is 1.2, this child scores about one standard deviation below the mean, and her performance might be interpreted as normal or low normal but not as cause for alarm. The description of the child's performance as one-year delayed creates a very different impression from the description of the child as scoring about one standard deviation below the mean for her age. Age norms often create a false impression of clinically significant delay.

***Relative Standing Scores.*** There are two types of scores that provide information about a child's performance relative to other children of the same age: percentile scores and standard scores. Percentile scores indicate the percent of scores or individuals that scored at or below a given raw score. These scores can be used with both ordinal and interval scales and do not require that scores be normally distributed.

There are a number of standard scores including z-scores and T-scores. Some tests give their standard score a unique name. For example, the IQ scores on the old *Peabody Picture Vocabulary Test* (Dunn, 1965) are standard scores with a mean of 100 and a standard deviation of 15; the Scaled Scores on the *Illinois Test of Psycholinguistic Abilities* (Kirk, McCarthy, & Kirk, 1969) are standard scores with a mean of 30 and a standard deviation of 6. All standard scores are derived scores in which raw scores are transformed so that the resulting set of scores always has the same mean and standard deviation. This allows comparison of performance across ages and often across subtests. In interpreting standard scores, the child's performance is always compared to other children of the same age, and the score is interpreted in terms of its distance and direction from the mean.

## Criterion-Referenced Tests

Criterion-referenced tests do not compare the performance of a child to other children of the same age but rather look at the degree to which a child has mastered a particular content area or subject matter. Criterion-referenced tests were first used in education to help teachers in planning a curriculum. They provided a description of the child's mastery of some aspect of the curriculum such as adding single digits or the spelling vocabulary of first grade. The specific items passed or failed on a criterion-referenced test are interpreted as indicating what the child does and does not know within a particular content area. These kinds of tests are sometimes called *content meaning* tests (Anastasi, 1968).

Both norm-referenced tests and criterion-referenced tests are objective measures of a child's behavior. The presentation of items and scoring of a criterion-referenced test should be standardized even though the test has no age norms. Both reliability and validity are important in criterion-referenced tests, though they may not be measured as they are on a norm-referenced test. A criterion-referenced test should provide a consistent (i.e., reliable) response from the child. If the pattern of errors is not the same on repeated testings of the same child, the reliability of the test would be questionable. The test should also be an accurate (i.e., valid) measure of the child's knowledge of the content area that is being evaluated. Criterion-referenced measures are of particular interest in the ongoing assessment of language within a therapy program, because they are used to examine knowledge of a content area and because responses are considered to reflect knowledge. In monitoring progress in therapy, the question to be answered by any assessment is how well the child has learned the information that was being taught.

## CHARACTERISTICS OF AN ONGOING ASSESSMENT

An assessment procedure designed to monitor progress in therapy and to determine when the goals of therapy have been met should have the following characteristics. First, it should reflect the theoretical model of language on which the teaching program is based. Second, the task used in the assessment should be a function of the particular aspect of language that is being taught, the model of language, and the goals of the teaching program. Third, the assessment procedure should sample enough language behavior to provide a statistically satisfactory measure of progress, and it should sample expected generalization to other linguistic or social contexts. This section considers the interrelationship that exists among the language model underlying therapy, the task or tasks used in assessment, and the size and scope of the language sample on which the assessment is based.

### Language Model

The assessment procedure used to monitor therapy should reflect the language model or the theory of language that underlies the teaching program. In some cases the language model is derived from the test or tests that were used in assessment to identify the child as language delayed. The clinician may not even recognize the language model that underlies, for example, the *Preschool Language Scale* (Zimmerman, Steiner, & Evatt, 1969) or the *Test of Language Development* (Newcomer & Hammill, 1982). It is particularly easy to accept the model of a test when related teaching materials have been developed, as was the case with the *Illinois Test of Psycholinguistic Abilities* (ITPA) (Kirk et al., 1969) and *Aids to Psycholinguistic Teaching* (Bush & Giles, 1969), or when an assessment procedure leads directly to therapy and training procedures, as with *Language Sampling, Analysis, and Training* (Tyack & Gottsleben, 1974). In other cases the relationship between what is being taught and the predicted outcomes of teaching may not be obvious, and the clinician, rather than specifying the expected outcome, may allow the available testing or assessment procedures to predict or anticipate change. Any model of language will make some particular claims about what is being taught and what kinds of changes are expected following teaching, and the clinician should be conscious of those claims. In the following example, three similar teaching programs would be monitored in three different ways, because they reflect three different models of what is being taught and, therefore, three different predicted outcomes.

Monitoring progress in therapy can be simple if the language model is simple. For example, if a child is being taught to produce word initial /t/ and if the language model is based on an autonomous phonological model (Postal, 1968) that predicts no generalization beyond that phonetic context, progress can be monitored with a list of words beginning with /t/. As therapy progresses, the child should produce word initial /t/ correctly in more and more of the words. When the child can produce some predetermined percent of the words correctly, that therapy program would be complete, and the child could proceed to another program or be dismissed.

While this is a simple example, it illustrates a number of points that are of concern in designing an ongoing assessment of language skills.

1. The skill to be taught must be specified—in this case, word initial /t/. The way the skill is specified will reflect the theoretical perspective of the teacher.

2. The measure of language change should assess generalizations predicted by the language model. Here the only generalization predicted is to other imitated words beginning with /t/.

3. The criteria for mastery will also reflect the language model. The criterion for mastery in this example is correct production of word initial /t/ in some percent of the words on a list when imitation is the task. The model predicts nothing more.

If the model of language is more complex, monitoring may become more complex. For example, if, rather than an autonomous phonological model, the child were being taught the contrast between voiced and voiceless sounds in the context of word initial /t/, expectations for the child's performance following teaching and the procedure for ongoing assessment of therapy would be very different. In this case the child would be assumed to be learning a distinctive feature contrast, and the theory predicts that training will generalize to the other phonetic contexts in which that contrast was missing. Voicing in all word initial obstruents (stops, fricatives, and affricates) might be assessed; the assessment might include obstruents in all phonetic contexts, depending on the child's error pattern and the clinician's expectations for generalization. If it is assumed that teaching should result in changes in the production of voicing in spontaneous speech, a sample of spontaneous speech should be included in the assessment. The criteria for mastery would then be described in terms of the percent of correctly voiced obstruents used in samples of imitated and spontaneous speech. If correct voicing were the goal, productions that were correctly voiced but incorrect in place or manner of articulation would be considered correct for this assessment.

To assess voicing in spontaneous speech one must know how voicing behaves in spontaneous speech. For any language skill, the formal description of the structure may not be an accurate description of how that structure is used in conversational speech. In this example voicing of /t/ varies with phonetic context. The /t/ in *batter* is usually a voiced tap, the /t/ in *mat* may be unreleased, and the /t/ in *mitten* may be a glottal stop. All of these are acceptable productions in conversational American English and should be considered correct in the speech sample.

Let's look at the effects of another theoretical model on the assessment of a program that includes the teaching of /t/. If the initial assessment described this child as using the phonological process of "stopping" (substituting stop consonants for fricative consonants), the teaching program might still include the phoneme /t/, in teaching an /s/–/t/ contrast, for example. Here the model would predict that, following teaching, fricative consonants would be produced as fricatives, and stop consonants should remain stops. Both fricatives and stops would be monitored, but continuancy rather than voicing would be of interest. The criterion for learning would be that continuant consonants are produced as continuants, and stop consonants are produced as stops some proportion of the time in a particular sample.

In summary, the language model that underlies a teaching program is reflected in the way language behavior is sampled and in the way that the sample of language is evaluated.

## Language Task

Language behavior must be evaluated by means of some task, and the nature of the task can affect the outcome of the assessment. For example, it is easier to sample expressive language than receptive language. However, the clinician has control of the contents of a sample of receptive language, while the contents of a sample of spontaneous speech, used to measure some expressive language skill, are largely under the control of the child. The problems of assessing receptive and expressive language are considered separately.

***Expressive Language*.** Evaluating language in a sample of spontaneous speech has a kind of face validity that no other procedure for sampling language behavior has. The ultimate goal in any language teaching program is to make the child a more effective communicator, and conversational speech would seem to be the ultimate measure of that goal. There are several good discussions of how to obtain a spontaneous language sample (Lund & Duchan, 1983; Miller, 1981) and how to analyze that sample (Crystal, Fletcher, & Garman, 1976; Lee, 1974; Miller, 1981; Muma, 1978; Tyack & Gottsleben, 1974). When monitoring progress in therapy, it would not be necessary to do a complete analysis of a language sample. Only the language structures that are being taught (and any related structures that might be expected to change) would need to be examined. If plurals are being taught, only plurals need to be monitored; if *wh*-questions are being taught, only the use of *wh*- questions needs to be monitored.

One problem with a spontaneous language sample is that it is only possible to evaluate those linguistic structures that occur in the sample. For example, Brown (1973) and de Villiers and de Villiers (1973) chose to study the acquisition of a particular set of syntactic forms, because those forms were obligatory and because the obligatory context occurred with some frequency in the speech of young children. Other language structures that children are learning during this period could not be assessed.

If the expressive language structure that is being taught has a frequent obligatory context, it may be best to monitor acquisition in samples of spontaneous speech. The index of acquisition would be some percent of correct use in a sample that contained at least a certain number of obligatory contexts, for example, correct use of regular plurals 9 of 10 times. Most single phonemes could be tested this way, though many consonant clusters and a few phonemes might not occur frequently enough to make this an efficient method of assessment. Acquisition of certain syntactic forms such as articles, *be* verbs, past tense and past and present progressive tense, and some prepositions could be monitored in an unstructured spontaneous speech sample. Some pragmatic functions might also fall into this category. In fact, some discourse measures such as topic maintenance and topic initiation may require a relatively free conversational sample to be measured at all.

However, sampling spontaneous speech in an unstructured situation is often an inefficient way to assess a particular expressive language behavior. The obligatory context for the behavior may occur infrequently, or the behavior may not have an obligatory context. For example, if children are being taught to make clear, accurate requests when they want something, they must want something for the behavior of interest to occur. Few obligatory contexts for requesting may occur in an unstructured sample of spontaneous speech. It may be more efficient to structure a situation in which the child wants something and to evaluate learning in that situation. Toys in a playroom, for example, could be placed in sight but out of reach. If children are learning the skills that are being taught, they should ask for the toys rather than gesture or cry.

A situation can be structured in a number of ways that vary in the degree of control that the clinician exercises. Some kinds of structure set the stage for the desired behavior. They increase the probability that that particular language form or language behavior will be produced by the child but do not guarantee its production. Presenting the child with objects with particular names is one way to increase the probability that certain phonemes will occur. The examples in the preceding paragraph were structured to increase the probability that requesting behavior would occur. In any case the child could choose to ignore the structure of the situation and talk about something else.

Some kinds of structure provide the child with examples of the behavior that is of interest and invite the child to reproduce the model through imitation or delayed imitation. Story retelling is such a task. A story can be constructed that has the phonological forms, syntactic forms, or sentence structures that are of interest. The story can be told to the child and the child asked to retell it. A direct imitation task adds even more structure and a Cloze task, where the child is asked to fill in the blank, still more. In each case the clinician's control over the content of the sample is increased, but the probability that the behavior is an accurate representation of the child's general behavior decreases. The child who can respond correctly to "This is a cup, here are two ______" may not use plurals in conversational speech. Still, knowing that the child can generate the plural form in this kind of task does provide some information.

Phonological, syntactic, and pragmatic skills are most often tested as expressive language skills. Samples of expressive language will vary in their structure or the degree of control that is exercised over the sample and in their face validity as accurate representations of the child's knowledge of language.

***Receptive Language.*** Often language skills cannot be assessed directly. This is particularly true for the comprehension of language. Here the child must do something to demonstrate that a particular aspect of language has been understood. There are a number of tasks that can be used to assess receptive language skills including picture pointing tasks, yes/no questions, and asking the child to follow directions. There are some tasks, for example, the completion of analogies (foot is to leg as hand is to ______) and Cloze tasks (Here the cat is on the chair; here the cat is ______), that are part receptive and part expressive. In every case, to respond correctly requires that both the task and the language skill be understood.

As an example, consider a child who does not use verb tense forms to indicate when an action happened. He doesn't use past, present, and future verb forms in spontaneous speech. This child also makes errors on items on the *Test of Auditory Comprehension of Language* (Carrow, 1973) and the *Northwest Syntax Screening Test* (Lee, 1971) that test the understanding of the temporal aspect of verb tense. The decision is made to teach the child the temporal meaning of verb forms before teaching him to produce them. The question here is how the child's learning of the meaning of verb forms can be monitored.

The task typically used to evaluate comprehension of verb tense is a picture pointing task (Broen & Santema, 1983; Carrow, 1973; Lee, 1971), though a Cloze task was used in the ITPA (Kirk et al., 1969). In monitoring the acquisition of the comprehension of a language structure such as verb tense, a picture pointing task has some drawbacks. Pictures are static representations. When some action is being illustrated, the child must interpret the picture or picture series as representing action. For example, the simple present tense has the meaning of "habitual action" (Palmer, 1974), but it is difficult to see how one can contrast in a picture the difference between "ongoing action that will come to an end" (present progressive) and "habitual action" (Palmer, 1974). The subtle difference between "The sun rises in the east" and "The sun is rising in the east" cannot be captured by a picture. Any time that a picture preference task is used, this problem should be recognized. Only gross differences can be assessed. The meaning of a picture also depends on the foils that are available. The meaning of *runs* that is being tested when the foils illustrate "crawls" and "walks" is different from the meaning of *runs* that is being tested when the foils illustrate a person crouched at a mark ready to run and a perspiring person in running clothes walking away from a track.

Two picture series (Broen & Santema, 1983) can serve as an illustration here (Figure 12.1). Pictures could be used to monitor the comprehension of the temporal aspects of past, present, and future tense forms. Using these pictures, the child would have to understand the meaning of the verb, in this case *throw* and *dress*, and its representation in the picture. The child would have to understand the left to right sequencing of the pictures. That is, the left-most picture indicates an action about to happen, the center picture an action that is happening, and the right picture a completed action. Understanding the meaning or implication of the left to right sequencing is more important in some cases than in others. The third picture in the *throw* series could be understood as representing "threw" or "was throwing" in the absence of the other two pictures, but the third picture in the *dress* sequence might not be understood as "dressed" or "was dressing" except in the context of the other two pictures.

The understanding of a set of verbs that differ in the form of the simple past could be monitored using picture sets similar to Figure 12.1. Two verbs representing each of the regular allomorphs /t/, /d/, and /ed/ and six irregular verbs would make a reasonable sample. The child could be tested on these 12 verbs periodically during the course of the remedial

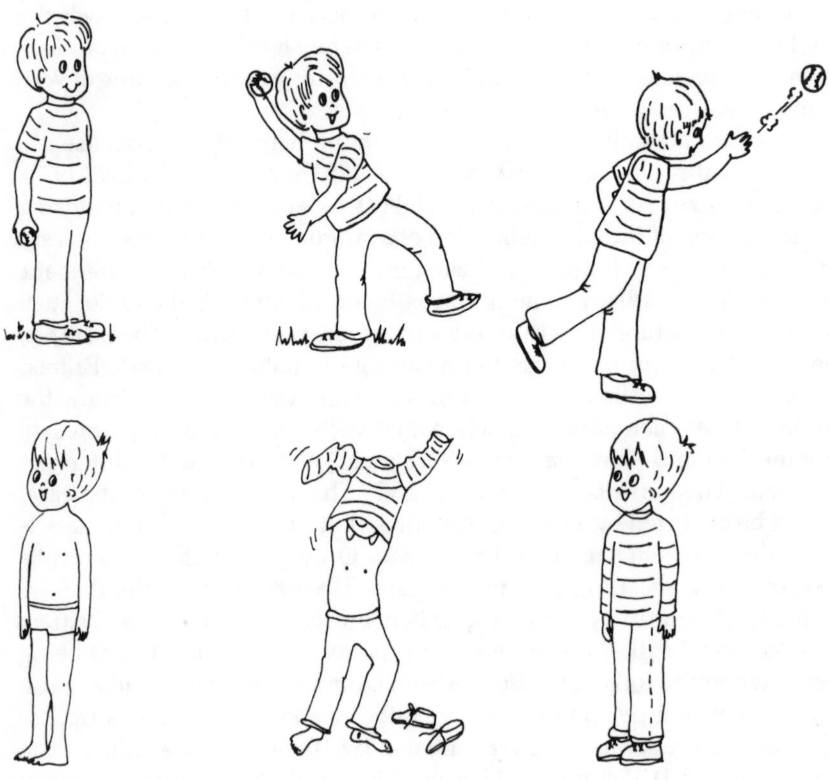

**Figure 12.1.** Illustration of the past, present, and future of the verbs *throw* and *dress.* Reprinted with permission of the publisher from "Children's Comprehension of Six Verb Tense Forms" by Patricia A. Broen & Susan A. Santema, *Journal of Communication Disorders, 16,* 85–97. Copyright 1983 by Elsevier Science Publishing.

program. The child would be expected to get more and more of the regular verbs correct as the teaching progressed. During this first teaching, it is not clear what would be expected to happen to the simple past tense form of the irregular verbs. Normally developing children learn some irregular verbs before regular verbs, but in this situation, where the child is being taught the regular form, the normal developmental progression might not occur. The past forms of the irregular verbs should behave like the other six verbs.

Vocabulary is the one skill that is almost always tested receptively. The receptive vocabulary of even a young or a language delayed child is too large to allow comprehensive testing, and so some subset of interest is usually tested. The subset may be a selected random sample, as with the PPVT (Dunn & Dunn, 1981), or it may be a sample that is of some particular interest like that tested by the *Boehm Test of Basic Concepts* (Boehm, 1971). As with verb tense, only a limited part of the meaning of a word can be captured in a picture. For example, the spatial meanings of prepositions can be assessed in a picture task, but other meanings are more difficult to capture visually. One can picture the meaning of *off* in "He fell off the wall," but the meaning of *off* in "He was off the job" is more difficult, and the meaning of *off* in "He is better off" is impossible to picture, yet it is the latter meanings that are most apt to cause the non-native speaker, the older retarded individual, or the hearing impaired teenager the most difficulty.

A child's response to requests for behavior can be used as a measure of the child's understanding of language. Such a procedure can be used at several levels. Mulligan and Guess (1984) describe a data sheet on which are recorded the responses of a child to a set of requests. Some of the requests are in the forms of statements. The clinician says, "It is time to clean up," and the child is expected to begin to move to clean up. Some requests are in an imperative form; the child is instructed "Touch block" and is expected to touch the block. In every case, the daily routine, the situational context, and the verbal stimulus cue the desired response. The child need not understand the specific words or the syntax of the sentence to respond appropriately. This represents an early stage of language comprehension in which routines and situational context provide cues for appropriate responding (Clark, 1973). The child may not respond appropriately to the same request in another context. The child who touches the block when only the block is on the table may touch the car when only the car is presented, even though the request is to touch the block. The same child may become confused when both the car and the block are present, because the request to touch the block is interpreted as a general request to touch the object on the table.

With some modification, this task can be used to assess a more sophisticated or complex understanding of language. For example, if the requested behavior is improbable in the context that is given, correct responding requires a more thorough understanding of the vocabulary being used and the syntax of the request (and perhaps the pragmatics of the request). If the request is "Put the cup on the plate," the sight of a plate and a cup and a verbal request may be enough to allow the child to respond correctly, If the request is "Put the plate on the cup" or "Put the cup under the plate," the correct response is less probable, and the child must have a better understanding of the vocabulary and the syntax to respond correctly. This kind of task can be used to assess children's understanding of passive sentences (e.g., Show me, "The dog was bitten by the boy"), embedded sentences (e.g., Show me, "The boy who bit the dog fell down"), and the difference between verbs such as *ask* and *tell* (e.g., "Ask me how old I am" vs. "Tell me how old I am").

Task plays a similar role in the testing and assessment of language skills regardless of the purpose of the assessment. The task, in a sense, is interposed between the child's knowledge of language and the clinician. If the child cannot or does not perform well in the task, the child's knowledge of language will be underestimated. If the child can master the task through some procedure other than knowing the language structure that is of interest, the child's knowledge of language will be overestimated. In designing procedures for monitoring the acquisition of linguistic understanding, the clinician needs to be sensitive to the demands of the task and must determine that the child understands the task so that failures can be attributed to a lack of linguistic knowledge (Broen, Strange, Doyle, & Heller, 1983).

## Language Sample Size

The sample of language behavior used to monitor progress must be large enough to provide an accurate indication of change but small enough to be used often. How big is big enough? That depends primarily on the nature of the task and the kinds of generalizations that are predicted by the language model.

***Nature of the Task.*** Some tasks allow the child to make a correct response without knowing the correct answer. This is particularly true for picture pointing and other multiple choice tasks. When the child is given a closed set of responses, there is some probability that the child will choose the correct response by chance. The number of choices will determine the size of that probability. In a two-choice task where both choices are equally likely, the child will be right by chance one out of two times or 50% of the time, in a three-choice task the child will be correct by chance 33.3% of the time, and with four choices the child who is performing randomly will be correct by chance 25% of the time. This assumes that all of the choices are equally likely. However, simply adding choices will not always decrease the likelihood of being correct by chance. Some foils are not real choices. For example, if the ability to understand the difference between active and passive sentences is being tested (e.g., "The boy pulled the girl" vs. "The boy was pulled by the girl"), it is unlikely that a third foil would represent an interesting or viable alternative. If the understanding of the difference between singular and plural nouns is being tested (e.g., *dog* vs. *dogs*), there is no equally likely third picture. The real probability in this case, even with a three-choice task, is 50%. Items that require a yes or no response can also be answered correctly 50% of the time by chance.

The sample of language behavior should be large enough to provide a statistically significant measure of the child's knowledge. If we want to allow at least one error due to inattention, we can use statistics to calculate the sample size that will be needed to rule out chance correct responding. As a rule of thumb, if a child can respond correctly 50% of the time by chance, the child must make no more than one error in nine responses (Siegel, 1956); if the child can respond correctly 33.3% of the time by chance, the child must make no more than one error in five responses; and if the child can respond correctly 25% of the time by chance, the child must make no more than one error in four responses.

In a spontaneous speech task there is less chance that a correct response will be made by chance. If a response is correct, it usually means that the child knows something about the structure being examined. However, speech samples have their own problems. Correct responses can be learned or memorized rather than reflecting knowledge of a linguistic rule. This is why overgeneralization is considered a good indication that a child knows the rule. The child who says "feet" may know only that plural form or may have learned that plural and several others as separate words. Use of the plural may not indicate knowledge of the plural rule. The child who says "foots" provides more evidence that the plural has been generated by a rule.

***Predicted Generalizations***. There are two questions to be addressed in designing the content of an ongoing measure of language: "How large should the sample be?" and "What should the scope of the sample be?" The size of the sample can be determined by the statistical requirements, but the scope of the sample is a direct reflection of the nature of the language skill being taught, the language model, and the kinds of generalizations that are predicted from that model. Some skills are very specific, and the assessment tool will examine the child's knowledge of the specific items that are being taught. If you are teaching the vocabulary used in an American history class to a group of high school–aged hearing impaired students, you want to test their knowledge of the specific vocabulary that is being taught. If you are teaching the same students to produce present perfect and future perfect verbs, you may want to test them on verbs that they have not encountered in class, because this is a skill that you expect to generalize, and the measure used should sample those generalizations. The broader the predicted generalization, the more items the monitoring procedure will need. If this creates a task that is too long, it may be possible to do a two-stage assessment. The first phase could assess the primary behavior that is being taught, and the second phase could test predicted generalizations. When the child shows some indication of learning the primary behavior, expected generalizations can be added to the assessment. This will make repeated measurement easier.

### Summary

In designing a procedure to monitor ongoing therapy and to determine when the expected learning has occurred, the clinician will want to ask the following questions.

1. What specific language skill am I teaching?
2. What changes do I expect to see following teaching?
3. What kind of task can be used to assess these skills?
4. What is my criterion for mastery?
5. How many items should be included in my assessment?

The process of designing and using an assessment tool should not only provide a good indication of progress in therapy, it should help the clinician specify and refine the goals of therapy.

## DEVELOPING AN ONGOING ASSESSMENT

Three major sources of materials for developing ongoing assessments of language are research projects designed to explore the acquisition of language, commercial materials that provide in-depth assessments, and the clinician's own creativity. In each case the particular goals of therapy need to be considered in adapting the materials to fit the needs of an ongoing assessment.

### Research as a Source of Materials

Both the speech pathology literature and the normal child language literature contain studies of the acquisition of all aspects of language by children. These are good sources of information for the clinician who is looking for materials to use in monitoring the language learning of a child. In some cases relevant research has already been identified. For example, Miller (1981), in his book, *Assessing Language Production in Children,* describes the use of a number of experimental procedures in the assessment of expressive or productive language. Many of the procedures suggested are nonstandardized in the formal sense, and many are drawn directly from research that explores the acquisition of language by normal children. This book is a good model for adapting research to initial assessment and to ongoing assessment. Lund and Duchan (1983) also describe the use of procedures drawn from research literature to assess all aspects of language. Again, they are talking primarily about the initial assessment of language skills, but the procedures suggested may be adapted to an ongoing assessment of language.

As an example of how an ongoing assessment might be developed from research procedures, consider a young teenage student who has a history of delayed language and now appears to be having difficulty with nonliteral language. When confronted with a metaphor or an idiom, he is apt to make a literal interpretation. When someone says "on the other hand," he tries to figure out which hand that is. When he is told that "the Constitution is the cornerstone of our government," he doesn't understand. He also fails items that test understanding of analogies, metaphors, and proverbs (Processing Relationships and Ambiguities subtest, *Clinical Evaluation of Language Function*, Semel & Wiig, 1980).

The decision was made to teach this individual to recognize and interpret figurative language. The ability to understand figurative language is a skill that develops gradually over late childhood and early adolescence (Pollio & Pollio, 1974; Winner, Rosenstiel, & Gardner, 1976). The literature on normal language development suggests that children are able to interpret some kinds of metaphor correctly in later childhood. This is particularly true for metaphor that describes the relationship of objects to physical characteristics of people (e.g., "Her feet were icy"). The ability to understand these terms when they are applied to the personal characteristics of an individual (e.g., "She was a cold person") is learned later, while the ability to interpret the nonliteral meanings of proverbs is not acquired until late in adolescence (Billow, 1975; Richardson & Church, 1959). In light of this, it would seem reasonable to teach metaphor first in relationship to personal physical characteristics, then personal characteristics, and then in relationship to the nonhuman world. Nippold and Fey (1983) describe the use of a task, first devised by Billow (1975), to assess the understanding of this range of metaphor by older normal and language delayed children. This task could be modified to monitor the acquistion of nonliteral or metaphorical understanding. It contains some sentences that apply to physical characteristics of an individual (e.g., "Her hair is spaghetti"), some that refer to personal characteristics (e.g., "Anger ate him up"), and some that refer to nonhuman metaphors (e.g., "The sun wakes the seeds").

In this case, the language skill that is being taught is the understanding of figurative language, specifically, the understanding of metaphorical language. It is assumed that there are at least three levels of difficulty that relate to the nature of the metaphor. Following teaching, we expect the child to be able to interpret metaphorical language in its nonliteral sense, first for metaphors referring to physical characteristics, then for personal characteristic metaphors, and last for nonhuman metaphors. To monitor the teaching process a task is used in which the child is asked to interpret a set of sentences that are metaphorical. The set of metaphors used contains some metaphors from each category.

The criterion for mastery is nonliteral interpretation of at least two of three novel metaphors at the particular level that is being taught. The assessment procedure would need to include at least nine metaphors, three from each category. The same set of metaphors could be used repeatedly in monitoring progress if the answers were not given, but the criterion for mastery or dismissal would be correct performance on six metaphors from a second set of nine that the child had never heard.

## Commercial Materials

Commercial materials are available that can be used to monitor progress in therapy. Often they are sold as assessment tools; they may or may not provide normative data. For the purposes of an ongoing assessment, normative information is interesting but not necessary. What is necessary is that the procedure provide a relatively large and interesting sample of the behavior that is of interest. *Language Sampling, Analysis, and Training* (Tyack & Gottsleben, 1974) is an example of a commercially available tool that could be used for the ongoing monitoring of language learning. This procedure provides a method or a framework for monitoring the acquisition of various syntactic forms. It is particularly useful for tracking the acquisition of obligatory forms such as articles, tense markers, *be* verbs, and plurals.

*A Deep Test of Articulation* (McDonald, 1964) is another example of commercially available material that can be adapted for the ongoing assessment of, in this case, phonological skills. Both the sentence version and the picture version of *A Deep Test of Articulation* provide repeated samples of the production of particular phonemes and subsets of sentences, or picture sets can be selected to test the particular phonemes that are of interest.

As an example here, consider again the child who fails to mark verbs for past tense. If this child demonstrates, on a set of receptive tests, that she understands the meaning of regular and irregular past tense forms, the goal of a remedial program will be the production of those forms. Progress toward that goal could be monitored in samples of spontaneous speech. While the final criterion for dismissal or for mastery of past tense production might well be the correct use of both regular and irregular past tense forms in at least 9 of 10 opportunities in a sample of spontaneous speech, a more efficient procedure might be used to monitor progress during therapy. If imitation is accepted as at least a reflection of productive speech, the *Oral Language Sentence Imitation Diagnostic Inventory* (OLSIDI) (Zachman, Huisingh, Jorgensen, & Berrett, 1977) provides sets of sentences, controlled for length, that can be used to monitor the child's acquisition of a number of syntactic forms including regular and irregular past tense. Each set of 10 sentences focuses on one particular syntactic or morphological structure. Within a sentence set, half of the sentences are eight morphemes long, and half are nine morphemes long. If past tense is the focus of the remedial program, the child can be given these two sentence sets prior to therapy and periodically during the course of therapy.

In this case what is being taught is the production of regular and irregular past tense forms. Following the teaching of regular past tense, the child should be able to imitate sentences containing past tense verbs; this form may generalize to irregular verbs. Following teaching of irregular past tense, the child should produce past tense correctly both in regular verbs and in those irregular past tense verbs that were taught. Ongoing progress will be monitored with a set of imitated sentences from OLSIDI. When these are imitated correctly 100% of the time, spontaneous speech will be sampled. The criterion for mastery will be at least 9 of 10 productions of regular and irregular past tense correct in a sample of spontaneous speech. The child was required to be correct 100% of the time in imitation, because this is assumed to be an easier task, while production of past tense in spontaneous speech is assumed to be more difficult and some margin of error is allowed.

## The Clinician's Creativity

Speech pathologists have always been clever at designing materials, but when language skills don't lend themselves to formal testing or formal assessment, they need to be particularly clever. For example, most pragmatic skills need to be measured in the context of an interpersonal interaction. This requires that the end goals of the program be carefully specified and that the ongoing assessment be relevant to those goals. Consider the mildly retarded young man who is employed in a sheltered workshop. His supervisor says that he could get a job as a yard worker at a local university if he could stay on topic when someone tries to talk with him. However, during conversations he changes the topic or introduces new topics without letting his listener know. He is disconcerting to talk with, even though he is a good worker. His supervisor has asked that he be taught to converse in a more acceptable fashion.

The language skill to be taught is "topic maintenance." The end goal is the ability to hold a conversation of some particular length with someone the young man does not know well. The situation in which progress is monitored should be similar to the situation in which the desired behavior is to occur. In this case the clinician needs to specify the situation and the criterion for mastery. Teaching may occur within the sheltered workshop, but monitoring progress probably requires a different context. The clinician might arrange with someone in a nearby building to spend 10 minutes with this young man each Friday afternoon. During that time they could talk about topics that are of mutual interest, with the goal being six exchanges of speaker/listener with no change of topic and appropriate introduction of new topics when they occur. It is unlikely that assessing topic maintenance in the therapy setting will provide a good measure of progress. It may not even be possible to do much teaching apart from contact with other workers and staff. Monitoring of ongoing therapy requires the clinician to be very specific about the desired outcome, and it requires that the clinician design a monitoring procedure that evaluates that outcome.

## SUMMARY

In this chapter I have defined some of the parameters of an ongoing assessment of language. This is an aspect of language remediation that has received relatively little attention in the past but one that needs some thoughtful consideration. Devising such an assessment is not easy, but it can be rewarding. The ongoing assessment of language learning is an important part of the therapy process. It provides the clinician with information about the effectiveness of the teaching process, and it provides a measure of the child's progress. In addition, the thought that goes into generating such a procedure will help the clinician define what is being taught and to be more effective in teaching.

## REFERENCES

American Psychological Association, American Educational Research Association, and National Council on Measurement in Education. (1974). *Standards for educational and psychological tests*. Washington, DC: American Psychological Association.

Anastasi, A. (1968). *Psychological testing* (2nd ed.). New York: Macmillan.

Billow, R. M. (1975). A cognitive developmental study of metaphor comprehension. *Developmental Psychology*, 11, 415–423.

Boehm, A. (1971). *Boehm Test of Basic Concepts*. New York: Psychological Corporation.

Broen, P. A., & Santema, S. (1983). Children's comprehension of six verb-tense forms. *Journal of Communication Disorders, 16*, 85–97.

Broen, P. A., Strange, W., Doyle, S. S., & Heller, J. H. (1983). Perception and production of approximant consonants by normal and articulation-delayed preschool children. *Journal of Speech and Hearing Research, 26*, 601–608.

Brown, R. (1973). *A first language: The early stages*. Cambridge, MA: Harvard University Press.

Bush, W. J., & Giles, M. T. (1969). *Aids to psycholinguistic teaching*. Columbus, OH: Charles E. Merrill.

Carrow, E. (1973) *Test for Auditory Comprehension of Language*. Evanston, IL: Northwestern University Press.

Clark, E. V. (1973). Nonlinguistic strategies and the acquisition of word meaning. *Cognition*, 2, 161–182.

Crystal, D., Fletcher, P., & Garman, M. (1976). *The grammatical analysis of language disability: A procedure for assessment and remediation*. London: Edward Arnold.

Darley, F. L., & Spriestersbach, D. C. (1978). *Diagnostic methods in speech pathology* (2nd ed.). New York: Harper & Row.

de Villiers, J., & de Villiers, P. (1973). A cross-sectional study of the acquisition of grammatical morphemes in child speech. *Journal of Psycholinguistic Research*, 2, 267–268.

Dunn, L. M. (1965). *Peabody Picture Vocabulary Test*. Circle Pines, MN: American Guidance Service.

Dunn, L., & Dunn, L. (1981). *Peabody Picture Vocabulary Test–Revised*. Circle Pines, MN: American Guidance Service.

Emerick, L. L., & Hatten, J. T. (1979). *Diagnosis and evaluation in speech pathology*. Englewood Cliffs, NJ: Prentice-Hall.

Kirk, S. A., McCarthy, J. J., & Kirk, W. D. (1969). *Illinois Test of Psycholinguistic Abilities*. Urbana, IL: University of Illinois Press.

Lee, L. (1971). *Northwestern Syntax Screening Test*. Evanston, IL: Northwestern University Press.

Lee, L. (1974). *Developmental Sentence Analysis*. Evanston, IL: Northwestern University Press.

Lund, N. J., & Duchan, J. F. (1983). *Assessing children's language in naturalistic contexts*. Englewood Cliffs, NJ: Prentice-Hall.

McCormick, L., & Schiefelbusch, R. L. (1984). *Early language intervention: An introduction*. Columbus, OH: Charles E. Merrill.

McDonald, E. (1964). *A Deep Test of Articulation*. Pittsburgh: Stanwix House.

Miller, J. (1981). *Assessing language production in children*. Austin, TX: PRO-ED.

Miller, J. F., & Chapman, R. S. (1981). Research note: The relationship between age and mean length of utterance in morphemes. *Journal of Speech and Hearing Research, 24*, 154–161.

Mulligan, M., & Guess, D. (1984). Using an individualized curriculum sequencing model. In L. McCormick & R. L. Schiefelbusch (Eds.), *Early language intervention: An introduction* (pp. 299–323). Columbus, OH: Charles E. Merrill.

Muma, J. R. (1978). *Language handbook*. Englewood Cliffs, NJ: Prentice-Hall.

Newcomer, P., & Hammill, D. (1982). *Test of Language Development*. Austin, TX: PRO-ED.

Newhoff, M., & Leonard, L. B. (1983). Diagnosis of developmental language disorders. In I. J. Meitus & B. Weinberg (Eds.), *Diagnosis in speech-language pathology* (pp. 71–112). Austin, TX: PRO-ED.

Nippold, M. A., & Fey, S. H., (1983). Metaphoric understanding in preadolescents having a history of language acquisition difficulties. *Language, Speech and Hearing Services in Schools, 14*, 171–180.

Owens, Jr., R. E., Haney, M. J., Giesow, V. E., Dooley, L. F., & Kelly, R. J. (1983). Language test content: A comparative study. *Language, Speech and Hearing Services in Schools, 14*, 7–21.

Palmer, F. R. (1974). *The English verb*. London: Longmans.

Pollio, M. R., & Pollio, H. R. (1974). The development of figurative language in children. *Journal of Psycholinguistic Research, 3*, 185–201.

Postal, P. M. (1968). *Aspects of Phonological Theory*. New York: Harper & Row.

Richardson, C., & Church, J. (1959). A developmental analysis of proverb interpretations. *Journal of Genetic Psychology, 94*, 169–179.

Salvia, J., & Ysseldyke, J. E. (1981). *Assessment in special and remedial education*. Dallas: Houghton Mifflin.

Semel, E. M., & Wiig, E. H. (1980). *Clinical evaluation of language functions*. Columbus, OH: Charles E. Merrill.

Siegel, S. (1956). *Nonparametric statistics for the behavioral sciences*. New York: McGraw-Hill.

Tyack, D., & Gottsleben, R. (1974). *Language sampling, analysis, and training: A handbook for teachers and clinicians*. Palo Alto, CA: Consulting Psychologists Press.

Winner, E., Rosensteil, A., & Gardner, H. (1976). The development of metaphorical understanding. *Developmental Psychology, 12*, 289–297.

Zachman, L., Huisingh, R., Jorgensen, C., & Berrett, M. (1977). *Oral Language Sentences Diagnostic Inventory*. Moline, IL: Linguisystems.

Zimmerman, I., Steiner, V., & Evatt, R. (1969). *Preschool Language Scale*. Columbus, OH: Charles E. Merrill.

13

# Selecting Augmentative Communication Interventions: A Critique of Candidacy Criteria and a Proposed Alternative

JOE REICHLE AND
GEORGE KARLAN

Within the past few years, several sets of decision rules have been posited that address the selection of augmentative communication systems (Chapman & Miller, 1980; Nietupski & Hamre-Nietupski, 1979; Sailor et al., 1980; Scheuerman, Baumgart, Sipsma, & Brown, 1976; Shane, 1980; Shane & Bashir, 1980). Most of these investigators have favored (if not advocated) the use of a two-tiered process in which the need for an augmentative system is quantified first and then further criteria are applied to select a specific system. An alternative involves sampling two modes before selecting a single augmentative system (Alpert, 1980; Kiernan, 1981). More recently, Keogh and Reichle (1985) have suggested that forcing a quick selection between

Preparation of this chapter was supported in part by Contract No.300-82-0363 awarded to the University of Minnesota from the Division of Innovation and Development, Special Education Programs, U.S. Department of Education. The opinions expressed herein do not necessarily reflect the position or policy of the U.S. Department of Education, and no official endorsement should be inferred. Portions of this chapter are reprinted with minor modifications, with permission, from J. Reichle and G. Karlan, 1985, "The selection of an augmentative system in communication intervention: A critique of decision rules," *The Journal of The Association for Persons with Severe Handicaps, 10*, 146–155.

signing and communication boards may create a "pseudo-issue" for the interventionist. Many learners may benefit from continued use of a "mixed" system—that is, one that combines the use of some signs/ gestures with other graphic symbols. Consequently, selecting a single augmentative system may not be the most critical initial issue.

## DESCRIBING EXISTING DECISION RULES

Four basic sets of decision rules for determining whether to implement a nonspeech communication system have been reported (Chapman & Miller, 1980; Nietupski & Hamre-Nietupski, 1979; Sailor et al., 1980; Scheuerman et al., 1976; Shane, 1980; Shane & Bashir, 1980). These decision-rule sets are not exclusive of one another and often overlap. Their commonalities and differences can best be understood by examining factors that each set of rules uses in assisting teachers and speech/ language pathologists to make decisions regarding the implementation of augmentative communication systems.

Three questions appear to guide the formation of decision rules under review (Reichle & Karlan, 1986).

1. When should nonspeech communication programs be initiated (Nietupski & Hamre-Nietupski, 1979)? Or alternatively, who is a good candidate for nonspeech communication systems (Chapman & Miller, 1980; Sailor et al., 1980; Shane & Bashir, 1980)?
2. Should the nonspeech system augment or substitute for spoken communication (Alberto, Garrett, Briggs, & Umberger, 1983; Chapman & Miller, 1980)?
3. Which nonspeech system is best suited for the individual (Chapman & Miller, 1980; Sailor et al., 1980; Nietupski & Hamre-Nietupski, 1979)?

The only question held in common by the decision-rule systems under review is the question of candidacy. Thus, the only outcome common among them is deciding the appropriateness of the use of nonspeech communication systems with an individual.

Reichle and Karlan (1986) have presented a detailed analysis of the variables that are included in each decision system; these variables fall into three general classes: (a) characteristics of the individual, (b) training history, and (c) environmental variables. A large portion of the decision systems consider some of these variables either implicitly or explicitly, but do not actually use them as a basis for a decision point. In other decision systems, these variables are used as a basis for questions and, hence, information gathering, but that information has no differential effect on decision outcome. Finally, all of the decision systems use certain variables as the basis for actual decision points. In those systems where actual decision points can be stated, Table 13.1 contains the actual decision-rule system or set of questions.

Scheuerman et al. (1976), later published by Nietupski and Hamre-Nietupski (1979), use the fewest decision points of any of the four decision-rule sets. Although the degree of language comprehension is considered as a criterion for augmentative system selection (see Reichle & Karlan, 1986, for details), only the degree of language production is used as a criterial factor. As a variable, the status of the speech production mechanism (the ability to produce and control speech sounds) in determining appropriate use of nonspeech systems appears to be subsumed under the consideration of training history. An inability to produce and control speech sounds undoubtedly would contribute greatly to the failure of past efforts at training speech production. It might also be assumed that an inability to learn verbal imitation even when an intact speech production mechanism exists will result in failure to acquire speech production. The obvious drawback to this system is that considerable time (5 to 8 years according to the rule) must be invested in trial speech production training. Further, this rule assumes that the intervention efforts implemented during the learner's first 5 to 8 years represent systematically implemented and logical procedures.

Chapman and Miller (1980) presume that successful acquisition of language, whether spoken or nonspoken, is predicated upon the development of a certain level of cognitive performance. Further, they suggest that there must be a language production problem before nonspeech intervention is appropriate. While they agree that the failure to develop productive speech commensurate with chronological age and failure of past speech production training to yield functional spoken communication are good reasons, Chapman and Miller argue that these are not sufficient reasons for instituting augmentative systems. The key to the decision rules (see Table 13.1) formulated by Chapman and Miller (1980) is the relationship among cognition, comprehension, and production. The inclusion of the alternate requirement of a deviant speech mechanism appears to be redundant with the requirements of unintelligible speech (it does not matter why language production is unintelligible, only that it is).

By far, the most complicated system of decision rules is that delineated by Shane (1980) and Shane and Bashir (1980), which yields three decision paths (see Table 13.1). Nine variables were considered and are apparently used in arriving at specific decision points. However, only five of these factors are used as specific decision points in deciding whether nonspeech communication is appropriate for an individual (Reichle & Karlan, 1986).

**TABLE 13.1**

**Characteristics Considered for Use and Used in Decision Rules for Determining Whether to Implement a Nonspeech Communication System with an Individual**

| | Age | Status of speech production mechanism | Etiology of language production problem | Past performance in speech production training | Degree of language development | | Level of cognitive development | Degree of pragmatic development | Evidence of emotional problems | Level of environmental support |
|---|---|---|---|---|---|---|---|---|---|---|
| | | | | | Comprehension | Production | | | | |
| Scheuerman et al. (1976) | Decision point | Considered | | Decision point | Considered | Decision point | | | | |
| Nietupski & Hamre-Nietupski (1979) | | | | | | | | | | |
| Chapman & Miller (1980) | Considered | Considered | | Considered | Decision point | Decision point | Decision point | Decision point | | |
| Shane (1980) | Used | Decision point | Used | Decision point | Used | Decision point | Decision point | Used[a] | Used | Decision point |
| Shane & Bashir (1980) | | | | | | | | | | |
| Sailor et al. (1980) | | Considered | | Considered | Considered | Considered | Decision point | Considered | | Considered |

[a]Though not considered explicitly, some aspects of this characteristic are included in the evaluation of language production capability.

One factor common to each of the paths delineated by Shane (1980) and Shane and Bashir (1980) is the status of the learner's cognitive development. If cognitive development is at or beyond sensorimotor stage 5 intelligence, then the decision process can continue. The other common factor is the willingness of significant others in the environment to implement the nonspeech systems. Following the determination of cognitive status, the status of the speech production mechanism as evidenced by persistent oral-motor reflex problems is examined. If problems are found and the environment is cooperative, implementation is undertaken. If, however, no evidence is found, then past speech production training is evaluated (Path 2); if previously unsuccessful training is demonstrated and the learner's current environment is cooperative, implementation is undertaken. On the other hand, if there has been no speech production training (Path 3), then the degree of speech or language production is examined together with the ability to imitate speech sounds or gross motor or oral motor movements. If deficiencies are identified and the environment is cooperative, then implementation is undertaken. All of the preceding paths apply to learners who have failed previously to emit verbal utterances.

Sailor et al. (1980) recommend a set of decision rules that separately address the identification of output as well as input modes for learners with severe oral/aural mode deficits. With respect to outputs the interventionist must first answer four questions: (a) Can the learner benefit from incoming auditory information? (b) Can the learner benefit from incoming visual stimuli? (c) Will the learner's oral/motor status support speech output? and (d) Is the learner vocally imitative? If the answer to these initial questions is "yes," a speech mode is selected. If, on the other hand, the answer is "no" (presumably to any of the questions), the interventionist is asked to complete a comparative evaluation of signing and boards based on environmental considerations (e.g., preference of parents, cost of system, etc.) in addition to the proficiency with which the learner might be able to use the available response modalities. Learners who point are determined to be candidates for communication boards (blind children who point are candidates for tactile stimuli on communication boards).

As was the case in Shane's (1980) decision rules, the failure to engage in generalized imitation serves as a criterion that allows the interventionist to opt for an augmentative system. Presumably, a learner would have to be enrolled in vocal imitation training for some (unspecified) amount of time without significant success before an augmentative mode would be implemented. Further, Sailor et al. (1980) appear to direct an augmentative user to sign as a preferable system to communication boards. That is, their decision rules focus the user on communication boards as a last resort, yet no clear explanation for this direction is provided.

In summary, no common approach to the issue of how the nonspeech systems should be used (whether in support or in place of spoken communication) has received a consensus of approval. Nietupski and Hamre-Nietupski (1979) simply advocate concurrent training so that spoken communication is always augmented. Chapman and Miller (1980) make a clear distinction between augmentative usage and usage as a substitute for spoken communication. They indicate that if there is clearly a deviant speech production mechanism with a poor prognosis for improvement, then nonspeech communication systems will be required to substitute for rather than to augment speech. Shane and Bashir (1980) state that a decision to elect nonspeech systems "designates that such a system be used to facilitate oral language production . . . to augment communication . . . to enhance oral speech intelligibility . . . or some combination of the above" (p. 140). One may, however, question how speech facilitation or enhancement results from the application of these decision rules. There is no option in the Shane and Bashir rules permitting spoken language production to continue during the implementation of nonspeech communication. The actual outcome points would appear to indicate that the nonspeech systems substitute for the oral systems.

The decision rules reviewed thus far have a common focus: determining when it is advisable to use a nonspeech system of communication. These decision-rule systems adhere to the same basic strategy of first establishing a certain severity of impairment that must be present prior to scrutinizing prerequisites required for entry into a specific augmentative communication system. As a result, a significant number of learners with severe handicaps become trapped in a "no man's land" of having a sufficiently severe impairment but failing to have the prerequisites (primarily cognitive). In the discussion that follows, we explore the difficulties in implementing existing augmentative decision rules.

## Can Existing Decision Rules Be Implemented Systematically?

Individual variability in language acquisition, as well as procedural vagueness, make it difficult to implement systematically the decision rules reviewed. All of the existing decision rules require the interventionist to identify a significant communication delay. Given the extreme variability in the communicative development even of normal preschoolers, it may be difficult to identify the point at which a communicative delay becomes predictive of a significant problem. Variability extends across phonological, semantic, pragmatic, and syntactic skills as well as across comprehension and production. With a very young child, it is difficult to conclude whether failure to produce a spoken word by 18 or 19 months represents a clinically/educationally significant delay when there is a reasonable possibility that the child in question will develop normal communication production. The identification of significant lags becomes even more difficult when the interventionist attempts to make relative comparisons between comprehension and production skills. This is true particularly in the case of decision rules such as Chapman and Miller's (1980), which require that direct comparisons be made.

In addition to comprehension-production comparisons, Chapman and Miller (1980) require that the interventionist compare the learner's current cognitive status with language comprehension and production. Unfortunately, they do not specify whether individual cognitive subscale data (i.e., means/end, causality, imitation, space, motor and vocal imitation, object permanency) or some combined "average" of subscale scores should be used in determining cognitive status. Rogers (1977) found that a severely intellectually delayed population exhibited less homogeneity across cognitive subscales than normal children. For example, a severely handicapped child might be operating at sensorimotor stage 3 (4–8 months) performance in motor imitation but stage 5 (12–18 months) in means-end. Available data continue to support the conclusion that individuals with severe handicaps are heterogeneous with respect to the level of cognitive development attained across several different areas of behavior at a given time (Karlan & Lloyd, 1985). Obviously, this heterogeneity when manifest across cognitive assessment scales casts considerable doubt on the usefulness of an overall cognitive stage score, which both Shane and Bashir (1980) and Chapman and Miller (1980) seem to recommend. In determining criteria for a significant cognitive and/or communicative delay, existing decision rules seem to have oversimplified the considerations involved.

## Cognitive Acquisitions as Prerequisites to Augmentative System Use

Rice (1983) stated that "there is a detectable sense of frustration regarding the elusiveness of cognition and its role in language impairment and the remediation process" (p.347). As yet, there are no empirical data supporting a causal relationship between cognitive and communicative behavior in either normal or intellectually delayed learners. That certain cognitive and language skills appear to develop at about the same time may be dependent on some underlying source common to both domains of development such as the more fundamental Piagetian processes of assimilation and accommodation. Or the developments in cognition and language may be interactive (i.e., there may exist a bidirectional influence).

Theoretical issues aside, one might ask whether the empirical evidence supports the position that particular cognitive skills facilitate the acquisition or use of specific communication skills or functions.

Reichle and Karlan (1986) provided a review of cognitive domains that included imitation, means-end, causality, and object permanency. They found a lack of compelling evidence that demonstrated a causal link between cognitive prerequisites and the acquisition of communicative behavior. Further, they suggested that there is little research exploring the issue of cognitive prerequisites with persons who exhibit severe handicaps. In spite of the sparse empirical bases for citing specific cognitive prerequisites to the communication acquisition process, many interventionists may pigeonhole the learner into a level of intervention in domains such as imitation that may not be necessary in order to implement a communication intervention program.

Some specifications of cognitive prerequisites in augmentative decision rules have been relatively vague. For example, Shane and Bashir (1980) suggested that learners functioning at a level commensurate with a normal 12-month-old are "probably not at an appropriate age for communication prosthesis, even one made out of the most iconic materials" (p. 314). To the contrary, Reichle and Yoder (1985) demonstrated that simple labeling skills could be taught before a child was functioning as a 12-month-old. In the signing modality, McIntire (1974) described the use of signed vocabulary by an 8-month-old hearing impaired child. Stillman, Alymer, and Vandivort (1983) have reported teaching severely and profoundly handicapped individuals to use communicative "signals" to control participation in certain gross motor activities. These individuals were taught to use abbreviated forms of the action, idiosyncratic gestures, or actual manual signs to initiate an activity, request recurrence of an activity, redirect to another activity, and terminate activities. These behaviors were not specifically directed to an audience. That is, given the proper context, the individual would signal the behavior whether or not the adult was attending. Thus, although these handicapped individuals did not recognize the role of the audience and, therefore, would not be considered to have "intentional" communication, they did demonstrate an ability to learn a contextually relevant action (the signals) to control some aspect of the activity (the goal). The key issue is whether "social agency" (recognition of the need to direct messages to an audience) must be present before communicative behaviors can be taught. There appears to be ample evidence to support a strategy that shapes intentional communicative behavior from preexisting perlocutionary signaling behavior (see Reichle, Sigafoos, Piché-Cragoe, & Doss, 1986).

In summary, there seems to be a lack of convincing evidence to demonstrate a causal link between particular cognitive prerequisites and the acquisition of communicative behavior. Although there does seem to be a fairly compelling logic to suggest that some classes of behavior may facilitate the acquisition of communicative behavior, the specificity with which authors of augmentative decision rules assign cognitive prerequisites does not appear to be warranted based on available empirical data.

## USE OF AUGMENTATIVE SYSTEMS FOR PREVENTION OF LATER PRODUCTION DEFICITS

One interesting by-product from the implementation of manual signing and communication board programs has been the apparent facilitating effect of the use of augmentative modalities upon acquisition of communicative behavior in the vocal modality. In the manual signing modality, Reichle, McQuarter, and Rogers (1983) reviewed a number of investigations that reported a positive effect of signing upon frequency and/or quality of vocal/verbal production. However, in most instances the effects were reported anecdotally.

Remington and Clark (1983) demonstrated that cross-modal transfer of training (sign to vocal mode) occurred with a learner who was capable of vocal imitation skills. Conversely, transfer did not occur for a learner who did not engage in vocal imitation. This finding suggests that learners who attended to the presentation of two elements of a complex stimulus (sign and a spoken word) benefited from both elements of the stimulus. That is, they were able to act differentially on each element. It does not necessarily suggest that signing was facilitative of the vocal mode.

The general conclusion of many investigations (Daniloff, Fristoe, & Lloyd, 1982; Konstantares, Oxman, & Webster, 1978) has been that signing often facilitates the production of vocal/verbal repertoires and that exposing or teaching learners to sign has no adverse effect upon the acquisition of vocal mode communication. At present, we hope that the former is true but have good evidence only to support the latter. In the realm of production, we support the point of view that the use of augmentative modes may be a useful preventive measure for avoiding later production deficits. Unfortunately, this potential benefit is minimized by decision rules which require a significant production delay prior to the implementation of augmentative communication intervention. More traditional decision rules that have been described require significant evidence of delay prior to such implementation. Decision rules offered by Nietupski and Hamre-Nietupski (1979) and Scheuerman et al. (1976) present the greatest problems in implementing a strategy using augmentative modalities to reduce the probability of later production deficits by waiting until the learner is between 5 and 8 years old before the decision to implement an augmentative system can be made.

In addition to the positive influence that they may have on communication production, augmentative communication systems may facilitate comprehension. Chapman and Miller (1980) and Shane and Bashir (1980) suggested that one criterion has been met for the implementation of an augmentative communication system when the learner's production significantly lags behind his or her comprehension skills. This criterion implies that augmentative communication systems are intended primarily to deal with production deficits. If one were to pursue this logic, an individual with a severe intellectual delay might never be a candidate for an augmentative intervention if his or her comprehension was sufficiently delayed so that a comprehension-production gap never developed.

Apart from any value in facilitating production, the use of augmentative techniques can benefit comprehension intervention. Several studies have demonstrated a direct effect of the use of manual signs upon comprehension skills exhibited by moderately and severely handicapped learners. Kohl, Karlan, and Heal (1979) demonstrated that severely handicapped children's ability to follow instructions was significantly better when spoken and manually signed instructions were combined as compared with the use of spoken instructions only. Additionally, Karlan and Lloyd (1983) found that comprehension recall (i.e., identifying the correct picture from an array of pictures) was significantly improved by the use of manually signed cues during the learning task.

Clearly, a rationale for the value of augmentative modalities in the generation of language comprehension programs can be built, and this rationale will find sufficient empirical support to justify its application.

## ALTERNATIVES TO TRADITIONAL DECISION RULES

Objectively comparing learner performance in each of several communicative modes (modality sampling) is not a particularly new idea (Alpert, 1980; Kiernan, 1977). Keogh and Reichle (1985) described several types of difficult to teach learners that we believe would best benefit from modality sampling procedures. Some of these learners seem to exhibit all of the motivational prerequisites to engage in an instructional task (e.g., they sit and seem to be attending, they reach and have unrestricted movement of fingers or gait, they readily accept food and praise), yet they fail to learn. Other difficult to teach learners seem to be passive participants in instructional activities. That is, they sit and allow the teacher to prompt or put them through targeted behaviors but do little else. For the most part, we do not believe that modality sampling will prove as beneficial with learners who exhibit severe motor impairment. For these individuals, augmentative system selection probably will be more straightforward.

The systematic comparison of augmentative communication modes could yield outcomes that include (a) the eventual selection of a single communicative modality or (b) two or more strong and durable alternative modes that are vocabulary specific, setting specific, or audience specific. To achieve these outcomes, procedures must be designed to maximize the learner's opportunity to succeed in each of the modes sampled while at the same time carefully considering the constraints that the environment places on each potential augmentative mode that might be used to represent a given vocabulary item. Within the past several years a variety of different modality sampling strategies that incorporate performance baselines has been proposed.

## Successive Modality Sampling Baselines

Alpert (1980) identified an assessment/training procedure for determining the optimal nonspeech mode to use with autistic children once the decision has been made to augment speech. Her procedure involves teaching specific language responses in each of two successively taught nonspeech modes. Reichle and Keogh (1986) suggested that this strategy might be thought of as a strategy of generating "performance baselines." By comparing respective acquisition rates between baselines, the interventionist may be able to identify, empirically, a single modality for long-term intervention. Alpert's (1980) strategy suggests making decisions using a preventative logic regarding the need for an augmentative system and the best type of augmentative system to use. That is, rather than specifying an arbitrarily imposed failure criterion, Alpert suggested utilizing learner generated data to stimulate the decision-making process. As such, there is no need to set specific selection criteria. Outcomes from Alpert's system would result in (a) the selection of a superior augmentative mode or (b) no clear evidence to support the selection of a single mode.

Although useful, there may be potential disadvantages in the successive implementation of different potential augmentative modes. Implementing only one mode at a time may delay the learner's acquisition of meaningful communicative skills, if the first mode to be sampled does not prove to be the mode of choice. If a concurrent sampling of potential augmentative modes could be achieved, the superiority of one augmentative system over another might become obvious at an earlier point. Additionally, although learner performance is critical, successive performance baselines may not be particularly sensitive to the communicative demands of the learner's environments.

## Concurrent Modality Sampling Baselines

Concurrent modality sampling may be implemented using one of several strategies. One strategy involves establishing the same vocabulary in each of two separate modes. That is, the vocabulary *apple* could be taught in sign/gesture during some targeted activities and in the graphic mode during other activities. Another alternative would involve teaching *different* vocabulary in each of two concurrently implemented modes. For example, *apple* might be taught in sign/gesture but not in the graphic mode. Concurrently, *orange* might be taught in the graphic mode but not in the sign/gesture mode. Advantages and disadvantages in using each of these two concurrently implemented alternatives require further consideration.

*Teaching the Same Vocabulary Concurrently in Two Different Modes.* Teaching the same vocabulary concurrently in each of two different modes has potential advantages as well as disadvantages. Acquisition of both the graphic symbol and the manual sign representing *apple* might allow an opportunity to determine which mode might be most likely to be used by the learner in contexts different from those used during acquisition.

On the other hand, teaching the same vocabulary concurrently in each of two modes may present a distinct disadvantage. The learner may have difficulty selecting a mode to use when presented with a situation that does not contain stimulus characteristics that were present during mode specific intervention activities. Second, and perhaps more important, one might argue that because a severely handicapped learner's communication repertoire is already sparsely populated, it would be more efficient to introduce the greatest number of different vocabulary items by dividing the available items between the modes being sampled. Teaching the same vocabulary concurrently in two modes may reduce the number of different vocabulary that could have been introduced in the same intervention period.

*Teaching Different Vocabulary in Each of Two Augmentative Modes.* The use of mode specific vocabulary during the implementation of a concurrent modality sampling strategy allows the interventionist to more sensitively consider the effect that the environment may play in the selection of the best augmentative mode. In part, the issue here is whether some settings better support the use of sign/gesture while others better support the use of graphics. If so, the mode that is most effective and efficient in meeting demands in the greatest number of environments or contexts in which a vocabulary item will be used should be selected as the mode of instruction for that vocabulary item.

If during the ensuing performance baselines the learner shows no widely discrepant pattern of acquisition between the two modes, the learner will be well on his or her way to the acquisition of what Reichle and Keogh (1986) referred to as a mixed mode system, which is sensitive to the communicative demands of different environments.

For example, the natural gestures of shaking one's head up and down, or from side-to-side, or holding one's hand up to signal "stop" are fairly universal responses. In terms of teaching, such gestures are easily modeled and prompted. Additionally, natural teaching opportunities arise often. These characteristics render certain natural gestures more efficient than the formal manual signs even for learners who may possess all of the physiological and imitative requirements for producing the formal signs for "yes" and "no." Further, gestures can be observed at some distance, while most graphic displays cannot. For example, assume that a communication board user is attempting to communicate that the listener should move away. Using a system that requires a close approach for the listener to read the message may result in the approach of the listener, which the communication board user is trying to prevent.

Other considerations in selecting specific signs or graphic symbols may be less environmentally oriented but nevertheless provide support for considering the use of mixed mode communication systems. There is a growing literature that suggests that iconic signs/gestures and logographs may be more easily acquired than less iconic signs/symbols. In the graphic mode, many agree that object logographs tend to be more iconic than logographs depicting actions (Karlan & Lloyd, 1985). If this finding is applicable to learners with severe handicaps and assuming that graphic and gestural modes were acquired at equal rates, an increased number of action vocabulary may be emitted in the gestural mode, whereas a greater proportion of object vocabulary may occur as graphic mode responses.

## Teaching Vocal Mode Production During Modality Sampling

At the same time that the learner is engaged in performance baselines in both graphic and gestural modes, concurrent intervention also may begin in the vocal mode. Because there is some evidence to suggest that vocal mode acquisition may be slower than acquisition in the augmentative modes (Schaeffer, 1980), we suggest that while different vocabulary items may be assigned to each augmentative mode, vocabulary taught in the vocal mode should replicate that taught in the graphic or gestural modes. That is, if vocabulary *a* and *b* are assigned to the gestural mode and *c* and *d* to the graphic mode, then *a* and *c* might be assigned to the vocal mode. Because the vocal mode represents such a powerful means of production, we believe that it is not subject to a direct comparison with the performance baselines established in the graphic and gestural modes. At present we believe that there is an insufficient empirical basis to suggest a decision point that addresses when to stop attempting intervention in the vocal mode. The strategy for vocal mode intervention presented here involves maximizing the number of different vocabulary items that are taught in the augmentative mode. At the same time, the interventionist refrains from assigning a significant vocabulary item exclusively into a communication mode that may require an extensive intervention period before it meets the communicative needs of the learner.

## Determining When to Begin Modality Sampling

Keogh and Reichle (1985) and Reichle and Keogh (1986) have suggested that early communication production targets should include the establishment of requesting, rejecting, and commenting/describing communicative intents. Consequently, the interventionist's early efforts can be aimed at determining whether the learner emits any discrete voluntary idiosyncratic behavior to (a) gain access to objects/events, (b) escape or avoid any objects/events, or (c) socially interact with others. If learners are not actively emitting voluntary behavior, then systematic attempts to stimulate the learner's overtures toward or away from objects/events in the natural environment should be undertaken. As soon as specific likes and dislikes can be identified, the process of modality sampling may begin. Reichle and Keogh (1986) have provided a detailed explanation of specific communication intervention procedures that might be used during the process of modality sampling.

## Determining When to End Modality Sampling

Determining when to terminate a modality sampling procedure is much like determining when to discontinue any baseline. Once a clear-cut advantage for one of the two augmentative systems is supported by data, the interventionist has a legitimate basis for discontinuing intervention in the less productive mode. However, with respect to clear-cut advantage, several issues or cautions must be addressed. At present little is known about the relationships among acquisition, maintenance, and generalization in comparing graphic and gestural mode performance.

It is possible that symbols might be acquired more quickly in one modality but maintained better and/or generalized more efficiently in another modality. In comparing any instructional practices, interventionists usually assume that trends found during acquisition will hold during maintenance and generalization tasks. Such has been the case in comparing logographic systems. Hurlbut, Iwata, & Green (1982) found that highly iconic line drawings were learned faster, maintained better, and generalized more readily than less iconic line drawings. Unfortunately, there are no such empirical comparisons that have been made *across* augmentative modalities. One could argue that because a graphic modality involves a closed set of response alternatives (while a gestural mode system involves an open set of response alternatives), the board user would have a more visible stimulus prompt to use logographics when encountering new contexts in which he or she could communicate. Alternatively, one could argue that because signing is quick and can be understood by a listener at some distance, fewer communicative attempts emitted in the natural environment would go unreinforced.

At present we can only speculate about these matters. There is a critical need to implement a modality sampling strategy for a sufficient time to generate a base of maintenance and generalization data to permit cross-mode comparisons. We know little about the applicability of maintenance and generalization results obtained for one vocabulary class (e.g., objects) to other classes (e.g., actions). Signs, for example, may provide more iconic representations of actions than graphics, thereby biasing a modality sampling strategy that used only action vocabulary in favor of signs. The superiority of signs when object vocabulary is taught may, however, disappear. Therefore, conclusions regarding the potential of each augmentative mode should be based upon a sampling of vocabulary from several classes. In some cases the superiority of one modality over another may be context specific, making it impossible to select a single most effective augmentative system. Finally, among learners who readily acquire vocabulary in either augmentative mode, context or setting variables may well be the primary factor in determining which mode to use in representing new vocabulary. In all likelihood, it seems that such a learner might well become a mixed mode user (using some sign/gestures and some graphic symbols).

## Distinguishing Between Modality Sampling and Total Communication

Moores (1974) pointed out that there are different interpretations of total and simultaneous communication as methodologies. However, Reichle and Keogh (1986) suggested that it is generally accepted that each is characterized by, at least, the concurrent presentation in one context of oral and nonoral symbolic forms for the same referents (Denton, 1972; Fulwiler & Fouts, 1976; Gustason, Pfetzing, & Zawolkow, 1972). The basis for advocating the simultaneous method is that a multimodal approach may maximize the probability of learning successes with low-functioning individuals (Hopper & Helmick, 1977). Thus, total communication involves the concurrent presentation in a single context of speech and sign, or gestures, or graphics as multisymbol equivalents. In contrast, modality sampling procedures as described previously attempt to establish the use of a single symbolic form during a specific communicative episode.

## Describing Duplicated Mode Use

Some learners who are now in their thirties originally learned sign/gestures as their primary augmentative mode. In the years that ensued, learners found it increasingly difficult to communicate in community environments because few individuals signed (Reichle & York, in preparation). This situation has resulted in the need for an augmentation of the original augmentative mode. That is, when in the community, the learner needed some viable substitute for sign. At the same time, because signing was quick to use and very portable, it seemed problematic to replace sign with a graphic augmentation. The program reported by Reichle and Ward (1985) taught the discriminative use of two different symbol systems for the same vocabulary. If, for example, a learner wanted to order a coke at McDonalds, he was taught to use the graphic mode. However, if he wanted his mother to fix him a coke, he was taught to sign. Although we do not view duplicated mode use as the intervention choice, we do recognize its value in instances in which the learner produces an extensive repertoire of signs but cannot communicate effectively in community settings.

## Summary

It is important to emphasize that in advocating modality sampling, we are not necessarily advocating the selection of a single augmentative mode. Many learners may do equally well in graphic or gestural modes. In a sense, many learners may become mixed mode communicators. If this is the case, then environmental conditions will exert an even greater impact on assignment of augmentative mode to vocabulary items. That is, it may be possible to implement a mixed augmentative system that enhances the advantages of gestural and graphic modes while at the same time minimizing the disadvantages inherent in each system. An examination of the sorts of communication exchanges that are possible in the learner's day-to-day environment often shows that, in some situations or activities, manual signing is the most effective, while in other situations or activities occurring in the same day, a graphic system or natural gestures is more effective. By utilizing recently developed assessment procedures for identifying learner opportunities for interaction (Brown et al., 1979; Iverson, Williams, Schutz, & Fox, 1983; Snell, 1983; Wilcox & Bellamy, 1982), a specific modality for expression (i.e., natural gestures) might be determined to be most efficient in one set of circumstances but not in others, providing the basis for a mixed modality system.

Use of a modality sampling strategy appears to provide a meaningful and useful method for quantifying decisions regarding the selection of an augmentative system. In the absence of any existing validated decision models, concurrent modality sampling offers the interventionist an opportunity simultaneously to address the question of whether some augmentative system is warranted while at the same time determining which system or systems, if needed, would be most desirable.

## REFERENCES


Alberto, P., Garrett, E. J., Briggs, T., & Umberger, F. (1983, March). Selection and initiation of a nonvocal communication program for severely handicapped students. *Focus on Exceptional Children, 15*(7), 1–15

Alpert, C. (1980). Procedures for determining the optional nonspeech mode with the autistic child. In R. L. Schiefelbusch (Ed.), *Nonspeech language and communication: Analysis and intervention* (pp. 389–420). Austin, TX: PRO-ED.

Brown, L., Branston, M., Baumbart, D., Vincent, L., Falvey, M., & Schroeder, J. (1979). Using the characteristics of current and subsequent least restrictive environments as factors in the development of curricular content for severely handicapped students. *AAESPH Review*, *4*, 407–424.

Chapman, R., & Miller, J. (1980). Analyzing language and communication in the child. In R. L. Schiefelbusch (Ed.), *Nonspeech language and communication: Acquisition and intervention* (pp. 159–196). Austin, TX: PRO-ED.

Daniloff, J., Noll, J., Fristoe, M., & Lloyd, L. (1982). Gesture recognition in patients with aphasia. *Journal of Speech and Hearing Disorders*, *47*, 43–49.

Denton, D. (1972). A rationale for total communication. *American Annals for the Deaf*, *51*, 53–61.

Fulwiler, R., & Fouts, R. (1976). Acquisition of American Sign Language by a noncommunicating autistic child. *Journal of Autism and Childhood Schizophrenia*, *6*, 43–51.

Gustason, G., Pfetzing, D., & Zawolkow, E. (1972). *Signing exact English*. Rossmoor, CA: Modern Signs Press.

Hopper, C., & Helmick, R. (1977). Nonverbal communication for the severely handicapped: Some considerations. *AAESPH Review*, *2*, 47–52.

Hurlbut, B., Iwata, B., & Green, J. (1982). Nonvocal language acquisition in adolescents with severe physical disabilities. Blissymbol vs. iconic stimulus formats. *Journal of Applied Behavior Analysis, 15,* 241–258.

Iverson, G., Williams, W., Schutz, R. & Fox, t. (1983). Burlington's making special friends project: Strategies for implementing model components (Vol. IV). *Center for Developmentally Disabled Monograph Series, 3,* University of Vermont.

Karlan, G., & Lloyd, L. (1985). Unpublished manuscript. Department of Special Education, Purdue University, West Lafayette, IN.

Karlan, G., & Lloyd, L. (1983, May). *Examination of recall comprehension by moderately retarded individuals responding to oral and manual cues.* Paper presented at the 107th annual meeting of the American Association on Mental Deficiency, Dallas, TX.

Keogh, W., & Reichle, J. (1985). Communication intervention for the "Difficult-to-teach" severely handicapped. In S. Warren & A. Rogers-Warren (Eds)., *Teaching functional language* (pp. 157–196). Austin, TX: PRO-ED.

Kiernan, C. (1977). Alternatives to speech. A review of research on manual and other alternative forms of communication in the mentally handicapped. *British Journal of Mental Subnormality, 23,* 6–28.

Kiernan, C. (1981). A strategy for research on the use of nonvocal systems of communication. *Journal of Autism and Developmental Disabilities, 11,* 139–151.

Kohl, F., Karlan, G., & Heal, L. (1979). Effects of pairing manual signs with verbal cues upon the acquisition of instruction-following behaviors and the generalization to expressive language with severely handicapped children. *AAESPH Review, 4,* 91–103.

Konstantares, M., Oxman, J., & Webster, C. (1978). Iconicity: Effects on the acquisition of sign language by autistic and other severely dysfunctional children. In P. Siple (Ed.), *Understanding language through sign language research* (pp. 213–237). New York: Academic Press.

McIntire, M. (1974). *A modified model for the description of language acquisition in a deaf child.* Unpublished master's thesis, California State University, Northridge.

Moores, D. (1974). Nonvocal system of verbal behavior. In R. L. Schiefelbusch & L. Lloyd (Eds.), *Language perspectives: Acquisition, retardation, and intervention* (pp. 377–417). Austin, TX: PRO-ED.

Nietupski, J., & Hamre-Nietupski, S. (1979). Teaching auxiliary communication skills to severely handicapped learners. *AAESPH Review, 4,* 107–124.

Reichle, J., & Karlan, G. (1986). The selection of an augmentative system in communication intervention: A critique of decision rules. *Journal of the Association for Persons with Severe Handicaps, 10,* 146–156.

Reichle, J., & Keogh, W. (1985). Communication intervention: A selective review of what, when and how to teach. In S. Warren & A. Rogers-Warren (Eds.), *Teaching functional language* (pp. 25–59). Austin, TX: PRO-ED.

Reichle, J., McQuarter, R., & Rogers, N. (1983). *Sign intervention with severely handicapped learners: A review.* Unpublished manuscript, University of Minnesota, Minneapolis.

Reichle, J., Sigafoos, J., Piché-Cragoe, L., & Doss, S. (1986). *Optimizing functional communication for persons with severe handicaps.* Unpublished manuscript, University of Minnesota.

Reichle, J., & Ward, M. (1985). Teaching discriminative use of signed English and encoding graphic modality to an autistic adolescent. *Language, Speech and Hearing Services in Schools, 16,* 146–157.

Reichle, J., & Yoder, D. (1985). Communication board use in severely handicapped learners. *Language, Speech and Hearing Services in Schools, 16,* 146–157.

Reichle, J., & York, J. (in preparation). *Issues in implementing communication aids.* Unpublished manuscript, University of Minnesota.

Remington, N., & Clark, S. (1983). The acquisition of expressive signing by autistic children: An evaluation of the relative effects of simultaneous communication and sign above training. *Journal of Applied Behavior Analysis, 16,* 315–328.

Rice, M. (1983). Contemporary accounts of the cognition/language relationship: Implications for speech-language clinicians. *Journal of Speech and Hearing Disorders, 48,* 347–359.

Rogers, S. (1977). Characteristics of the cognitive development of profoundly retarded children. *Child Development, 48,* 837–843.

Sailor, W., Guess, D., Goetz, L., Schuler, A., Utley, B., & Baldwin, M. (1980). Language and severely handicapped persons: Deciding what to teach whom. In W. Sailor, B. Wilcox, & L. Brown (Eds.), *Methods of instruction for severely handicapped students* (pp. 71–108). Baltimore: Paul H. Brookes.

Schaeffer, B. (1980). Spontaneous language through signed speech. In R. L. Schiefelbusch (Ed.), *Nonspeech language and communication: Analysis and intervention* (pp. 421–446). Austin, TX: PRO-ED.

Scheuerman, N., Baumgart, D., Simpsa, K. & Brown, L. (1976). Toward the development of a curriculum for teaching nonverbal communication skills to severely handicapped students: Teaching basic tracking, scanning and selection skills. In L. Brown, N. Scheuerman, & T. Crowner (Eds.), *Madison's alternative for zero exclusion: Toward an integrated therapy model for teaching motor, tracking and scanning skills to severely handicapped students* (Vol. 6, pt. 3). Madison, WI: Madison Metropolitan School District.

Shane, H. (1980). Approaches to assessing the communication of nonoral persons. In R. L. Schiefelbusch (Ed.), *Nonspeech language and communication: Analysis and intervention* (pp. 197–224). Austin, TX: PRO-ED.

Shane, H. & Bashir, A. (1980). Election criteria for the adoption of an augmentative communication system: Preliminary considerations. *Journal of Speech and Hearing Disorders, 5,* 408–414.

Snell, M. (1983). *Systematic instruction of the moderately and severely handicapped.* Columbus, OH. Charles E. Merrill.

Stillman, R., Alymer, J. & Vandivort, J. (1983, June). *The functions of signaling behaviors in profoundly impaired, deaf-blind children, and adolescents.* Paper presented at the 107th annual meeting of the American Association on Mental Deficiency, Dallas, TX.

Wilcox, B., & Bellamy, G. T. (1982). *Design of high school programs for severely handicapped students.* Baltimore: Paul H. Brookes.

SECTION VI

# *Intervention*

LYLE L. LLOYD AND
RICHARD L. SCHIEFELBUSCH, EDITORS

# 14

# *Augmentative and Alternative Communication Issues*

Mary Ann Romski, Lyle L. Lloyd, and Rose A. Sevcik

Based on demographic figures, it is estimated that there are 1,225,000 children in the United States alone who are nonspeaking, or severely speech impaired, as a result of a neurological, physical, or psychological disability (Yoder, 1980). During the past quarter century, and especially during the past decade, augmentative and alternative communication systems have emerged as viable means of expression for persons with severe oral communication impairments.[1] Antecedents to the current use of nonspeech communication systems include the use of manual communication with retarded children who evidenced significant hearing impairments (e.g., Berger, 1972; Hall & Talkington, 1970; Hoffmeister & Farmer, 1972), language relevant research with nonhuman primates (e.g., Gardner & Gardner, 1969; Premack, 1970;

Preparation of this chapter was supported in part by National Institutes of Health grants NICHD-06016 and RR-00165 to the Yerkes Regional Primate Research Center, Emory University, Atlanta, Georgia, and United States Office of Special Education grant G00-8300868 to Purdue University, West Lafayette, Indiana. The contents do not necessarily represent the policy of these agencies or the endorsement of the federal government. The authors wish to thank Dr. George R. Karlan for his suggestions in the early development of parts of this chapter.

[1] Nonspeech communication systems have a variety of uses. They can be used to augment speech, to facilitate speech, or to substitute for it. A number of terms have been used to refer to these communicative systems including *augmentative* and *alternative* (Lloyd, 1984). In this chapter we use the term *nonspeech communication* to refer to all of the uses of these systems.

Rumbaugh, 1977), and advances in electronic technology (e.g., Vanderheiden & Grilley, 1977). (See Lloyd & Karlan, 1984, for a complete review.) Case studies and controlled investigations alike support the use of nonspeech communication approaches with individuals who do not speak (e.g., Berger, 1972; Brookner & Murphy, 1975; Carrier, 1974; Duncan & Silverman, 1977; Linville, 1977; Miller & Miller, 1973; Reich, 1978).[2]

When the first volume of *Language Perspectives* (Schiefelbusch & Lloyd, 1974) was published, the modern use of nonspeech communication was in its infancy. The inclusion of a section on the topic in that volume was considered a major advance from previous books on language acquisition and intervention. Since 1974, nonspeech communication has received increasing attention from occupational therapists, psychologists, physical therapists, rehabilitation engineers, special educators, and speech/language clinicians, among others, concerned with the needs of persons who evidence severe oral communication impairments (e.g., Kiernan, Reid, & Jones, 1982; Lloyd, 1976; Musselwhite & St. Louis, 1982; Schiefelbusch, 1980a; Schiefelbusch & Hollis, 1979; Siiverman, 1980; Vanderheiden & Grilley, 1976). In this chapter we provide a brief overview of the currently available nonspeech communication systems, discuss suggested reasons for their success in communication intervention, and consider the clinical and research issues that have emerged as these nonspeech systems are employed in intervention programs with persons who exhibit severe oral communication impairments.

## NONSPEECH COMMUNICATION SYSTEMS

A nonspeech communication system is the total functional communication system of an individual; it includes the communicative technique used, the symbol set or system, and the communicative interaction ("Nonspeech Communication," 1980). The communication technique serves to transmit the message, while the symbol system is the representational means through which that message is conveyed. While these two components (technique and symbol system) are both integral parts of the complete system, the communicative interaction or the interindividual exchange is necessary for the message to be transmitted and received.

---

[2] This chapter focuses on those persons with severe oral communication impairments but with primary etiologies other than hearing impairment (e.g., autism, mental retardation).

## Aided and Unaided Symbol Systems

Communicative symbol systems can be divided into two types: unaided and aided (Fristoe & Lloyd, 1979; Lloyd & Fuller, 1986; Lloyd & Karlan, 1984). The range of available systems is provided in Table 14.1. In the right column of Table 14.1 are the unaided symbol sets (e.g., manual signs). These symbol sets do not require a physical aid for access. Aided non-speech symbol sets (e.g., Blissymbols) use some type of external device (i.e., a board or display) to access them (see left column of Table 14.1)

Speech is an unaided arbitrary communication system that employs an auditory channel for input and a vocal channel for output. It is temporally based, dynamic, and, once it has been produced, exists only in the sender's and the receiver's memories (Hockett, 1960). Other unaided, as well as aided, symbol systems can differ from speech in a number of characteristics including the input and output channels, the user's response, the memory for the signal, and the signal's structure, permanency, and arbitrariness (Romski, Sevcik, & Joyner, 1984).

Unaided symbol sets share some of the signal characteristics of speech. The structure of the signal is transitory in form and frequently involves movement or change. In many instances, the change conveys much of the meaning; therefore, the symbols may be considered dynamic. When used without speech accompaniment, the modality of input (visual) and output (manual) is different from speech. Like speech, however, the communicator must produce the message utilizing recall memory.

Aided symbol sets differ from speech and from unaided symbol sets in terms of the communicator's response and the characteristics of the signal. In addition to writing and drawing, there are three general methods of response with aided symbol sets: direct selection, scanning, and encoding (see Vanderheiden & Harris-Vanderheiden, 1976, for a complete description of these alternatives). With the exception of synthetic speech, all of these methods employ graphic symbols that typically are structured along spatial dimensions and remain fixed or static. In contrast to unaided systems, the user is not required to recall a symbol; instead, the user relies on recognition memory to select a symbol for communication.

Another dimension along which unaided and aided symbol systems vary is arbitrariness. In Table 14.1 unaided and aided symbols are arranged in a general hierarchy of arbitrariness. This hierarchy represents the relationship characteristic of the symbol sets as a whole; slight variations within the hierarchical schema do exist, however, for specific subsets of some symbol systems.

From an adult language user's perspective, the symbols located at the top of each column in Table 14.1 are more concretely related to their referents that those that appear at the bottom of the column. While mime,

TABLE 14.1

**Communication Symbols and Symbol Systems**[a]

| Aided | Unaided |
|---|---|
| Objects | Pointing |
| Pictures (photographs and line drawings) | Yes/no gestures |
| Simple Rebus | Mime |
| Sigsymbols | Generally understood gestures |
| Picsyms | Amer-Ind |
| Pictogram Ideogram Communication (PIC) | Other gestures |
| Blissymbols | Esoteric signs |
| Graphic representation of manual signs and/or gestures (e.g., HANDS, Sign Writer, Sigsymbols, Worldsign) | Gestuno |
| Complex Rebus | Natural Sign Languages (e.g., ASL, BSL, etc.) |
| Other logographs | Manually coded English (e.g., Signed English, PGSS, SEE-1, SEE2) |
| Lexigrams | Manual alphabet |
| Plastic Manipulable symbols (e.g., Non-SLIP) | Gestural Morse Code |
| Writing and Printed Words (TO) | Eye blink codes |
| Modified Orthography | Vocal codes |
| Braille and other vibrotactual codes | Hand cued speech (e.g., cued speech, Danish Mouth Hand) |
| Linear printing (WRITE) | Speech |
| Synthetic Speech (e.g., SAL, SPEEC) | |

[a] These are "formal" or conventionalized symbols; informal nonverbal behaviors have not been included.

Reprinted from "Nonspeech Communication Symbols and Systems" by L. L. Lloyd & G. W. Karlan, 1984, *Journal of Mental Deficiency Research*, *28*, 6.

generally understood gestures, Amer-Ind, and other gestures are more obviously related to their referents, a degree of arbitrariness is still found with some gestures. The Amer-Ind gesture for television, for example, conveys information about what a television looks like and what you do with it (e.g., look, listen) (Skelly, 1979). Competent spoken language users find Amer-Ind gestures approximately 50% identifiable, even if presented out of context (Daniloff, Lloyd, & Fristoe, 1983; Kirschner, Algozzine, & Abbott, 1979). The adult or child with a severe oral communication impairment must possess some nonlinguistic knowledge of what constitutes an Amer-Ind representation to associate the gestures with their appropriate meanings. Even pictures that are relatively representative of their referents may depict action in a somewhat arbitrary fashion. For example, a picture of an individual with one foot on the ground and the other foot raised and pointing back, with one arm pointing forward and the other arm pointing backward, is a common way to pictorially represent the verb *run*. While Blissymbols, PIC, Picsyms, and Sigsymbols possess a number of items that are concrete visual representations, they also have many items that require considerable abstraction. In addition, for some visual-graphic systems such as Blissymbols a person must be able to differentiate complex spatial representation such as ground and skyline placements of geometric forms (Chapman & Miller, 1980).

All of the remaining unaided and aided systems utilize primarily arbitrary symbols. Some individual signs, however, may be considered iconic, that is, they resemble the meanings for which they stand. Studies of American Sign Language (ASL) with normal hearing adults indicate that it is typically difficult to discern what a sign means from simply seeing it produced (Klima & Bellugi, 1979). Although few signs are transparent, many signs are translucent, that is, there is a visual relationship between the sign and its referent. Such a relationship is typically not found in speech (Lloyd, Loeding, & Doherty, 1985).

Clearly, the level of arbitrariness varies within, as well as between, symbol sets. To date, its role in facilitating learning is not clearly understood. Chapman & Miller (1980), for example, have questioned whether nonspeech systems function as a means to teach representational skills, or whether they actually require representational skills in order to be learned. Little attention has been given to the prerequisite representational behaviors necessary to use any given nonspeech system.

## Explanations for Nonspeech Communication Success

As positive reports on the implementation of these nonspeech systems emerge, it is important to consider why they have been successful when other oral approaches have failed. For some individuals, particularly those who evidence severe dysarthria with relatively intact cognitive skills and language comprehension skills, the reason is obvious: Nonspeech systems provide an alternative output mode (Beukelman & Yorkston, 1982). For those persons with oral communication impairments related to language difficulties, however, the reasons for success are not as clear. Fristoe and Lloyd (1979) and later Lloyd and Karlan (1984) have suggested a number of factors that could account for the facilitative effects reported in the literature. These factors, listed in Table 14.2 and briefly recounted and discussed in the following paragraphs, focus on the potential advantages for both the users and their teachers when a nonspeech communication system is employed.

***Signal Input Advantages.*** When information is presented to an individual in a nonspeech form, the input signal is altered. The visual input signal is typically produced at a slower rate than the speech signal. When speech is paired with the visual signal, the dual signal is generally of a longer duration (Shane, Lipschultz, & Shane, 1982) and less complex than when a spoken communication is presented alone. The amount of "verbiage" the person hears is, therefore, both decreased and simplified

***Signal Output Advantages.*** The motor acts necessary to produce a nonspeech communication are different from those required for speech production, because the output mode is manual rather than vocal. The fine motor coordination necessary to use unaided symbols (e.g., manual sign), however, is frequently more complex than that required for aided symbols. Using an alternative output mode for communication may also decrease the pressure to speak. In addition, there are instructional advantages in the nonspeech response mode, because the intervention approach utilized to teach production also changes. The clinician can physically manipulate the child's or the adult's hands to produce a sign or select a symbol from an array. Cueing and prompting may also be enhanced. Analysis of the characteristics and topography of response approximations and incorrect forms of desired nonspeech productions is more obvious than it is for speech.

***Advantages for Persons with Severe Handicapping Conditions.*** For those persons with severe intellectual impairments, additional advantages are possible. Vocabulary to be taught can be limited by focusing on functional items in the person's environment (e.g., drink, eat, more, bathroom). Deficits in attention are one consistent difficulty evidenced by mentally retarded persons (Zeaman & House, 1979). With visually presented symbols, evaluation and maintenance of on-task attention may be easier to monitor and control than when speech is employed.

**TABLE 14.2**

## Explanations for Nonspeech Communication Success

1. Signal input advantages
   a. Verbiage is reduced
   b. Rate is adjustable
2. Signal output advantages
   a. Pressure for speech is removed
   b. Physical demands are decreased
   c. Physical manipulation of the response is possible
   d. Clinician's observation of shaping is facilitated
3. Advantages for persons with severe handicapping conditions
   a. Vocabulary is limited and functional
   b. Individual's attention is easier to maintain
4. Receptive language/auditory processing advantages
   a. Structure of language input is simplified
   b. Auditory short-term memory and/or auditory processing problems are minimized
5. Stimulus processing/stimulus association advantages
   a. Figure-ground differential is enhanced.
   b. Stimulus consistency is optimized
   c. Temporal duration is greater
   d. A unimodal rather than cross-modal relationship exists between nonspeech symbols and visual referents
6. Symbolic representational advantages
   a. Supplemental representation is possible
   b. Visual representation is possible

Adapted from "Nonspeech Communication Symbols and Systems" by L. L. Loyd & G. W. Karlan, 1984, *Journal of Mental Deficiency Research*, *28*, 10-13.

***Receptive Language/Auditory Processing Advantages.*** For some persons who do not learn to talk, one overriding problem is processing the auditory information. Altering the input modality can circumvent this difficulty. Even when a visual communication system is employed in conjunction with speech, the visual information is frequently presented in telegraphic form. These symbols, then, may represent only the semantically relevant or meaningful information in the message; only the critical information is then highlighted, minimizing the need to process and remember auditory information.

*Stimulus Processing/Stimulus Association Advantages.* The use of the visual medium may facilitate the processing of symbolic information by enhancing the difference between figure and ground. The visual form of the stimulus is consistent in representation and production. The duration of the stimulus can be adjusted without altering what the individual perceives to be the form of the stimulus. In the case of aided symbols, static representations allow the user to refer once again to the communication after it has been produced. Further, there is a unimodal, rather than a cross-modal, relationship between nonspeech symbols and their visual referents. Learning that a symbol represents a referent may be easier when both exist in the same stimulus modality.

*Symbolic Representational Advantages* These nonspeech symbols can be employed to supplement the spoken word (Moores, 1974). Since the representations are visual, there may be some type of visual relationship between the symbols and their referents. This type of relationship, known as iconicity, may serve to facilitate recall and learning.

## CLINICAL AND RESEARCH CONSIDERATIONS

While potential reasons for success in nonspeech communication are intriguing, research directed toward experimental validation of these hypotheses has, to date, been limited. The implementation of augmentative/alternative communication systems requires consideration of a number of issues. Motoric, cognitive, language intervention, sociocommunicative, and technological variables are some domains that must be examined (Lloyd & Karlan, 1984; Romski, Sevcik, & Joyner, 1984).

### Motoric Issues

The choice between unaided and aided nonspeech systems has typically been based on the physical abilities of the potential user. Goodman, Wilson, and Bornstein (1978) reported that speech/language clinicians and special educators who responded to a national survey on sign language programs used manual signs with persons who had "sufficient manual dexterity" (p. 105). Kiernan (1981), in a review of nonvocal system use in the United Kingdom, also reported that manual signs were used for the majority of persons with upper limb integrity; most other individuals were assigned to aided symbol sets. There is, however, an increasing tendency to use aided systems with individuals who do not exhibit physical handicaps and, conversely, to use unaided systems with persons who have physical disabilities,

Kiernan (1980), for example, has described individual differences in nonspeech vocabulary acquisition for three severely retarded children. One child received manual sign + speech treatment after he experienced difficulty suppressing positional responses to symbols on a communication board. Another child demonstrated substantial difficulty discriminating signs and accurately producing them; he, therefore, received instruction using an aided symbol set. The third child responded equally well to unaided and aided symbol systems, and a multimodal approach (i.e., speech + sign + graphic symbols) was employed with her. While physical abilities play a role in determining the symbol system a person uses, other factors, such as learning, memory, and communication skills, may also influence the efficiency and effectiveness of a given augmentative communication system.

A person's motoric skills when considering the selection of a symbol system may be evaluated along a number of parameters. Topper-Zweiban (1977) reported that the manual expression subtest of the *Illinois Test of Psycholinguistic Abilities* (Kirk, McCarthy, & Kirk, 1968) was the most reliable indicator of success in her gestural language program in which subjects were institutionalized nonverbal profoundly retarded adolescents and adults, aged 14 to 30 years. Age at the onset of teaching and number of years of institutionalization were also cited as important factors in the amount of instruction required to learn manual sign. Alpert (1980) has described an approach for determining the optimal nonspeech mode for autistic children. She compared vocabulary learning in three ambulatory autistic children who received instruction using both manual signs and plastic manipulable symbols. She found that individual differences were the rule rather than the exception.

Assessment for assistive device use and the interface between the device and the symbol system are other motoric considerations (McDonald, 1980; Vanderheiden & Grilley, 1976). Coleman, Cook, and Meyers (1980) have developed systematic assessment procedures that consider physical parameters such as activation force, range and resolution of motion, reaction time, and repetition of response coupled with prelanguage and language skills. The efficacy of such assessment procedures/measures and their reliability and validity are future concerns for this particular area.

As described earlier in this chapter, unaided symbol sets place greater fine motor demands on the user than aided symbol sets, because the user must produce a sign configuration rather than select a symbol from an existing display. The production must be clear and intelligible to a communicative partner, since signs possess articulatory features (e.g., *tab* or location, *sig* or movement, and *dez* or handshape) that are similar to speech. If an individual cannot produce an intelligible sign due to sign articulatory errors, his or her ability to communicate in the environment is affected (Dennis, Reichle, Williams, & Vogelsberg, 1982). So although a person has upper limb integrity, he or she may still encounter difficulty producing clear unaided communications. In fact, some unaided systems may require less complex motor coordination for sign production than others. Daniloff and Vergara (1984) compared Amer-Ind signals and ASL signs with respect to the motor coordination necessary to execute both systems. ASL signs were judged more complex in terms of changes of hand orientation during production, the use of two hands rather than one, the number of different handshapes used, and the total amount of movement required. When the two systems were compared with respect to normal development of finger, hand, and arm movements, it was found that more Amer-Ind signals than ASL signs were within the range of physical competence for infants at both the 6-month and the 12-month developmental levels. Amer-Ind may offer some motoric advantages over ASL to individuals functioning within this developmental period.

Clearly, upper limb integrity is not the only consideration in determining the appropriateness of unaided or aided symbol sets. Each person's motoric strengths and weaknesses must be evaluated with respect to his or her cognitive and communicative skills and matched to the characteristics of the individual symbol systems.

## Cognitive Issues

A number of minimum cognitive skills, some similar to those related to spoken language acquisition, have been suggested as important in the decision to employ an augmentative communication system (Chapman & Miller, 1980; Shane, 1981). Among these skills are stage V sensorimotor intelligence (Shane, 1981), a developmental age of at least 18 months (Chapman & Miller, 1980; Shane, 1981), matching-to-sample skills (Keogh & Reichle, 1985; Woolman, 1980), and the ability to recognize photographs (Shane, 1981). While these skills may be important, the specific prerequisite role they play in any type of language intervention, regardless of the modality, has not been specified. (See Reichle & Karlan, Chapter 13 of this volume, for a discussion of decision-making processes specific to augmentative communication use.)

***Sensorimotor Intelligence.*** The development of Piagetian sensorimotor intelligence has been linked to language learning success. Kahn (1975) found a strong positive relationship for profoundly retarded children between meaningful expressive language (regardless of the modality) and stage VI functioning on the Uzgiris-Hunt scales. In a more recent investigation, performance on scale 5 (causality) and learning to sign or to speak were significantly correlated (Kahn, 1981). Such a finding suggests that the relationship between sensorimotor performance and early language learning may be much more specific than previously indicated. Reichle and Yoder (1985), however, demonstrated that children who exhibited stage 4 means-end performance could learn to label symbols prior to the use of an adult as an agent. This type of information has important implications for augmentative communication decision-making processes. Reports of young deaf children's first signs suggest that they begin to sign prior to the acquisition of advanced sensorimotor skills (Bonvillian, Orlansky, & Novack, 1983; Holmes & Holmes, 1980; McIntire, 1977; Orlansky & Bonvillian, 1984; Prinz & Prinz, 1979). As reported in much of the literature on the relationship between language and cognition, general cognitive skill may not always precede language comprehension and production. (See Rice, 1980; Rice, 1983; Rice & Kempler, 1984, for more complete discussions of the relationship between cognition and language.)

***Matching Skills.*** Another element identified as important in early communication training is the establishment of matching-to-sample skills. Keogh and Reichle (1985) suggest that identity and nonidentity matching-to-sample skills are important steps toward learning to use visual-graphic communication systems. They liken the importance of these skills to the importance of motoric and vocal imitation skills for spoken language learning. In a longitudinal study of visual-graphic communicative symbol learning, Romski, Sevcik, and Pate (1986) found a significant correlation between pretraining identity matching-to-sample skills for three dimensional objects and colors and subsequent success in the intervention program.

***Arbitrariness of Symbols.*** Symbol arbitrariness, an issue discussed in an earlier section of this chapter, has also been identified as a possible cognitive factor that affects symbol learning. Iconic signs, for example, have been found to facilitate vocabulary learning (Dennis et al., 1982; Goossens, 1983; Griffith & Robinson, 1980; Nietupski & Hamre-Nietupski, 1979; Reichle, Williams, & Ryan, 1981). More specifically, iconic signs that visually represent the function of the referent, or action patterns evoked by the referent, appear easier to learn than signs that visually represent the static features of the referent. Knudson (1980), however, found an interaction between the severity of individuals' intellectual handicaps and their ability to learn these two types (i.e., dynamic and static) of iconic signs. Dynamic signs were easier for the more severely intellectually handicapped persons to learn than static signs.

Aided symbol sets employ a variety of different media, from photographs to line drawings and abstract geometric shapes. A common belief has been that pictographic symbols may facilitate learning because they, like iconic signs, allow the child to call to mind a referent. Comparisons of aided symbol systems that vary in arbitrariness have suggested that differences in learning rates do exist in favor of pictographic symbols (Clark, 1981; Green, Hurlbut, & Iwata, 1982). Although pictographic symbols may be easier to learn for some persons, Kuntz, Carrier, and Hollis (1978) found that experience with arbitrary symbols (i.e., Non-SLIP symbols) fostered transfer (i.e., decreased the trials to criterion) to traditional orthography better than pictographic symbols did.

Differences in learning rates, however, may not be attributable to the arbitrariness of the symbol systems alone. Persons with severe mental retardation who are learning language for the first time may not possess the pictorial referents, experience, and/or speech comprehension vocabulary to which they can attach meaning. In such cases, the iconic sign or the pictographic symbol may not conjure up a visual image for the person, although these signs or symbols may be essentially equivalent to the arbitrary symbol in the person's mind. In an assessment of representational matching using different media (e.g., real objects, photographs, line drawings), Sevcik and Romski (1986) reported that individuals with "functional language skills" (at least 10 words, signs, or graphic symbols) performed significantly better than persons lacking such skills. In addition, within the nonfunctional language group, a hierarchy across conditions was discovered, with real objects being easier to match than photographs, which were in turn easier to match than line drawings. The results of this study address the issue raised by Chapman and Miller (1980) concerning the potential prerequisites to nonspeech symbol usage. If the goal of intervention is to teach symbolic representational skills, then the symbol system chosen may be different from that chosen if the user is expected to be a symbolic communicator at the onset of nonspeech communication system usage.

## Language Teaching Issues

As suggested above, many of the persons for whom nonspeech communication systems are appropriate also require a program of language intervention. As with any language intervention program, a number of areas must be considered.

***Vocabulary.*** Several papers have discussed initial vocabulary selection in language intervention (Holland, 1975; Lahey & Bloom, 1977) as well as concerns specific to nonspeech communication systems (Fristoe & Lloyd,

1980; Karlan & Lloyd, 1983; Parnes, 1980; Wilson, 1980). All of these papers stress the importance of the functional value of the chosen vocabulary items. Signs/symbols with a functional value in sociocommunicative situations are more likely to be used than those without such a value. The sign for a highly preferred food, for example, might be more readily employed than the sign for a body part. Systematic investigations of vocabulary acquisition have typically focused on the use of unaided systems, with little information available about variables that affect vocabulary acquisition using graphic symbols.

Signs with high functional utility are acquired more rapidly and maintained longer than signs that are not functional (Dennis et al., 1982; Reichle et al., 1981). Likewise, signs representing objects familiar to the child are also learned more quickly than those representing unfamiliar objects (Dennis et al., 1982; Nietupski & Hamre-Nietupski, 1979). While teaching verb + noun Signed English phrases to moderately and severely handicapped children, Karlan et al. (1982) reported that verbs were more difficult for the children to learn than nouns and suggested that this finding may be due to the dynamics and shorter duration of verb signs. Konstantareas, Oxman, and Webster (1978) found that autistic children learned nouns and verbs with equal difficulty. Knudson (1980) and Snyder-McLean (1978) found that signs involving action as part of their production were learned more readily than signs lacking this component. It is important, then, to distinguish between signs that represent verbs and signs that have an action component to their production. The salient feature of the signs that seems to increase their learnability is action or movement during production.

In one report of initial visual-graphic (lexigram) vocabulary acquisition by three severely retarded adults, Romski and Sevcik (1986) described a phenomenon similar to the overextensions seen in the speech of young typical children. They suggested that perhaps for such adults initial vocabulary meanings should be broader than some previous studies have recommended. For example, a symbol for *drink* might be used to refer to the act of drinking—for example, a glass, a can or bottle of soda, or water.

Meyers, Andersen, and Liddicoat (1984) quantitatively defined the communicative needs of 25 developmentally delayed nonspeaking school children via interviews and questionnaires completed by persons familiar with the nonspeaking individuals. Four major dimensions of need were identified: interpersonal/academic needs, recreational activities/special events, basic needs, and apperceptive content. They suggested that these categories may be beneficial for defining clusters of communicative need and then individually specifying the content items for each cluster.

Some important considerations relating to vocabulary have been identified. Additional specification is needed concerning the acquisition of different word classes and the interaction of these word classes with both unaided and aided symbols. Differences between comprehension and production must also be recognized. These issues are important for children and adults who come to the language learning task with different degrees of spoken language comprehension.

*Teaching Modes.* Teaching in the receptive and expressive modes has been an issue of interest in the language intervention literature for some time (e.g., Guess, Sailor, & Baer, 1974; Ruder, Hermann, & Schiefelbusch, 1977; Ruder, Smith, & Hermann, 1974). Systematic investigations within this area suggest that at specific times and for specific language components each mode may promote better generalization and use than the other. Investigations concerning these different teaching modes have emerged for nonspeech communication systems as well.

Teaching manual sign comprehension does not always lead to sign production (Kohl, Karlan, & Heal, 1979; Romski & Ruder, 1984). Conversely, teaching production does not automatically generalize to comprehension for visual-graphic symbols (Romski, Sevcik, & Pate, 1986). Specification of the strengths and weaknesses of each mode in teaching both unaided and aided nonspeech communication systems will lead to the most efficient and effective intervention programs.

*Teaching Approaches.* One important consideration concerning teaching approaches is time of initiation. Research has demonstrated that early language intervention can facilitate language learning within a communicative context (e.g., Schiefelbusch & Bricker, 1981). Schiefelbusch (1980b) suggested that for chiidren who are at risk for speech and language development for any number of reasons, nonspeech communication systems might be part of the language intervention program from birth. Employing such an approach, the nonspeech communication system would essentially be used as input during early parent-child interactions. With the exception of early manual sign intervention with young deaf infants, systematic investigations employing nonspeech communication systems with children who have other types of disabilities have not been undertaken as yet. This type of intervention approach holds promise for use with other children who are at risk for speech and language development. As Schiefelbusch (1980b) points out, such an intervention approach would decrease the level of communicative frustration for both child and parents, perhaps facilitating the course of the parent-child interaction.

The setting in which nonspeech language intervention takes place is also an important consideration. Kohl, Wilcox, and Karlan (1978) taught manual signs to three severely handicapped children in two settings. Signs taught within the classroom environment were learned more rapidly (i.e., fewer trials to criterion) than signs taught in an individual therapy setting. Extending these findings, Oliver and Halle (1982) found that signs learned in a classroom setting resulted in initiation of sign use and in generalization to another teacher. Instruction within natural communicative settings seems to be the method of choice when the end goal of intervention is functional use of the nonspeech symbol system. For some persons, however, structured individual instruction within a communicative paradigm may be necessary to establish basic communicative skills prior to use in daily environments (Romski, Sevcik, & Pate, 1986; Stoddard, 1982).

***Generalization.*** Since a person cannot be taught every communicative behavior that he or she needs to know, generalization of acquired communication skills is essential to the success of any language intervention program. The literature, although sparse, suggests that nonspeech systems do facilitate maintenance and generalization of communication skills. Romski, Sevcik, and Rumbaugh (1985) reported the successful retention and maintenance of a nonspeech communication system by four severely retarded individuals 18 months after teaching had ceased. Porter and Schroeder (1980) reported maintenance of learned communication skills 3 years after Non-SLIP training ceased. Each of these reports concerned arbitrary symbols. Perhaps the more general representation skills required with the use of arbitrary symbols promote long-term generalization and use.

***Facilitation of Speech.*** One of the most encouraging by-products of augmentative communication use is the facilitation of speech comprehension and speech production. Case studies observe the onset of, or increase in, vocalizations and/or word approximations (Berger, 1972; Brookner & Murphy, 1975; Carr, 1979; Fulwiler & Fouts, 1976; Grinnel, Detamore, & Lippke, 1976; Miller & Miller, 1973; Stremel-Campbell, Cantrell, & Halle, 1977). Other researchers report increases in the comprehension of speech (Bricker, 1972; Linville, 1977; Romski, Sevcik, & Pate, 1986). To date, factors contributing to the facilitative effects of these systems have not been specified. These factors are likely to include characteristics of the nonspeech symbols and physical, cognitive, and social characteristics of the user.

## Sociocommunicative and Environmental Issues

Individuals who demonstrate an interest in communication or attempt to communicate prior to the initiation of teaching are more likely to succeed than those who do not (Romski, Sevcik, & Pate, 1986; Song, 1979). Some persons do not exhibit this desire because of social, cognitive, and/or emotional deficits; others have not been placed in situations where it is necessary to communicate. Differentiation of these two sorts of reasons (an individual vs. an environmental deficit) for not communicating is essential. Once the desire to communicate is established, a way to communicate can be provided, and sociocommunicative interactions with peers and adults can be fostered.

As alluded to earlier in this chapter, nonspeech communication systems can remove the pressure to talk. While the removal of this burden can facilitate communicative exchanges, such exchanges present new and different communicative challenges for their users.

The implementation of the communication system with familiar and unfamiliar communicative partners is a critical component of any intervention program. Clients and their communicative partners must first accept the nonspeech system (Lloyd & Karlan, 1984). For example, some clients may not understand that their speech is unintelligible to others. Some parents may think that a nonspeech communication system interferes with their child's potential for speech. Descriptive measures of acceptance rates with unaided and aided symbol systems and reasons for hesitancy or nonacceptance are needed in order to understand the factors that contribute to acceptance or denial on the part of clients and the communities in which they live.

Once a person actually acquires a nonspeech communication system, the expectation is that the he or she will use it to communicate. Unfortunately, this expectation is not always met. While reports of sign language acquisition describe spontaneous usage, aided symbols frequently present a different situation. Calculator and Dollagan (1982) and Harris (1982) report that nonspeech communicators using communication boards are more likely to respond to a message than to initiate a communication. Calculator and Dollagan speculated that lack of success in the initiator's role fostered the respondent's role. In their study, students elicited more acknowledgment from their teachers and received fewer requests for clarification when they responded to teachers' communication. Here the aided communication system interacted with the students' communicative partners to determine the type and form of the communicative exchanges.

As persons who are nonspeaking learn to use a nonspeech communication system, their communicative partners must understand and be able to use the system for communication as well. While manual signs have been popular, their implementation in the environment requires that communicative partners learn a new communication system or that an interpreter be available to gloss the English meaning of the signs at all times. Visual-graphic symbols on a board may, and often do, place the printed English word above or below the symbol. A literate communicative partner should be able to understand the communication without additional interpretation. Synthetic speech, employed with computerized communication systems, can add auditory output to the visual symbol, thus making the communication approximate the spoken word.

The use of unaided or aided nonspeech communication systems alters the typical communicative exchange, because a number of characteristics of the system are different from spoken language (Higginbotham & Yoder, 1982). Although a great deal is known about the components of successful oral conversation (Duncan & Fiske, 1977; Payotos, 1980), the components of successful communicative exchanges when an unaided or aided nonspeech communication system is employed have not been identified. Turn taking, topic maintenance, and communicative functions, to name a few, may be altered from what is observed in the typical spoken communication exchange. This area of need has been identified (Yoder & Kraat, 1983), and some clinical assessment and intervention tools are available. Bolton and Dashiell (1984) have developed a clinical observation tool to assess interactive behavior using nonspeech communication systems. Strategies for the prevention and repair of communication breakdown in interactions with communication board users have been offered by Fishman, Timler, and Yoder (1985).

## Technological Issues

Electronic and microcomputer technology has advanced rapidly in recent years. Rehabilitation engineers have devised access modes to microcomputers for even the most severely physically involved persons. While these achievements are encouraging, operating microcomputers requires a certain level of cognitive skill. For persons with severe mental retardation, modifications in hardware and software are necessary if basic instructional approaches are to be developed.

One of the most promising technological advances is the development and use of synthetic speech. Synthetic speech can function as a "speech prosthesis" for persons with severe oral communication impairments (Lloyd & Karlan, 1984). Text-to-speech processors receive data from a computer software program and function to translate standard English text (orthography) into a phonetic code that allows the synthesizer to articulate the pronunciation of the text. Computers can be programmed so that when a letter- or symbol-embossed "key" is accessed (via direct selection, scanning, or encoding), the synthesized word is produced. For individuals with severe mental retardation who evidence concomitant productive and/or receptive language deficits, an individual may not necessarily need to comprehend the synthesized word. With a communication board, for example, an individual may use the graphic symbol that represents the actual referent while his or her communicative partner hears and decodes the synthetic word. The effect that the introduction of this medium will have on communicative exchange is not yet known. As this technology advances, research directed toward an understanding of its strengths and limitations in nonspeech communication system intervention is needed.

## SUMMARY AND CONCLUSIONS

The field of augmentative and alternative communication has progressed considerably in the past quarter century. Demonstrating that these systems were feasible for a broad range of individuals was a necessary first step toward the specification of important clinical and research issues. Although the clinical implementation of aided and unaided nonspeech communication systems has advanced, there has been relatively little published empirical research on the topic. Of the research available, unaided communication systems have received more attention than aided systems. Future research directions should include comparisons of both aided and unaided systems on a number of dimensions. Comparisons with spoken language learning and use are essential. In addition, investigations highlighting the similarities and differences of symbol sets, both aided and unaided, with respect to a user's ability to efficiently and effectively use them are necessary.

Technological advances that can change the course of service delivery for nonspeaking persons are being realized. Our excitement over technological advances must be balanced by an experimental examination of the variables (such as those addressed in this chapter) that affect the use of nonspeech communication systems by children and adults with a variety of disabilities.

## REFERENCES

Alpert, C. L. (1980). Procedures for determining the optimal nonspeech mode with the autistic child. In R. L. Schiefelbusch (Ed.), *Nonspeech language and communication: Analysis and intervention* (pp. 389–420). Austin, TX: PRO-ED.

Berger, S. L. (1972). A clinical program for developing multimodal language responses in atypical children. In J. E. McLean, D. E. Yoder, & R. L. Schiefelbusch (Eds.), *Language intervention with the mentally retarded* (pp. 212–235). Baltimore: University Park Press.

Beukelman, D. R., & Yorkston, K. M. (1982). Communication interaction of adult communication augmentation system use. *Topics in Language Disorders, 2,* 39–53.

Bolton, S. O., & Dashiell, S. E. (1984). *Interaction checklist for augmentative communication*. Huntington Beach, CA: Inch Associates.

Bonvillian, J. D., Orlansky, M. D., & Novack, L. L. (1983). Developmental milestones: Sign language acquisition and motor development. *Child Development, 54*, 1435–1445.

Bricker, D. D. (1972). Imitative sign training as a facilitator of word-object association with low-functioning children. *American Journal of Mental Deficiency, 76*, 509–516.

Brookner, S. P., & Murphy, N. O. (1975). The use of a total communication approach with a nondeaf child: A case study. *Language, Speech and Hearing Services in the Schools, 6*, 131–139.

Calculator, S., & Dollagan, C. (1982). The use of communication boards in a residential setting: An evaluation. *Journal of Speech and Hearing Disorders, 47*, 281–287.

Carr, E. G. (1979). Teaching autistic children to use sign language: Some research issues. *Journal of Autism Developmental Disorders, 9*, 345–359.

Carrier, J. K. (1974). Nonspeech noun usage training with severely and profoundly retarded children. *Journal of Speech and Hearing Research, 17*, 510–517.

Chapman, R. S., & Miller, J. F. (1980). Analyzing language and communication in the child. In R. L. Schiefelbusch (Ed.), *Nonspeech language and communication: Analysis and intervention* (pp. 159–196). Austin, TX: PRO-ED.

Clark, C. (1981). Learning words using traditional orthography and the symbols of Rebus, Bliss, and Carrier. *Journal of Speech and Hearing Disorders, 46*, 191–196.

Coleman, C. L., Cook, A. M., & Meyers, L. S. (1980). Assessing non-oral clients for assistive communication devices. *Journal of Speech and Hearing Disorders, 45*, 515–526.

Daniloff, J., Lloyd, L., & Fristoe, M. (1983). Amer-Ind transparency. *Journal of Speech and Hearing Disorders, 48*, 103–110.

Daniloff, J., & Vergara, D. (1984). Comparison between the motoric constraints for Amer-Ind and ASL sign formation. *Journal of Speech and Hearing Research, 27*, 76–88.

Dennis, R., Reichle, J., Williams, W., & Vogelsberg, R. T. (1982). Motoric factors influencing the selection of vocabulary for sign production programs. *Journal of the Association for the Severely Handicapped, 7*, 20–32.

Duncan, S., & Fiske, D. W. (1977). *Face-to-face interaction: Research, methods, and theory*. Hillsdale, NJ: Lawrence Erlbaum.

Duncan, J., & Silverman, F. (1977). Impacts of learning Amer-Ind on mentally retarded children: A preliminary report. *Perceptual and Motor Skills, 44*, 1138.

Fishman, S., Timler, G., & Yoder, D. E. (1985). Strategies for the prevention and repair of communication breakdown in interactions with communication board users. *Augmentative and Alternative Communication, 1*, 38–51.

Fristoe, M., & Lloyd, L. L. (1979). Nonspeech communication. In N. R. Ellis (Ed.), *Handbook of mental deficiency: Psychological theory and research* (pp. 401–430). Hillsdale, NJ: Lawrence Erlbaum.

Fristoe, M., & Lloyd, L. L. (1980). Planning an initial expressive sign lexicon for persons with severe communication impairment. *Journal of Speech and Hearing Disorders, 45*, 170–180.

Fulwiler, R. L., & Fouts, R. S. (1976). Acquisition of American Sign Language by noncommunicating autistic child. *Journal of Autism and Childhood Schizophrenia, 6*, 43–51.

Gardner, R. A., & Gardner, B. T. (1969). Teaching sign language to a chimpanzee. *Science, 165*, 664–672.

Goodman, L., Wilson, P. S., & Bornstein, H. (1978). Results of a national survey of sign language programs in special education. *Mental Retardation, 16*, 104–106.

Goossens, C. (1983). *The relative iconicity and learnability of verb reference differentially represented by manual signs, Blissymbols, and rebus symbols: An investigation with moderately retarded individuals*. Unpublished doctoral dissertation, Purdue University, West Lafayette, IN.

Green, J. D., Hurlbut, B. I., & Iwata, B. A. (1982). Nonvocal language acquisition in adolescents with severe physical disabilities: Blissymbol versus iconic stimulus formats. *Applied Behavior Analysis, 15*, 241–258.

Griffith, P., & Robinson, J. (1980). Influence of iconicity and phonological similarity on sign learning by mentally retarded children. *American Journal of Mental Deficiency, 85*, 291–298.

Grinnel, M., Detamore, K., & Lippke, B. (1976). Sign it successful: Manual English encourages expressive communication. *Teaching the Exceptional Child, 10*, 123–124.

Guess, D., Sailor, W., Baer, D. M. (1974). To teach language to retarded children. In R. L. Schiefelbusch & Lyle L. Lloyd (Eds.), *Language perspectives—Acquisition, retardation, and intervention* (pp. 529–563). Austin, TX: PRO-ED.

Hall, S. M., & Talkington, L. M. (1970). Evaluation of a manual approach to programming for deaf retarded. *American Journal of Mental Deficiency, 75*, 378–380.

Harris, D. (1982). Communicative interaction processes involving nonvocal physically handicapped children. *Topics in Language Disorders, 2*, 21–37.

Higginbotham, D., & Yoder, D. E. (1982). Communication within natural conversational interaction: Implications for severely communicatively impaired persons. *Topics in Language Disorders, 2*, 1–19.

Hockett, C. F. (1960). The origin of speech. *Scientific American, 203*, 88–96.

Hoffmeister, R. J., & Farmer, A. (1972). The development of manual sign language in mentally retarded deaf individuals. *Journal of the Rehabilitation for the Deaf, 6*, 19–26.

Holland, A. L. (1975). Language therapy for children: Some thoughts on context and content. *Journal of Speech and Hearing Disorders, 40*, 514–523.

Holmes, K., & Holmes, D. (1980). Signed and spoken language development in a hearing child of hearing parents. *Sign Language Studies, 28*, 239–254.

Kahn, J. V. (1975). Relationship of Piaget's sensorimotor period to language acquisition of profoundly retarded children. *American Journal of Mental Deficiency, 79*, 640–643.

Kahn, J. V. (1981). A comparison of sign and verbal language training with nonverbal retarded children. *Journal of Speech and Hearing Research, 46*, 113–119.

Karlan, G. R., Lentz, A., Brenn-White, B., Hodur, P., Egger, D., & Frankoff, D. (1982). Establishing generalized, productive verb-noun phrase usage in a manual language system with moderately handicapped children. *Journal of Speech and Hearing Disorders, 47*, 31–42.

Karlan, G. R., & Lloyd, L. L. (1983). Consideration in the planning of communication intervention: I. Selecting the lexicon. *Journal of the Association for Severely Handicapped, 8*, 13–25.

Keogh, W. J., & Reichle, J. (1985). Communication intervention for the "difficult-to-teach" severely handicapped. In S. F. Warren & A. K. Rogers-Warren (Eds.), *Teaching functional language* (pp. 157–194). Austin, TX: PRO-ED.

Kiernan, C. C. (1980). *Preverbal communication schedule (PVC)*. London: Thomas Coram Research Unit, University of London Institute of Education.

Kiernan, C. C. (1981). A strategy for research on the use of nonvocal systems of communication. *Journal of Autism and Developmental Disorders, 47*, 31–42.

Kiernan, C., Reid, B., & Jones, L. (1982). *Signs and symbols: A review of literature and survey of the use of nonvocal communication*. London: Heinemann Educational Books.

Kirk, S., McCarthy, J., & Kirk, W. (1968). *The Illinois Test of Psycholinguistic Abilities*. Urbana, IL: University of Illinois Press.

Kirschner, A., Algozzine, B., & Abbott, T. B. (1979). Manual communication system: A comparison and its implications. *Education and Training of the Mentally Retarded, 14*, 5–10.

Klima, E., & Bellugi, U. (1979). *The signs of language*. Cambridge, MA: Harvard University Press.

Knudson, C. A. (1980). *Rate of enactive vs. iconic manual sign acquisition by retarded learners*. Unpublished master's thesis, University of Kansas, Lawrence, KS.

Kohl, F., Karlan, G., & Heal, L. (1979). Effects of pairing manual signs with verbal cues upon the acquisition of instruction-following behavior and the generalization to expressive language with severely handicapped students. *AAESPH Review, 4*, 291–300.

Kohl, F., Wilcox, B., & Karlan, G. (1978). Effects of training conditions on the generalization of manual signs with moderately handicapped students. *Education and Training of the Mentally Retarded, 13*, 327–335.

Konstantareas, M. M., Oxman, J., & Webster, C. D. (1978). Iconicity: Effects on the acquisition of sign language by autistic and other severely dysfunctional children. *Understanding Language Through Sign Language Research, 8*, 213–237.

Kuntz, J., Carrier, J., & Hollis, J. (1978). A nonvocal system of teaching retarded children to read and write. In C. E. Meyers (Ed.), *Quality of life in severely and profoundly mentally retarded people: Research foundations for improvement* (pp. 145–191) (American Association on Mental Deficiency Monograph No. 3). Washington, DC: AAMD.

Lahey, M., & Bloom, L. (1977). Planning a first lexicon: Which words to teach first. *Journal of Speech and Hearing Disorders, 42*, 340–349.

Linville, S. (1977). Signed English: A language teaching technique for totally nonverbal severely mentally retarded adolescents. *Language, Speech and Hearing Services in the Schools, 8*, 170–175.

Lloyd, L. L. (1976). *Communication assessment and intervention strategies*. Baltimore: University Park Press.

Lloyd, L. L. (1984). Comments on terminology. *Communication Together, 2*, 19–21.

Lloyd, L. L., & Fuller, D. R. (1986). Toward an augmentative and alternative communication symbol taxonomy: A proposed superordinate classification. *Augmentative and Alternative Communication, 2*, 165–171.

Lloyd, L. L., & Karlan, G. R. (1984). Nonspeech communication symbols and systems: Where have we been and where are we going? *Journal of Mental Deficiency Research, 28*, 3–20.

Lloyd, L. L., Loeding, B., & Doherty, J. E. (1985). The role of iconicity in sign language. *Journal of Speech and Hearing Disorders, 50*, 299–301.

McDonald., E. T. (1980). Early identification and treatment of children at risk for speech development. In R. L. Schiefelbusch (Ed.), *Nonspeech language and communication: Analysis and intervention* (pp. 49–79). Austin, TX: PRO-ED.

McIntire, M. (1977). The acquisition of American Sign Language hand configurations. *Sign Language Studies, 16*, 247–266.

Meyers, L. S., Andersen, C., & Liddicoat, C. M. (1984). Perceived communication needs of developmentally delayed nonspeaking children. *The Psychological Record, 34*, 55–68.

Miller, A., & Miller, E. (1973). Cognitive-developmental training with elevated boards and sign language. *Journal of Autism and Childhood Schizophrenia, 3*, 65–85.

Moores, D. F. (1974). Nonvocal systems of verbal behavior. In R. L. Schiefelbusch & L. L. Lloyd (Eds.), *Language perspectives—Acquisition, retardation, and intervention* (pp. 377–417). Austin, TX: PRO-ED.

Musselwhite, C. R., & St. Louis, K. W. (1982). *Communication programming for the severely handicapped: Vocal and nonvocal strategies*. San Diego: College-Hill Press.

Nietupski, J., & Hamre-Nietupski, S. (1979). Teaching auxiliary communication skills to severely handicapped students. *AAESPH Review, 4*, 107–124.

Nonspeech communication: A position paper. (1980). *American Speech and Hearing Association, 22*, 267–272.

Oliver, C., & Halle, J. (1982). Language training in the everyday environment: Teaching functional sign use to a retarded child. *Journal of the Association for the Severely Handicapped, 7*, 50–62.

Orlansky, M., & Bonvillian, J. (1984). The role of iconicity in early sign language acquisition. *Journal of Speech and Hearing Disorders, 49*, 287–292.

Parnes, P. (1980). *Use of BCI flashcard vocabulary*. Unpublished manuscript, Ontario, Canada: Blissymbolics Communication Institute.

Payotos, F. (1980). Interactive functions and limitations of verbal and nonverbal behaviors in natural conversation. *Semiotica, 30*, 211–244.

Porter, P. B., & Schroeder, S. R. (1980). Generalization and maintenance of skills acquired in nonspeech language initiation program training. *Applied Research in Mental Retardation, 1*, 71–84.

Premack, D. (1970). A functional analysis of language. *Journal of Experimental Behavior Analysis, 14*, 107–125.

Prinz, P., & Prinz, E. (1979). Simultaneous acquisition of ASL and spoken English: Phase I: Early lexical development. *Sign Language Studies, 25*, 283–296.

Reich, R. (1978). Gestural facilitation of expressive language in moderately/severely retarded preschoolers. *Mental Retardation, 16*, 113–117.

Reichle, J., Williams, W., & Ryan, S. (1981). Selecting signs for the formulation of an augmentative communication modality. *The Journal of the Association for Severely Handicapped, 6*, 48–56.

Reichle, J., & Yoder, D. (1985). Communication board use in severely handicapped learners. *Language, Speech and Hearing Services in the Schools, 16*, 146–157.

Rice, M. (1980). *Cognition to language: Categories, word meanings, and training*. Baltimore: University Park Press.

Rice, M. (1983). Contemporary accounts of the cognition/language language relationship: Implications for speech-language clinicians. *Journal of Speech and Hearing Disorders, 48*, 347–359.

Rice, M., & Kempler, S. (1984). *Child language and cognition*. Austin, TX: PRO-ED.

Romski, M. A., & Ruder, K. F. (1984). Effects of speech and sign on oral language learning in Down's syndrome children. *Journal of Speech and Hearing Disorders, 49*, 293–302.

Romski, M. A., & Sevcik, R. A. (1986). *Symbol meaning boundaries in adults with severe retardation: Two case profiles*. Manuscript submitted for publication.

Romski, M. A., Sevcik, R. A., & Joyner, S. (1984). Nonspeech communication systems: Implication for language intervention with mentally retarded children. *Topics in Language Disorders, 5*, 66–81.

Romski, M. A., Sevcik, R. A., & Pate, J. (1986). *The establishment of symbolic communication in persons with severe retardation*. Manuscript submitted for publication.

Romski, M. A., Sevcik, R. A., & Rumbaugh, D. M. (1985). Retention of symbolic communication in five severely retarded persons. *American Journal of Mental Deficiency, 89*, 441–444.

Ruder, K., Hermann, P., & Schiefelbusch, R. L. (1977). Effects of verbal imitation and comprehension training on verbal production. *Journal of Psycholinguistic Research, 6*, 59–72.

Ruder, K., Smith, M., & Hermann, P. (1974). Effects of verbal imitation and comprehension on verbal production of lexical items. In L. McReynolds (Ed.), *Developing systematic procedures for training children's language* (ASHA Monograph No. 18, pp. 15–29). Rockville, MD: American Speech and Hearing Association.

Rumbaugh, D. M. (1977). *Language learning by a chimpanzee: The LANA Project*. New York: Academic Press.

Schiefelbusch, R. L. (1980a). *Nonspeech language and communication: Analysis and intervention*. Austin, TX: PRO-ED.

Schiefelbusch, R. L. (1980b, August). *Speech, language, and communication disorders of the multiple handicapped*. Paper presented at the International Association of Logopedics, Washington, DC.

Schiefelbusch, R. L., & Bricker, D. D. (1981). *Early language: Acquisition and intervention*. Austin, TX: PRO-ED.

Schiefelbusch, R. L. & Hollis, J. (1979). *Language intervention from ape to child*. Baltimore: University Park Press.

Schiefelbusch, R. L. & Lloyd, L. L. (1974). *Language perspectives—Acquisition, retardation, and intervention*. Austin, TX: PRO-ED.

Sevcik, R. A., & Romski, M. A. (1986). Representational matching skills of persons with severe retardation. *Augmentative and Alternative Communication, 2*, 160–164.

Shane, H. C., (1981). Decision making in early augmentative communication system use. In R. L. Schiefelbusch & D. D. Bricker (Eds.), *Early language: Acquisition and intervention* (pp. 389–425). Austin, TX: PRO-ED.

Shane, H. C., Lipschultz, M. S., & Shane, C. L. (1982). Facilitating the communicative interaction of nonspeaking persons in large residential settings. *Topics in Language Disorders*, 73–84.

Silverman, F. (1980). *Communication for the speechless*. Englewood Cliffs, NJ: Prentice-Hall.

Skelly, M. (1979). *Amer-Ind gestural code based on universal American Indian Hand Talk*. New York: Elsevier.

Snyder-McLean, L. (1978, November). *Functional stimulus and response variables in sign training with retarded subjects*. Paper presented at the American Speech-Language-Hearing Association Convention, San Francisco.

Song, A. (1979). Acquisition and use of Blissymbols by severely retarded adolescents. *Mental Retardation, 17*, 253–255.

Stoddard, L. T. (1982). An investigation of automated methods of teaching severely retarded individuals. *International Review of Research in Mental Retardation, 11*, 163–208.

Stremel-Campbell, K., Cantrell, D., & Halle, J. (1977). Manual signing as a language system and as a speech initiator for the nonverbal severely handicapped student. In E. Sontag, J. Smith, & W. Certo (Eds.), *Educational programming for the severely and profoundly handicapped* (pp. 335–347). Reston, VA: Council for Exceptional Children.

Topper-Zweiban, S. (1977). Indicators of success in learning a manual communication mode. *Mental Retardation, 15*, 47–49.

Vanderheiden, G., & Harris-Vanderheiden, D. (1976). Communication techniques and aids for the nonvocal severely handicapped. In L. L. Lloyd (Ed.), *Communication assessment and intervention strategies* (pp. 607–652). Baltimore: University Park Press.

Vanderheiden, G. C., & Grilley, K. (1977). *Non-vocal communication techniques and aids for the severely physically handicapped*. Austin, TX: PRO-ED.

Wilson, K. D. (1980). Selection of a core lexicon for use with graphic communicative systems. *Journal of Children's Communication Disorders, 4*, 111–123.

Woolman, D. H. (1980). A presymbolic training program. In R. L. Schiefelbusch (Ed.), *Nonspeech language and communication: Analysis and intervention* (pp. 325–356). Austin, TX: PRO-ED.

Yoder, D. E. (1980). Communication systems for non-speech children. *New Directions in the Exceptional Child, 2*, 63–78.

Yoder, D. E., & Kraat, A. (1983). Intervention issues in nonspeech communication. In J. Miller, D. E. Yoder, & R. Schiefelbusch (Eds.), *Contemporary issues in language intervention* (pp. 27–51). Rockville, MD: American Speech-Language-Hearing Association.

Zeaman, D., & House, B. J. (1979). A review of attention theory. In N. R. Ellis (Ed.), *Handbook of mental deficiency, psychological theory and research*. Hillsdale, NJ: Lawrence Erlbaum.

# 15

# *Classroom Text: The Next Stage of Intervention*

Marion Blank

In the past two decades, the field of child language research has been marked by an explosion of knowledge with profound practical effects. Many groups of language impaired children, including deaf, aphasic, autistic, and mentally retarded, are now treated in markedly different and more effective ways than had previously been available (Blank, 1983; Lund & Duchan, 1983; Schiefelbusch, 1980). When advances occur in an area, however, it is not uncommon to find that the problem has not been "solved"—if by solved, one means that the issues are fully understood and can thereby be laid to rest. Instead, a new, higher level of understanding often reveals unforeseen complexities that in turn call out for solutions. It is true that many children who heretofore would have been severely limited have been able to make major strides in the acquisition of language. Yet it is equally true that much about such children's language is strange and inappropriate. Of even greater importance is the fact that the strangeness and inappropriateness seem to be a direct result of the teaching experience.

An anecdote reported by Norma Rees (1978) captures some undefined, but clearly present, problems. Describing "a mentally retarded girl" who had received "psycholinguistic training," she reports that when handed a cup, the girl responded "It's a cup, it's pink, it's plastic, you drink out of it." Rees concludes the example with the statement, "While no one would quarrel with either the accuracy of the content or with the grammar, the response has a "bizarre quality" (p. 193). She then goes on to say that the bizarre quality does not represent failure in the structures that the child has been taught but rather failures in the functions of language. The teaching experiences have somehow led the student to use language in ways that are not simply different, but inappropriately different, from those of the average person. Clearly something is wrong—but what?

Given the intricacies of language, the effort of defining what is awry must be complex. The task is made even more difficult by the fact that it requires a major conceptual shift in the units of analysis to which we have been accustomed. Regardless of theoretical approach, language has generally been viewed as a system composed of words, clauses, and sentences. While these units exist, they are far from the complete story. The focus now is on communication. In the majority of cases, this means that we must extend the units of analysis to go beyond even complex, multiclausal sentences. Verbal communication consists of related sets of utterances which can best be subsumed under the rubric of *text*.

According to Halliday and Hasan (1976), *text* refers to "any passage, spoken or written, of whatever length, that does form a unified whole" (p. 1). Text represents

> [a] unit of language in use. A text is not something like a sentence, only bigger. It is something that differs from a sentence in kind. A text is best regarded as a semantic unit; a unit not of form but of meaning . . . a text does not consist of sentences; it is REALIZED BY, or encoded in sentences. If we understand it in this way, we shall not expect to find the same kind of structural integration among the parts of a text as we find among the parts of a sentence or clause. The unity of a text is a unity of a different kind. (Halliday & Hasan, 1976, p. 2. See Halliday & Hasan, 1980)

> Conversations are everyday examples of the fact that . . . participants can jointly produce coherent texts; utterances and parts of utterances relate back and forwards, place certain restrictions on what can occur and affect how preceding or succeeding items are interpreted. (Sinclair & Coulthard, 1975, p. 2)

The sum and substance of these remarks is that most talk is not confined simply to words or sentences. Rather, it is contained in sequenced sets of words and sentences which ultimately serve to create the text of a conversation.

In highlighting the idea of text, I do not mean to imply that this aspect of verbal communication has gone unrecognized. Commonly used terms such as *discussion*, *interchange*, and *discourse* are predicated on the notion of a sustained text. However, as frequently occurs with omnipresent phenomena, the textual component of language seems to have been taken for granted. This unquestioning acceptance has permitted the educational system to create, with good intentions but unfortunate results, texts that lead directly to the "pink, plastic cup" interchange cited above. The remainder of this chapter is devoted to the elaboration of the idea that traditional approaches to education have created such problems in communication. In addition, the chapter offers proposals for a more constructive alternative to teaching children to communicate, thus providing a promising approach to language intervention in the future.

## CURRENT CLASSROOM TEXTS

A major consequence of focusing on text is a fundamental shift in the behavior to be analyzed. Typically, when one's focus is on words and sentences, the logical beginning step is to examine the language of the children and determine the skills that they do and do not possess. But texts are joint enterprises involving—in the case of the school—both children and teachers.

Accordingly, the examination of language from a text point of view will begin by studying the language of teachers and children rather than that of children alone. Further, it will not be the language used with handicapped children, but rather the language used with normal, well-functioning children that will be studied. While its power has often not been recognized, school language with normal children has profoundly influenced the teaching of handicapped children—and, ultimately, the problems handicapped children have encountered in mastering communication. Recognition of the structure and role of school language is vital in determining the ways in which intervention efforts can and should change.

### An Example of School Language

The segment of school language that follows is part of a dialogue between a teacher and a small group of well-functioning 4-year-old children. The recording was made in Scotland. Consequently, some of the words and phrases may sound a bit strange. The selection of a non-American classroom was not made by chance. The overwhelming impression created by the interaction is not one of cultural difference, but rather one of similarity. As such, the dialogue serves to illustrate the remarkably strong and pervasive patterns that are found in classroom dialogues across a variety of nations.

The teacher has set as her goal the teaching of the concept of texture. She plans to achieve this goal by having the children group rough objects in one circle (the circle that belongs to Mr. Rough) and smooth ones in another (the circle that belongs to Mr. Smooth). At the outset, the objects (all common objects such as balls, soap, brushes, etc.) are in a box, and each child is given a turn to select one item. The dialogue proceeds as follows:

**Teacher**: Well, let's see, Steven. Would you like to go into the box and pick out something?

**Steven**: (selects a ball)

**Teacher**: What's that? You just look at it. What's that?

**Steven**: A ball.

**Teacher**: What do you use a ball for, Peter?

**Peter**: Bouncing up and down and throwing up.

**Teacher**: And would it just be boys and girls that use the ball?

**Peter**: Yes.

**Teacher**: Is it? No one else at all?

**Peter**: Nope.

**Teacher**: No? What colors are in the ball, Pauline?

**Pauline**: Blue and yellow and red and orange.

**Teacher**: Pauline, Mr. Rough (referring to a puppet) wants you to decide if that ball is smooth like Mr. Smooth or is it rough like Mr. Rough? Would you like to feel it against your cheek? Put it up against your cheek with your hands.

**Pauline**: (rubs ball against cheek)

**Teacher**: Is it smooth or is it rough?

**Pauline**: Smooth.

**Teacher**: It's smooth. Well. Mr. Rough has a rough ring here and Mr. Smooth has a smooth ring here, and he wants Peter and Steven and Laura Ann to put the articles that are either smooth or rough into the right one. Pauline, you said it was smooth—so what one are you going to put it in?

**Pauline**: (puts ball in smooth ring)

**Teacher**: The smooth one! So Mr. Smooth has got one. Right. Peter, would you like to get into the box please?

**Peter**: (takes out grater) (Laura Ann spontaneously says, "That one's for Mr. Rough.")

**Teacher**: Now, what's that? Can you tell us what that is?

**Laura**: A grater.

**Teacher**: A grater. What do you use a grater for?

**Pauline**: Grating cheese.

**Teacher**: Grate cheese. Anything else?

**Steven**: Carrots.

**Teacher**: What do you grate carrots for?

**Steven**: Eat.

**Teacher**: What foods would you be eating if you were grating carrots?

**Laura**: Soup?

**Teacher**: Soup. Oh, we have lovely soup in the wintertime. Well, who does the grater belong to?

**Steven**: (pointing to an object in the box) That's for the winter.

**Teacher**: For the winter and that's when we have soup as well.

**Laura**: Mr. Rough! Mr. Rough!

**Teacher**: Well, are we going to put it in Mr. Rough's ring?

**Peter**: (puts it in the circle for Mr. Rough)

**Teacher**: So each one has one thing each. Right. Mr. Rough (puppet is on hand) is going in and he's picking out this and he wants Pauline to tell him what this is.

**Pauline**: A polishing brush.

**Teacher**: A polishing brush. And what do you polish with that?

**Pauline**: Shoes.

**Teacher**: Your shoes—anything else?

**Children**:(talking together) Just shoes.

**Teacher**: Well, who do you think it belongs to? Is it Mr. Rough's or Mr. Smooth's?

**Pauline**: Mr. Rough's.

**Teacher**: It's Mr. Rough's. So which one are you going to put it in?

**Pauline**: (puts it in Mr. Rough's circle)

The dialogue then continues, with the children selecting and sorting a number of additional objects (e.g., a rolling pin, a bar of soap, etc.). Even from this restricted segment, however, it is clear that the teacher and children are not engaged simply in the production of utterances. Rather, the utterances are embedded in extended sequences which have a distinctive organization. These sequences are what are referred to as texts.

Further, the segment of dialogue just presented contains a pattern that encompasses the range of utterances. The pattern is a recurring one that is applied to each and every child. The teacher starts by requesting a label for the object that has been chosen; she then asks a series of questions which may vary in order but which consistently involve the identification of color (e.g., What colors are in the ball?), function (e.g., What do you use a ball for?), category association (e.g., What foods would you be eating if you were grating carrots?), and finally texture (e.g., Is it rough or smooth?).

This type of dialogue is so familiar in classrooms that it takes on the quality of most familiar patterns; that is, it feels both appropriate and comfortable. Yet it is nearly identical to the language intervention dialogues that led the mentally retarded girl to produce the "pink, plastic cup" example cited earlier. Her bizarre response was not the result of poor learning, but rather of effective learning. Like the children in Scotland, and like the children in hundreds of classrooms around the world, for years she had been told to cite the name, size, color, shape, and composition of objects; and she now quite reasonably believes that this type of label and attribute description form the core of a conversation.

Better functioning children fortunately do not arrive at a similar conclusion. Their ability to avoid this pitfall, however, ought not to be taken as a sign that the teaching is more profitable for them. Admittedly, since they can answer almost all the questions that are asked, the teaching may reinforce in them the feeling that they are competent and successful. But this should not be taken to mean that the teaching provides a model of effective verbal communication. Rather, their skill in dialogue seems likely to derive from their ability to perceive and interpret the wide array of nonschool discourse that they experience. This sensitivity leads them to recognize that language is, and must be, far more important than what is taught in school (Blank, Rose, & Berlin, 1978).

## Limitations of School Language

Recognition of the limitations of school language is, of course, far from new. The efforts to change, however, have been seriously limited by the failure to extend the unit of analysis beyond the level of the sentence. For example, one line of intervention currently being pursued is based upon concepts from the study of pragmatics. Analysis of language from this perspective leads to an emphasis on the social appropriateness of one's utterances (Bryan & Pflaum, 1978). Accordingly, it has been suggested that abstract, nonsocial concepts such as size and shape be replaced by more relevant, social concepts such as knowing how to formulate requests, knowing how to ask questions, and so forth.

The limitations of this approach are highlighted in the following anecdote. A clinician who adopted a focus on pragmatics decided to take one of her students on a walk. As they opened the school door to go outdoors, the child called out—with no one in sight— "Who is it? What is it? Where is it?" Admittedly, the content is different from the labels of "pink" and "plastic" and "cup." Yet the underlying process is identical. The child has been taught an inappropriate and inadequate text which is of service to him in no setting other than the classroom.

One source of the difficulty is that school texts contain highly structured, repetitive routines. Given the wide array of functions that language serves, routinized texts certainly have a place. For example, social routines such as greeting and leave taking are expedited by having set dialogues that can be conducted with little conscious thought or effort (e.g., Hello, how are you? Fine, etc.). Indeed, the absence of thought and effort is precisely what make these dialogues so useful—they allow predictable, recurring patterns to proceed without requiring undue attention. But if they are to be useful, automatized, effortless routines must be limited to appropriate contexts. They ought not form the sum and substance of one's verbal repertoire.

Further, such routines are far from what teachers hope, and have been mandated, to accomplish in their classroom dialogues. Indeed, the goals that teachers have been assigned and that they have taken on are opposed to such thoughtless behavior. Teachers' ambitions are to stimulate thinking, imagination, and flexibility—all of the cognitive processes that are seen as the ultimate in human intelligence (see Stevenson et al., 1978, pp. 1–2). If these goals are to be attained, it is essential to specify the characteristics of productive dialogue and to develop a structure that can serve as an effective vehicle for these characteristics.

## ESTABLISHING PRODUCTIVE DIALOGUE

Three issues that are essential for the delineation of a meaningful text are considered in the following paragraphs. All revolve about the *content* of school texts. Content is a difficult domain, because it represents a virtually limitless field whose parameters seem to defy definition (McTear, 1984). Nevertheless, there is a set of relationships that determine the way in which content and text mesh with one another. These relationships are found in how content relates to (a) the relevance of an utterance in a text, (b) the usefulness of an utterance in a text, and (c) the connections between the successive utterances in a text. These issues will be analyzed primarily from the perspective of discussions with young children. However, many of the ideas are applicable to discussions with older students as well. Each issue is dealt with in two parts: It is first considered as it applies to current school texts; then it is considered from the point of view of its implications for intervention.

### The Relevance of an Utterance: The Role of Topic

***Applications to Current School Texts.*** A meaningful text is not simply an extended sequence of language. If the text is to be comprehensible, all the components must somehow relate to one another. In turn, topic is a key factor in determining whether the relationships in the text are meaningful.

Topic is the overriding variable that essentially determines the ideas that can be raised and, equally important, the ideas that ought *not* to be raised in any particular discussion. Thus, one would, and should, quite reasonably expect that a conversation about the conflict in the Middle East will be markedly different from one concerned with shopping for food. In the former, one could imagine hearing a host of issues including the length of time the conflict has gone on, the possibility of peace, and the forces that led to the tension; in the latter, one might hear about the price of particular items, the availability of certain foods, and the way in which the bags ought to be packed for taking home. The specifics are not important—the key idea is that the topic essentially determines the relevance or irrelevance of any bit of information raised.

The issue of relevance (i.e., the meaningfulness of an idea) should not be confused with the issue of validity (i.e., the truth of an idea). This sort of confusion is common regarding school dialogue, and it is often the factor responsible for inappropriate conversation. The Mr. Rough–Mr. Smooth dialogue presented earlier is an example of the failure to make the distinction between relevance and validity. The teacher has ostensibly set the concept of texture as the topic. In this context, all of the questions that she asks represent valid characteristics of the objects being discussed (i.e., each object does have a color, a function, etc.); but almost none of the questions are relevant to the topic of texture. The ball's smoothness does not depend upon its being red or blue or any other color; similarly, the fact that carrots can be put into soups has nothing to do with the roughness of the grater.

The linking of irrelevance and validity is responsible for providing children with incorrect information about the organization and purpose of dialogue. Its importance can be gauged from the fact that it is probably the key factor in determining our feelings about the inappropriateness of the "conversation" about the pink plastic cup. Pink and plastic and cup are all valid characteristics of the cup, but that fact does not make them relevant items for conversation. In indiscriminately pointing out each and any component of an object, we essentially have no topic of conversation; rather, we have an assortment of unrelated ideas bearing no connection to a unifying topic.

The schism in school dialogue between relevance and validity is largely the inevitable consequence of the "topics" that have been selected for discussion. For a number of reasons, schools have placed great weight on verbal categories, particularly those that lend themselves to superordinate organization. From preschool on, texts (lesson plans) abound with topics such as *vehicles*, *community helpers*, *holidays* and *weather*. Further, this mode of characterization forms the basis of dialogue. The classroom conversation presented earlier is clearly of this type. The teacher selected the category of texture as the one to teach, but she could just as easily have chosen *color* or *toys* or *tools*.

These sorts of categories are useful in a number of ways such as in the storage and retrieval of information. For example, if one goes to a library for material on birds and finds no classification system for locating the material, chaos would exist. Such classification systems, however, are not what conversation is about. Admittedly, this mode of structuring talk is so common in schools that it has come to feel "right" and "appropriate." Nevertheless, verbal categories of the sort generally used in schools cannot form the basis of meaningful interchange.

For example, if one looks back at the Scottish dialogue cited earlier, it is interesting to note that questions on texture occupy only about one-sixth of the dialogue and certainly are no more frequent or compelling than questions on color or function. This attribute of school dialogue is not a weakness of the teacher, but an unavoidable consequence of the topic that has been selected. There is not much one can say in conversation about texture as an isolated attribute other than to ask if it is "rough" or "smooth." The teacher senses this, and, in an effort to flesh out the conversation, she falls back on the standard set of questions about color, function, association, and so forth. Thus, the consequence of basing a conversation on an unsuitable topic is that all conversations begin to sound alike. The result for the children is that they are given models that mislead them as to the true diverse nature of dialogue.

The limitations just discussed are by no means restricted to the topic of texture. They apply equally to most of the discussions set up for young children, whether they are concerned with colors, trips, or foods. The weaknesses of these conversations would be even more apparent if they involved only a teacher and a single child rather than what is more commonly the case, namely, a teacher and a group of children. The presence of several children allows the same series of questions to be raised with each child, thereby giving the appearance that something in the nature of a sustained dialogue is taking place. If only one child were present, the paucity of ideas in the topic the teacher has selected would rapidly become evident. The material is not inherently interesting, it provides no organization as to how ideas ought to be developed, and it thereby leaves the children with no sense as to how conversation is constructed.

***Implications for Intervention*.** The statements in the preceding paragraphs do not mean that traditional school topics are without value. Traditional school topics have been selected to represent concrete, sensory experiences that young children can comprehend. As such, these topics are a vital first step in allowing children to talk about a world they understand. But if the material is to realize its potential value, it must be adapted to the vehicle of conversation.

The adaptation can be achieved by a process that might best be termed *predicting the concept*. In brief, this process means that the topic selected for discussion is represented not simply by a noun (e.g., colors, numbers, food, etc.), but rather by a relevant predicate that modifies the noun. Newspaper headlines offer useful illustrations as to how a predicated concept constrains a text. For example, imagine a headline involving the concept of *baby*. Like all concepts, this one involves a rich set of associations (e.g., helplessness, pregnancy, gender, family planning, etc.). If the headline states, however, "Baby Receives Baboon Heart," one's line of reasoning is immediately restricted and organized. The associations with *baby* stated above would fade, and one would expect to receive quite different information (e.g., information concerned with an operation, the likelihood of survival, the ethical implications, etc.).

Just as our thinking is focused by the predication of a concept in a headline, it is also focused when this restraint is applied to the language of the school. For example, if one were to predicate the common topic of foods, one might have a lesson on *going to buy food* or one on *cooking a food* and still another on *setting up a table to serve food*. While food is common to the three topics, the different predicates automatically lead to different conversations. Thus, the issues that are likely to be raised with regard to purchasing food include the money that is necessary, a shopping list to aid recall, the place where one can obtain the items, and so forth. By contrast, a discussion on preparing food might include information such as the utensils one would need, the ingredients one plans to combine, or the preparation of the ingredients.

Of course, these examples are by no means exhaustive. They serve solely to illustrate the dramatically different ways in which a concept or category is treated in conversation when an appropriate constraining predicate is introduced. Just as one would be unlikely to discuss the color of the uniforms or the shape of the soldiers' hats in a discussion on the war in the Middle East, so too would one be unlikely to discuss the texture of the jar in a discussion on how to make peanut butter sandwiches. The conceptual level of the two dialogues may be quite different (i.e., the Middle East war and the preparation of sandwiches), but the constraining and structuring effects of an appropriate predicate are similar. Predication of an idea, theme, or topic is central to the development of meaningful conversation (see Blank & Marquis, 1987, for examples of predicated topics).

Even if this idea is accepted, one may feel that conversations along these lines can take place only after the more traditionally taught concepts have been acquired. In this view, concepts such as color, name, size, and function are seen as the essential "building blocks" of later discourse. This position raises a host of complicated issues which cannot be given adequate consideration here (e.g., what range and number of concepts a child must possess; whether concepts are ever learned effectively when they are presented in an abstract, decontextualized manner; etc.). Further, the question is basically an empirical one that can truly be addressed only by comparing the development in language impaired children when they are taught—as they generally are now—through the use of decontextualized categories and when they are taught through the use of predicated concepts.

There does, however, appear to be a realm where the "building block" argument has validity. For children with minimal language (those who have few words and little or no ability to formulate meaningful word groupings), it would be impossible to conduct conversations along the lines outlined above. In these cases, the focus of the intervention would have to be on the development of the building blocks. It should be noted, however, that it would be equally impossible to conduct a conversation along the more traditionally accepted lines. If a child were so poor in verbal skills as to be unable to create meaningful phrases, it is almost certain that he or she would also have difficulty in understanding and therefore in answering typical questions such as those found in the rough-smooth dialogue (e.g., "Where does this one go?" and "Who uses this?"). (Those readers interested in developing beginning conversational skills may refer to Blank and Milewski, 1981, for an alternative strategy to current teaching techniques.)

## The Usefulness of an Utterance: Going Beyond the "Given"

*Applications to Current School Texts.* The aberrant quality of school dialogue is not caused solely by the topics that have been selected for discussion. Co-existing with the unpredicated concept is another significant feature. The content of many school discussions is concerned with salient, readily apparent physical attributes such as size, shape, and color. It seems likely that this form of conversation evolved in an effort to cater to the limitations of young children. Their acknowledged difficulties with higher-level conceptualization preclude the discussion of abstract ideas. In turn, the avoidance of abstraction seems to have been operationally translated to mean a focus on concrete, salient physical attributes.

Discussions about concrete objects and salient attributes automatically contain a central characteristic—that is, they focus on the obvious. Meaningful conversation, however, is rarely about the obvious. When things are obvious, they do not require discussion. Indeed, in many cases, discussion of the obvious is not only unnecessary, but unsuitable. For example, if someone is directing you into his car, it would be bizarre were he to say, "Well, you'll find it in the lot. You'll know it because it has wheels, windows made of glass, and a body made of metal." In repetitively focusing on the obvious properties of labels, sizes, shapes, and colors, schools are often teaching children to talk in ways that violate the basic nature of meaningful conversation. (Readers familiar with the playwright Harold Pinter will recognize that he has made his career on capturing the emptiness and lack of communication that is felt in conversations about the obvious such as endless discussions of one's choice of breakfast cereals.)

The comments above might be questioned on the grounds that adult criteria are being used to assess children's conversations. In this view, a discussion of the "givens" in a situation, while inappropriate with adults, might be seen as necessary and useful with young children. While this line of reasoning has some intuitive appeal, its validity is questionable. Examination of spontaneous conversations involving even quite young children indicates that the language is not confined to describing a few obvious, stable, unchanging characteristics.

The following segment of dialogue between a 3-year-old and her mother illustrates the level of conversation that occurs. Both are at lunch, and the mother has just set out a plate of applesauce for her daughter. The conversation proceeds as follows:

**Child**: Where's my spoon?

**Mother**: (offering a spoon) Here you go!

**Child**: Is this (referring to the applesauce) from the red apples?

**Mother**: No.

**Child**: What apples?

**Mother**: The yellow ones.

**Child**: Mommy, when are they going to come in red apples?

**Mother**: Actually, you know what Nancy?

**Child**: What?

**Mother**: I think that this may be from the red apples. I think the peels, the red peels, are taken off. The inside of the red apple is yellow, right?

**Child**: No response—(pause) Did you make this yourself?

**Mother**: No, I bought it at the store.

**Child**: When are you going to make it?

**Mother**: We'll make it someday.

(This excerpt is from Blank & Franklin, 1980. Additional examples of comparable interchanges with 3-year-olds can be found in that paper.)

While this conversation revolves around concrete attributes, the attributes do not concern anything immediately in front of either the parent or child. Rather, the presence of the applesauce has led to a discussion that might be given the title, "How Applesauce Comes to Be." Within this predicated concept, the attribute of color is relevant not because it exists, but rather because there is a discrepancy between the color of the applesauce in front of the child and the color of most apples with which she is familiar. Not one of the utterances on the part of either the child or the mother is limited to, or focused upon, a description of what is immediately evident to both.

One might maintain that, while conversations with a normal young child are not concerned with a description of the evident, conversations with a handicapped child must have this focus. This viewpoint is based on the assumption that discussions of the obvious represent the compensatory pathway upon which later, more mature, conversations can be based. There is little evidence to support this claim, and upon reflection it seems questionable. It is valid only if the children are capable of enormous generalization (i.e., it assumes that they will spontaneously adapt and extend the limited format they have been taught to situations of far greater complexity). The children's difficulties in language and cognition strongly suggest that this sort of extension is highly unlikely. This type of generalization becomes even less probable given the fact that we are considering language at the level of text rather than at the level of the utterance. The pattern of any text will and should vary greatly with the topic (i.e., different types of information will be raised in different texts). The repetitive, routinized patterns of school language work in direct opposition to the recognition of the variability of text. Regardless of topic (e.g., "show and tell," discussions about class trips, holidays, conversations about ongoing activities such as making cookies, etc.), the same set of questions appears and reappears—What is it? What color is it? What do we do with it? Instead of recognizing the difficult, but fundamental, principle that different aspects of the nonevident are discussed in different types of conversations, children are being taught that all topics can be handled by the same linguistic routine of describing the obvious.

Another quite different line of reasoning might be used in defense of current school texts. The assertion could be made that children's intellectual limitations require them to be restricted to the present; anything more would confuse and overwhelm them. This strategy might be valid if the language training were designed primarily to allow the children to talk with their teachers, since it is mainly in schools that one hears conversations in which what is evident to all is systematically repeated in a ritualized manner. If children have intellectual limitations, it does not seem productive to have them use their restricted capacities to master a type of conversation that has little functional utility outside the school setting.

***Implications for Intervention***: While there are limitations to "conversations" about obvious physical properties, this type of dialogue does represent an attempt to accommodate the intellectual level of children. Although one might question the form of the accommodation, the need for the accommodation remains. The question is, "What form might a relevant accommodation take?" Some clues to an answer can be found by turning to the well-known distinction of "here and now" versus "there and then" conversations. The former term refers to conversations about events and materials that are immediately at hand, while the latter refers to conversations where the ideas under discussion extend to nonpresent events (i.e., the domain of the past, future, speculation, etc.).

"Here and now" conversations possess inherent limitations if the goal is to help a child master sustained verbal exchange. When all or most of the material is at hand, so much can be taken for granted that there is little need for explicit verbalization. Perceptual information and gestures can carry the bulk of whatever interchange takes place. Hence, the conversation can ramble on, at times noting the material at hand and at other times venturing into unrelated domains.

For example, imagine two people chatting while in the process of making a cake. Over the course of the activity, there could well be utterances that relate to the cake (e.g., "Do you think two eggs are enough?" "Could you light the oven?" or "I don't think we should use icing this time."). But these utterances are likely to co-exist with and possibly be submerged, both in number and interest, by the many other utterances likely to be raised during the dialogue (e.g., commenting on new clothes one has bought, plans for the weekend, etc.). Given the availability of the materials and the understanding that is shared by the participants, there is no need for the "here and now" discussion to be other than what it is. At the same time, it is important to recognize that the organization of a "here and now" discussion prevents it from serving as a vehicle for teaching sustained dialogue.

The picture changes dramatically if the conversation is in the "there and then" mode. Imagine, for example, describing to a person who had not been present the activity of having made a cake for a friend. Regardless of the various forms the conversation may take (e.g., speaking to an intimate will be different from speaking to a more distant figure), all will invariably contain a much more explicit and sequenced set of utterances than would a "here and now" conversation. One sample dialogue might be, "Well, you know it was Jim's birthday and he was coming over for dinner. I know he loves chocolate cake; and, even though I don't like baking that much, I thought it would really please him to have a homemade cake," etc.). The description in a "there and then" conversation, of necessity, must be more elaborated and detailed than one in a "here and now" dialogue.

This discrepancy in two conversations about the same topic raises some interesting problems. On the one hand, a "here and now" setting offers the simpler cognitive situation that many language disabled children require (Friel-Patti & Conti-Ramsden, 1984). At the same time, it is a situation that does not demand the type of language one hopes they will acquire. On the other hand, "there and then" conversations present situations that may exceed the children's cognitive capacities. Simultaneously, such dialogues facilitate the use of meaningful, connected utterances.

In this apparent dilemma, the lunchtime discussion between the 3-year-old and her mother becomes particularly relevant, because it occupies a locus somewhere between a "here and now" and a "there and then" discussion. As such, it contains, or more accurately can be molded to contain, the advantages of each type of conversation (i.e., the concrete, physical cues of a "here and now" discussion and the need for the extended verbalization of a "there and then" discussion). It can therefore serve as a model for the text of intervention work. To facilitate communication, this midway type of dialogue will henceforth be termed a "here to then" text.

Space does not permit delineating the full range of characteristics of a consciously created "here to then" text (i.e., a text designed to teach text). However, the following paragraphs describe its central features.

First, in line with the discussion above, a motivating topic involving a predicated concept must be selected. Further, the topic must permit sufficient elaboration so that children can be meaningfully occupied for 15 to 30 minutes. Unless children can experience a sustained text and participate in its development, they are unlikely to understand the processes involved. The time restriction is not overly confining since a wide array of lessons can be designed to draw on the play activities and games that children enjoy (e.g., building a doll house, repairing broken toys, making food, constructing a box to hold a gift, etc.) (see Blank, 1985; Blank & Marquis, 1987).

Next, the relevant material must be present. This permits children to experience situations that they can readily understand (e.g., making orange juice, building a toy house,etc.). The text accompanying the materials, however, need not and should not be confined to a discussion about the obvious. Having the material available permits one to lead the discussion so that a wide range of ideas is raised. The result is that a highly explicated text is offered to the child. In other words, a "here to then" conversation has the materials of a "here and now" text and careful delineation of ideas characteristic of a "there and then" text.

Finally, the issues raised at any point should be reasonable and appropriate to the context; however, they should not be totally predictable. These are the same constraints that obtain for any interesting and informative text. A text that has absolute predictability is boring, because it has no new information. On the other hand, total unpredictability is difficult to handle, since the material cannot be incorporated or interpreted.

The range between total predictability and total unpredictability is determined by the context. Any context establishes certain expectancies. For example, ordering food in a restaurant leads to one type of text, while purchasing food in a supermarket leads to another. Even though food is a major factor in both situations, the different contexts result in quite different dialogues. In the same way, conversations with young children ought to have different content and patterns depending on the context that the adult has created (e.g., a dialogue on making a dress for a doll would be different from one involved in setting up a game of tag).

As in any program of language intervention, a "here to then" text is far more controlled and structured than the language that children encounter in the nonschool world. The goal is to have the adult construct a situation whereby children can begin to extract the intangible, yet nevertheless definite, organization underlying elaborated texts. Just as children are not expected to verbalize the rules of syntax that underlie the sentences they construct, neither are they expected to be able to verbalize the organizational rules of coherent text. Rather it is anticipated that the repeated experience of participating in these texts will lead children to internalize the rules and gradually to use them both in comprehending texts created by others and in producing texts they themselves create.

## Linkages Between Utterances: The Coherence of a Text

Coherence is another feature that is central to creating unity in a text. That is, although individual utterances exist in a text, they somehow hold together in a meaningful way. As is so commonly the case with language, coherence is a complex, intricate attribute that is commonly taken for granted. Thus, if we see an acquaintance and greet him or her with some opening exchange such as, "How are things?", we are open to a variety of responses (e.g., "Fine," "Wish I could say everything is all right," "Just the same," etc.). Without conscious thought, we have also excluded a range of other possibilities. As a result, we would be disconcerted were the person to reply, "You know, women in Japan don't wear kimonos very much any more." The response may represent a valid idea and even, at some level, a possible interpretation of the first speaker's question (e.g., the change in kimono-wearing patterns may be seen as relating to current events and hence a reasonable reply to the query, "How are things?"). Nevertheless, the response is clearly perceived as alien and inappropriate. It violates the assumption that governs our participation in conversation—namely, that when we speak to one another, the utterances will relate or cohere. For the most part, our expectations are met. Indeed, were they not, communication would be impossible because the various utterances would be a jumble of random ideas.

While coherence of text is a feature of effective communication among sophisticated language users, its attainment is by no means either easy or assured. There is growing evidence that this aspect of communicative skill requires long and complex development (Dorval & Eckerman, 1984; Friel-Patti & Conti-Ramsden, 1984; Westby, 1984). Some insight into the reasons for the difficulty can be gained by examining even a relatively simple text. The segment that follows is from an English nursery story entitled "Squirrel Goes Skating" (Uttley, 1980). In the story Hare, who lives with Grey Rabbit, is speaking about his chilblain (a form of frostbite).

> "Ow, ow!" exclaimed Hare, rubbing his toe. "Do think of something Grey Rabbit, you don't know how it hurts."
>
> "Moldy Warp once told me to use some snow" said Grey Rabbit. "I'll get some." She ran outside and scraped the frost from the grass. Then she rubbed Hare's foot till the chilblain disappeared. (Uttley, 1980)

Because this text has been written for young children, it is not overly complex. Nevertheless, it contains a feature that is characteristic of any meaningful sustained text: Although there is an overall unity to the ideas, the actual language itself is marked by enormous changes from one sentence to the next. These changes are reflected in the variations in syntactic structures, in the number of words, in the specific concepts covered, and in the basic message of each sentence. For example, in terms of speaker intent—a major pragmatic variable—the first utterance is a complaint, followed by a direct request, which is then followed by an implied request. The second speaker responds by reporting some information that has been obtained from another party ("Moldy Warp once told me . . ."). From a purely logical point of view, it seems unnecessary at best, and foolish at worst, for a listener to respond to a request for help by reporting a bit of information representing a third person's idea. Nevertheless, the reply is not seen as illogical, but as sensible and possibly interesting.

For people who are fluent in language, the rapid shifts across sentences go almost unnoticed, and the text seems coherent. The reason for the coherence, however, is based not on anything that is said in the text, but rather on what is not said—what is invisible. Unstated, implicit ideas are available to the sophisticated language user, and they serve to unify the great variation of form and content in the information actually stated. The sense of text paradoxically comes as much, if not more, from the unstated as from the stated.

Although coherence between utterances is expected and understood by skilled language users, children who are poor in language face a markedly different situation. Those who lack mastery of sequenced texts do not possess the skills by which to connect the endless variety of utterances in the material they confront. In the absence of unstated organizing themes, these children have little expectancy as to how the text will proceed. For example, if one could ask the nonverbally sophisticated child, "Which sentence is a more logical one in the exchange between Hare and Grey Rabbit, 'She ran outside and scraped the frost from the grass' or 'She ran outside and made some snowballs for throwing,' " it is unclear whether the child would see one as preferable to the other. Indeed, the latter might be seen as better, since it both connects more directly to the word *snow* in the previous sentence and reflects a more desirable activity.

The absence of tests for assessing coherence means that there are no precise measures of the children's limitations. Nevertheless, clinical experience leads me to believe that many, if not most, children with language deficits have great difficulties in this sphere, and the difficulties may remain even through adulthood. Upon reflection, it seems that the problems are almost unavoidable. These children are plagued by confusion in dealing with the explicit language they must produce and comprehend. When it comes to the implicit aspect, they may not even recognize that this component exists; or, if they do recognize its existence, they are not eager or able to deal with it. Yet the perception of coherence relies on a subtle and complex meshing of explicit and implicit information. For instance, the request by Hare and the response of Grey Rabbit can be meaningfully linked only if the reader interpolates a range of unstated ideas such as: Grey Rabbit has recognized that Hare is complaining and that his complaint has a basis in reality; he plans to grapple with the problem; the way he is going to offer help is to rely on some information provided by another animal; that animal is Moldy Warp, and so on. For those readers who do not make these implicit connections, the two sentences stand as separate ideas that happen to be close, either in time (when the words are spoken) or in space (when the words are written).

Any difficulties that an individual experiences in this sphere can easily go unrecognized. For example, many tests of children's knowledge of what they have heard or read are in the form of questions (placed at the end of a reading or asked by the teacher) that demand recall of specific bits of information. Failure to perceive coherence is generally not revealed in this manner. Further, the formulation presented here suggests that the children may not distinguish between coherent and incoherent texts. However, since most texts are designed to be coherent, the children are rarely confronted by incoherent material. Hence, their problems in discerning coherence are not likely to be exposed.

There are some instances where the demands on the child are greater; significantly, language disabled children do display major difficulties in these circumstances. One such situation occurs when the child is asked to formulate the main idea in a passage or to produce stories such as telling the theme of a wordless book (i.e., a book where the pictures are sequenced to create a story without words) (Westby, 1984). Here, isolated details are of no help. Indeed, details may be misleading if they are seen as occupying the center stage rather than as small bits of a larger, albeit implicit, organization. Should the child be unable to perceive how the various bits link together, a unifying organization cannot be attained.

The request to create well-structured oral narratives is similar to the request to create written texts (e.g., asking children to write about an experience they have had). Teachers are long accustomed to the difficulties that children show in this latter area. Unlike most reading situations (where a coherent organization is presented to the reader), in writing one must create the organization. Again, children's difficulties in perceiving the way in which verbal information chains together make the writing task one that is often beyond their capabilities.

***Implications for Intervention*.** The creation and comprehension of coherence require considerable skill on the part of the child. One of the major demands stems from the amount of inferencing that must be carried out. Consider, for example, the first two sentences in the text about Hare's chilblain. The first is " 'Ow, ow!' exclaimed Hare, rubbing his toe," and the second is, "Do think of something Grey Rabbit, you don't know how it hurts." The connection between these two sentences may seem obvious to a sophisticated language user, and, relative to the range of texts one may encounter, these two sentences are indeed tightly linked. Nevertheless, an awareness of their ties still requires that the person receiving the message recognize that Hare is in pain, that the pain has something to do with his toe, that he feels he can rely on Grey Rabbit for help, and that it is sufficient to restrict his request for help to the relatively undefined, "Do something." If these implicit connections are not made, then the two sentences are perceived simply as random ideas that happened to follow one another and that could have been replaced by any other set of ideas.

*Making the implicit explicit*. In helping children gain a sense of the vital, but elusive, component of coherence, it is useful to employ a technique that might best be termed making the implicit explicit. Essentially, it involves the adult filling in the missing links so that the language disabled child is offered a model of how connected discourse is constructed. Of course, no text can be totally explicit. If the gaps are fairly small, however, children can cope more effectively. A narrow gap might be exemplified by the following: After Hare says, "You don't know how it hurts,"

Grey Rabbit might have said, "Oh, it does hurt and I will help you so that it stops hurting." The redundancy of the information and the closer semantic links (hurt-help) allow the child to avoid dealing with high levels of implicit information.

Even were one to choose not to make all implicit connections explicit, the text ought to be adaptable to implementation of the technique if one chooses to do so. If the text does not lend itself to this procedure, then the text probably is not suitable for the purpose of conducting discourse. In other words, the potential for making the implicit explicit can serve as an operational principle for judging the adequacy of a text.

To see this principle in action, one would find it useful to return to the classroom dialogue presented earlier. Examination of the interchanges indicates that few of the teacher's queries can be connected to each other. For example, at one point she asks, "What colors are in the ball?" After receiving a reply, she goes on to say, "Mr. Rough wants you to decide if that ball is smooth like Mr. Smooth or is it rough like Mr Rough?" The juxtaposition of a question about color with a question about texture implies that the two ideas are in some way related—that is, if the ball had been green, purple, and black rather than blue, yellow, red, and orange, the decision about its texture would have been different. (Just as one's actions would be affected by the answer received to the question, "What color is the traffic light now? I can't see it.") Similar comments hold throughout the text, such as when the teacher asks about the time of year one makes soup and then requests a decision about the texture of the grater.

We are accustomed to hearing unconnected sequences in classroom discourse. As so often occurs with familiar patterns, they feel comfortable. As a result, it may be difficult to accept the fact that these models of conversation are confusing and misleading. Were we to experience this type of incoherent text in any setting other than the school, the problems that it presents would be more readily perceived. For example, imagine a situation where you have just found a cup that you had been seeking. As you pick it up, a person who is with you asks, "What are cups used for?" As with any utterance, with some inventiveness one could create a rationale for the posing of the question (Goffman, 1981)—for example, perhaps the person asking the question has a joke in mind, and his or her query represents the opening line. However, at the very least, the question seems bizarre and out of place.

Interestingly, classroom dialogues with older children are generally more coherent than those with younger students. The nature of the topics selected for discussion leads the teacher to sense (even if only intuitively) that certain ideas are more relevant to the development of a topic than others. For example, in a discussion on the war in the Middle East (such as that to be presented below), it would not cross the teacher's mind to ask questions such as, "What is the color of the men's uniforms?" or "What is the shape of their hats?" Although the topic has not been predicated explicitly, it has been so constrained implicitly. Thus, while the explicit topic may be "The War in the Middle East," the implicit topic may be "The Renewal of Fighting in the Middle East" or the "Diminished Chances for Peace in the Middle East." Within these predicated concepts, it is intuitively clear that questions about the details cited above would render the dialogue incoherent.

*Teachers asking questions.* Although greater coherence is present in discussions with older students, the organization of the dialogues still may cloud one's recognition of the coherence. It has long been pointed out that classroom dialogues are organized so that teachers ask questions (Dillon, 1982). What is most relevant to our purposes here, however, is that the questions are presented one after the other in a rapid-fire fashion. Minimal information is given as to why the question is being asked, why some answers are accepted, why some are rejected, and why the issues seem to change in the way they do with no apparent predictability. This organization can be seen in the following teacher-pupil dialogue with high school students.

**Teacher**: O.K. Current events. Glen?

**Student**: Pablo Casals, the well-known cellist, died at age 96.

**Teacher**: O.K., shush, Jim?

**Student**: The war in the Middle East is still going on.

**Teacher**: Is it going on in the same way? Frank?

**Student**: Egypt asked Syria to intervene. They want a security meeting or quick meeting of the U.N. Security Council.

**Teacher**: O.K. For what reason? Do you know? Anyone know why Egypt has called a meeting of the Security Council of the U.N.? What has the Security Council just initiated?

**Student**: A cease fire.

**Teacher**: A cease fire? So what is Egypt claiming?

**Student**: Israel violated . . .

**Teacher**: Israel violated the cease fire. And what is Israel claiming?

(Peshkin, 1978, p. 102)

The value of this form of dialogue is questionable even when the students are adept at language. The teacher's utterances are formulated in a stripped-down, somewhat telegraphic manner that places great demands upon the listener's inferential skills. These demands occur because much of the important information is implicit rather than explicit. For example, the teacher chose not to pursue the issue about Pablo Casals, while he did choose to pursue the one concerning the war in the Middle East. We can conclude this not because he told us so, but rather because this is what occurred (i.e., nothing further was said about Casals, while a great deal more was said about the war). In other words, the teacher's reasons were never stated. Hence, for the flow of the dialogue to be understood, the student would have to engage in a form of inferencing such as the following: The teacher offered lukewarm approval for the Casals response, which was not followed by any further questioning. In some way, the teacher must have found that topic less than satisfactory. By contrast, continued questioning occurred after the response about the war in the Middle East. This must mean that the Middle East response was somehow more acceptable and worthy of elaboration.

A sophisticated language user might be willing and able to engage in this sort of problem solving—problem solving that is necessary simply to understand what is being said. It is almost certain, however, to represent a process that is beyond the capabilities of language disabled children. Even were these children able to engage in this much analysis, it is questionable that they would have the motivation to do so. Tasks that incur repeated failure are not likely to stimulate curiosity and interest.

*Guessing game.* From this vantage point, a question naturally arises as to why the teacher did not give clear, rather than implicit, cues to support his behavior. For instance, he might have said something to the effect, "Oh, when I asked about current events, I really had in mind some of the major international tensions that we are currently experiencing. While Casals was an important figure, I think these other issues are larger, and I'd like to pursue them at this time." In the absence of this type of explicit elaboration, the understanding of school dialogue—even coherent school dialogue—becomes a guessing game, with the prizes going to the children who can continue playing in the face of minimal cues. There may well be isolated situations where this type of code breaking is useful and necessary. However, language disabled children are not likely to be expected to deal with such situations. At the very least, there seems little justification for having the school situation marked by an enormously complex and possibly undecipherable code.

*Altering teacher behavior.* Were teachers to modify their behavior to make explicit what is typically implicit, the children's task would be greatly eased. For example, to continue with the dialogue just offered, had the teacher been interested in having the students consider the war in the Middle East, he could have bypassed what turned out to be a diversion about Pablo Casals by directly opening the exchange with a statement to the effect, "Remember, last week we discussed the situation in the Middle East? Well, lately there have been some important changes. What have some of them been?" If, on the other hand, the teacher had been genuinely interested in having the students set the topic, then he ought to have pursued the response about Casals by avoiding the unrelated command ("Shush, Jim") by offering some comment that would extend the response (e.g., "Yes, he was a very famous cellist. Is anyone else familiar with his work?").

At this point, the actual details of the expansion of the implicit to the explicit are not central. What is central is the idea that teachers ought to be aware of the dialogue they wish to pursue and be able to give clear expression to their goals so that students will be more likely to understand the evolving conversation. Naturally, the content and style of the expansion of the implicit to the explicit would vary according to the age of the students and the topic under discussion (e.g., the formulations would need to be simpler for younger students). Nevertheless, the basic principles, as outlined in the following paragraphs, would apply.

1. The teacher's verbalizations would be elaborated and would contain a number of comments surrounding any question or problem that is posed. For example, rather than asking the terse, albeit connected, questions, "Why has Egypt called a meeting? What has the Security Council initiated?", the teacher might have said, "Yes, Egypt does want a meeting. They've made this request because the Security Council has initiated a move that has altered the situation. What has the Security Council done?"

2. The teacher's elaborating comments would give explicit formulation to the ideas underlying the topic being pursued. The formulations would help the students connect what the teacher has been saying, as well as connect what they themselves have been saying, so that a much more integrated discussion takes place.

3. The teacher's utterances should contain considerable redundancy. Each statement builds slowly on the preceding one, and there should be frequent restatements of bits of information in slightly varying form (e.g., "Egypt does want a meeting. They made a request for a meeting," etc.).

These characteristics by themselves are not particularly striking. Nevertheless, their implementation effects dramatic changes in the overall dialogue. For instance, one consequence concerns the amount of language used by teachers. In contrast to the frequent suggestion that teachers ought to reduce their language output, the ideas proposed here lead to a substantial increase in teacher utterances. However, if their effects are to be positive, the increase cannot be indiscriminate; rather, the greater verbalization occurs primarily through the introduction of information in comment as opposed to question form. As a result, the rate of questioning should dip dramatically relative to the total amount of teacher verbalization.

The alteration in the teacher's pattern of language has definite advantages, particularly for language disabled children. As noted above, the expanded verbalization is largely redundant. As a result, if children attend, they have the opportunity to have the information reinforced. By contrast, if their attention waivers, they still have the opportunity to hear the message that might have been missed. In addition, the expanded messages provide children with more time between questions, thereby meeting their need to have longer periods in which to process information. Finally, in making the implicit explicit, the demands for inferential reasoning on the children's part are reduced, thereby bringing the conversation within manageable proportions.

## CONCLUDING NOTES

As is often the case in a field as complex and value-laden as language intervention, there is almost certain to be controversy about the approach that has been offered here. At this point, however, the prescriptions themselves are less important than the issue that led to their development. We are now at the stage where significant advances in therapeutic work require us to move beyond analyses focused on words and utterances and instead develop techniques that allow us to understand language at the level of the text. From this perspective, text is not simply one additional variable, but rather an overriding variable that critically affects all other components of verbal communication.

Typically, intervention work has relied on the idea that research with the normal population is the essential foundation for understanding what ought to occur with the impaired population. For example, if normal children achieve certain types of utterances in a particular sequence, then we ought to direct our teaching so that handicapped children acquire the same sequence of skills. The current chapter evolved from a different perspective. Its impetus was the "errors" produced by language disabled children. These errors, in turn, appeared to be directly linked to the intervention that the children had experienced. The next logical step was to engage in an analysis of teaching practices to determine how these errors arose.

A focus on the behavior of normal children would not have led to the same type of inquiry, because there would have been less concentration on examining the weaknesses in current teaching methods. This omission would have occurred, not because the teaching normal children experience is fruitful, but rather because normal children are less vulnerable to the limitations of current teaching practices.

With regard to future research, this situation contains interesting implications. While the traditional reliance upon using results from the normal population to benefit the abnormal is undoubtedly of value, the converse is probably equally true. In the words of Kurt Goldstein (1939)—a scientist who pioneered in studying impaired populations—"the observation and analyses of pathological phenomena often yield greater insight into the processes of the organism than that of the normal" (p. 9). Viewed from this perspective, work with language disabled children should no longer depend on waiting for new data based on the normal population. Rather, it should function as an equal partner in the research endeavor, with both branches serving to help us understand the enormously rich and powerful tool that we possess when we have mastered our verbal communication system.

## REFERENCES

Blank, M. (1985). Classroom discourse: The neglected topic of the topic. In M. M. Clark (Ed.), Helping communication in early education. *Educational Review, 11*, 13–20.

Blank, M., & Franklin, E. (1980). Dialogue with preschoolers: A cognitively-based system of assessment. *Applied Psycholinguistics, 1*, 127–150.

Blank, M., & Marquis, A. (1987). *Directing discourse: Teaching meaningful conversation to children*. Tucson, AZ: Communication Skill Builders.

Blank, M., & Milewski, J. (1981). Applying psycholinguistic concepts to the treatment of an autistic child. *Applied Psycholinguistics, 2*, 65–84.

Blank, M., Rose, S. A., & Berlin, L. (1978). *The language of learning: The preschool years*. New York: Grune & Stratton.

Bryan, T., & Pflaum, S. (1978). Linguistic, cognitive and social analyses of learning disabled children's interactions. *Learning Disabilities Quarterly, 1*, 70–79.

Dillon, J. T. (1982). The effect of questions in education and other enterprises. *Journal of Curriculum Studies, 14*, 127–152.

Dorval, B., & Eckerman, C. O. (1984). Developmental trends in the quality of conversation achieved by small groups of acquainted peers. *Monographs of the Society for Research in Child Development, 49* (2, Serial No. 206).

Friel-Patti, S., & Conti-Ramsden, G. (1984). Discourse development in atypical language learners. In S. A. Kuczaj (Ed.), *Discourse development: Progress in cognitive development research* (pp. 167–194). New York: Springer-Verlag.

Goffman, E. (1981). *Forms of talk*. London: Blackwell.

Goldstein, K. (1939). *The organism*. New York: American Books.

Halliday, M. A. K., & Hasan, R. (1976). *Cohesion in English*. London: Longman.

Halliday, M. A. K., & Hasan, R. (1980). Text and context: Aspects of language in a social-semiotic perspective. *Sophia Linguistica, 6*.

McTear, M. F. (1980). Structure and process in children's conversational development. In S. A. Kuczaj (Ed.), *Discourse development: Progress in cognitive research development* (pp. 37–76). New York: Springer-Verlag.

Peshkin, A. (1978). *Growing up American: Schooling and the survival of community*. Chicago: University of Chicago Press.

Rees, N. (1978). Pragmatics of language: Applications to normal and disordered language development. In R. L. Schiefelbusch (Ed.), *Bases of language intervention*. Austin, TX: PRO-ED.

Schiefelbusch, R. L. (Ed.). (1980). *Nonspeech language and communication: Analysis and intervention*. Austin, TX: PRO-ED.

Sinclair, J. McH., & Coulthard, R. M. (1975). *Towards an analysis of discourse: The English used by teachers and pupils*. Oxford: Oxford University Press.

Stevenson, H. W., Parker, T., Wilkinson, A., Bonnevaux, B., & Gonzalez, M. (1978). Schooling, environment and cognitive development: A cross-cultural study. *Monographs of the Society for Research in Child Development, 43* (3, Serial No. 175).

Uttley, A. (1980). *Squirrel goes skating*. Great Britain: Collins Colour Cubs.

Westby, C. E. (1984). Development of narrative language abilities. In G. P. Wallach & K. G. Butler (Eds.), *Language learning disabilities in school-age children*. Baltimore: Williams & Wilkins.

# 16

# *Pragmatics and Generalization*

ANN P. KAISER AND
STEVEN F. WARREN

The fields of language acquisition and language intervention are moving toward a more functional approach to communicative competence. Increasing emphasis has been placed on the study of how functional language is actually used in the environment. Within this context, pragmatics and generalization have been prominent in child language and language intervention. To those primarily interested in normal acquisition, *pragmatics* represents a renewed emphasis of the purposes or functions of language as determined by the communication context. Certainly, a pragmatic perspective in language is not novel (deLaguna, 1927; Morris, 1938); but within recent linguistic history, the focus on the pragmatics of language use represents a departure from a primary concern for the structure (syntax) or referential meaning (semantics) of children's language.

For some language interventionists, a key term of recent years has been *generalization*. The emphasis on generalization has arisen from the development of a behavioral technology to teach new skills and from the resulting widespread use of programs for changing behavior. Increased concern for extending behavior change to settings outside of those used in training and maintaining therapeutic changes has emphasized generalization in all areas of behavior modification. Generalization has been

Preparation of this chapter was supported in part by two grants from the Special Education Program in the U.S. Department of Education (USOE G0079-05112 and USOE 300-77-0408). Appreciation is extended to Richard L. Schiefelbusch and Betty Hart for their comments and suggestions on the basic ideas contained in this chapter.

recognized as an especially critical aspect of language intervention because of the nature of the target behavior and intended outcome. The purpose of language intervention is to provide a language deficient individual with a generative communicative repertoire to be used across settings, persons, and events to describe familiar and novel stimuli (Warren & Rogers-Warren, 1980). Some language interventionists (Hart, 1980; McLean & Snyder-McLean, 1978) have been influenced by the current emphasis on pragmatics in normal development and have related the concerns for generalization to recognition of the pragmatic functions of language. However, for the most part generalization has not been considered in relation to pragmatic theory or research.

Almost intuitively, one would assume a relationship between the focus of child language researchers and that of language interventionists. Although generalization and maintenance of language in the natural environment imply appropriate pragmatic use, the relationship between pragmatics and generalization has not been explored extensively. This chapter considers the theoretical and practical intersect of pragmatics and the process of generalization.

The purpose of this chapter is to point out certain basic points of intersect emerging from research on pragmatics and on generalization representing a confluence of developmental and behavioral research models during the last 20 years. This chapter is not intended to resolve theoretical differences or to argue for the relative integrity of one body of theory and research or the other. Rather, the merit of this discussion is that despite differences in focus, terminology, and response units, the two approaches share some essential views of language acquisition and use.

Pragmatics refers to both a theoretical viewpoint in child language research and to a specific characterization of language use. Generalization refers to a process and outcome of learning, but is not a theoretical viewpoint itself. Pragmatics and generalization are not parallel constructs. However, either construct can be employed to examine the functional use of language. In this chapter, pragmatics and generalization are primarily considered as descriptors of processes related to language acquisition and use. Pragmatic and functional approaches to the study and description of language use are delineated. This focus offers the occasion for the discussion of potential intersects between these perspectives.

## A FUNCTIONALIST PERSPECTIVE

The theoretical approach inherent in this chapter emanates from a functionalist perspective (Fodor, 1980). Contemporary functionalism draws from radical behaviorism (cf. Skinner, 1953), social learning theory (cf. Bandura, 1977), and to some extent operational approaches to information processing (Reitman, 1964). A common position derivable from these approaches is that overt human behavior is often the immediate product of organized systems of covert cognitive activity. These systems are themselves the resulting combination of simpler systems derived from the interaction of behavior and the environment (Whitehurst & Zimmerman, 1979). Such an approach allows, to some extent, behavioral (i.e., functional) and cognitive (i.e., structural) approaches to co-exist within the parameters of the traditional functionalist emphasis on empiricism and the establishment of demonstrable controlling relationships (Hilgard & Bower, 1975).

It is particularly difficult to deal with the functional issues of communicative competence using only one frame of reference (i.e., cognitive, behavioral, or psycholinguistic) at this time. Therefore, a functionalist perspective is particularly suitable for the study of language acquisition and use. Like behaviorism, it is a conservative approach; its practitioners are generally unwilling to extend their theory beyond the boundaries of their data. However, unlike behaviorism, it is not bound to a particular theoretical perspective, but to a set of scientific-methodological guidelines (Hilgard & Bower, 1975). A functionalist perspective is implicit throughout this chapter.

## SOME PRELIMINARY ASSUMPTIONS

This chapter begins with the assumption that language is not inherently different from other forms of behavior. Although it is structurally more complex, the processes underlying language acquisition and use are assumed to be similar to those supporting acquisition and use of other behavior. This approach is specified by three basic tenets.

1. *Language is behavior*. It is subject to the same contingencies as other types of behavior. It affects and is affected by the environment. It functions as a stimulus and response, and in conversation frequently serves both functions simultaneously. Language, by definition (Skinner, 1957), mediates the behavior of others.

2. *The meaning of language is not in the words themselves, but in how they are used* (Wittgenstein, 1953). Form and function cannot be meaningfully separated, and both must be accounted for in an adequate explanation of how language works and how it is acquired or taught. Further, language cannot be understood separate from its particular context.
3. *Form usually follows function* (e.g., Hart, 1980; Moerk, 1977; Nelson, 1973; Ratner & Bruner, 1978; Skinner, 1957). Form develops as the child's needs, wants, and intentions become more specific, thus requiring an

increasingly sophisticated communication system. These assumptions are implicit to the following discussion.

The remainder of this chapter is organized into five sections. First, an overview of the theory and research on pragmatics is presented. In the second section, theory and research on generalization, primarily from a behavioral perspective, are discussed. Next, possible points of intersect between the two areas are considered. In the fourth section, a communication model is proposed with the intention of integrating certain aspects of both behavioral and pragmatic perspectives. The goal of this model is to show how some of the subsystems of the communication system might relate and to provide a direction for intervention with deficient populations that facilitates the development of a generalized communication repertoire. In the fifth and final section, the implication of the proposed model and other proposals made are discussed in terms of theory, research, and intervention issues.

A thorough discussion of a functional perspective toward language would require more space than we have available here. Thus, many issues would have been mentioned briefly or omitted. The reader is encouraged to seek the cited primary sources for complete analyses of the issues being discussed. This chapter emphasizes generalization and mentions other relevant processes. This relative emphasis, although intentional, does not strictly presume proportional importance of generalization as a process in language learning and use.

## PRAGMATICS

Pragmatics has become a familiar term in child language only during the last decade. Its current use in child language is traditionally traced to the field of semiotics, in which pragmatics is the study of the relationship between signs or linguistic expressions and their users. In both the semiotic definition and current child language use, *pragmatics* still carries its original meaning, derived from the Greek word *pragmatikos* ("deed"). Currently, pragmatics assumes language use to be a deed, an action.

Pragmatics does not have a strict technical definition. Possibly, such a definition will develop in the course of child language work dealing with pragmatic issues. Specific and implicit definitions abound, however, and the range of definitions is indicative of the state of the art: relatively young, somewhat disparate, and lacking a succinct taxonomy of the behaviors or topics under study. A few of the most frequently cited definitions and perspectives on pragmatics are discussed here to characterize the common assumptions in pragmatics and the concerns of child language workers approaching children's language from a pragmatic perspective. These definitions are not exhaustive, but taken together they characterize the emergent perspective on children's language that is unique in its concerns.

## Definitions of Pragmatics

Austin (1962) frequently is credited with the contemporary introduction of the pragmatic focus in child language. Austin's theoretical description of locutionary, illocutionary, and prelocutionary acts posited that action occurs in the saying of an utterance. Utterances achieve outcomes because they are demands, protests, assertions, and so forth. The very saying of an utterance (with appropriate force and content) acts upon the individuals who hear the utterance. Austin introduced the notion of speech acts; and the traditional Greek definition of pragmatics, words as deed, was given a modern linguistic context.

Searle (1969) proposed the term *speech acts* and applied a pragmatic theoretical framework to modern studies of child language. Three aspects of his analysis have had particular impact on the current conceptualization of pragmatics. First, Searle posited that speaking a language is performing speech acts. The speech act thus became the unit of analysis in examining child conversation. Second, Searle suggested that the speech act, as the basic unit of linguistic communication, is shaped by rules for the use of its linguistic elements. The third aspect of Searle's conceptualization of language proposed that each utterance has a proposition (conceptual content) and an illocutionary force (how the utterance is to be taken). In sum, Searle offered a definition of language as a deed and as action, proposed that speakers have specific intentions that are considered in addition to the conceptual content of the utterance, and suggested that there are rules that govern the use of linguistic elements in particular context to convey meanings. Notably absent from Searle's account was the traditional emphasis on the specific forms of language. An important shift from form to function had been proposed.

Dore (1974) further explored the issue of intention in child language, focusing in particular on young children's communication prior to the development of complex grammar. He proposed a set of primitive speech acts, rudimentary referring expressions, and primitive forces. Dore expanded Searle's (1969) analysis in two important ways. He elaborated the issue of intention by proposing that intention derives from a cognitive-pragmatic basis and is distinct from grammatical categories that serve to express it. Intentions were posited to be functions of utterances as opposed to their meanings or forms. Thus, Dore further extended the study of child language from its predominantly semantic focus of the early 1970s. Dore also proposed that communicative intentions (rudimentary forces) exist prior to formal language. In keeping with the contemporary psychological developmental analysis of child behavior (cf. Bruner, 1968; Piaget, 1926), Dore suggested that communicative behavior is based in prelinguistic, nonverbal social, interactive behavior. Although Dore approached language from the perspective of linguistics, he reiterated the view of the developing child's repertoire of social and linguistic behavior as a continuation of earlier cognitive and social behaviors.

Halliday (1975) also contributed to the definition of pragmatics and the redefinition of early childhood communication. Halliday explored the issue of context in the syntigmatic (i.e., limited to the analysis of items within a given linguistic structure) sense in his earlier analyses of the development of syntax and rules governing its use in child and adult speakers. In his later work, Halliday approached the issue of context in the paradigmatic sense, exploring the relationship between utterances and the larger social context. Although the early and late portions of Halliday's work initially seemed somewhat disparate, his attempts to describe the comprehensive linguistic-communicative system in terms of multiple contexts of differing ranges was innovative and important to the developing perspective of child language as context determined. In his analysis of social context, Halliday defined "learning to mean" as acquiring skills at interpreting the social context of the utterance and expressing intentions (probably learned from the culture) within the rules defined by the particular social group and setting. Although Halliday's attempts at providing a model expressing the continuity of the linguistic communicative system from its smallest phonological constituent to its large conversational units were not entirely successful, or perhaps not clearly understood, he influenced both the implicit and explicit definitions of pragmatics. Possibly, his attempts will form the basis for the expansion of current experimental work in the direction of integrating previous syntactic, semantic, and communicative systems analysis into a comprehensive model.

Bates (1976) and her colleagues (Bates, Camaioni, & Volterra, 1979) addressed prelinguistic communication more specifically, attempting to verify its roots in Piaget's sensorimotor stages. Bates suggested that developmental progression signals intention and that performatives have a developmental history prior to speech itself. At first, children use signals (cries, regularized nonword vocalizations) to indicate intention. These performatives may be gestural or minimally verbal. Subsequently, propositions are added in the form of words used in a manner that is increasingly referential. Gradually, the child begins to acquire knowledge of the presuppositions of conversation (what the speaker assumes the listener already knows or what information is shared by speaker and listener). As presuppositions are refined, conversational postulates are formalized and emerge as guiding forces in social communication.

One of Bates' primary contributions was the description of the gradual differentiation of signals from context in the process of developing referential speech. Bates traced the development of communication acts through the prelocutionary stage (in which vocalizations have an effect on their listener, but the speaker does not necessarily recognize or actively control the communicative function; the child is not aware of the social conventions that make the vocalization interpretable to the listener), through the performative stage (in which signals are used intentionally, but the signals are not yet regularized word forms or sentences with specific propositional content). Finally, Bates examined the progressive introduction of regular structures with propositions having a specified referential value and an illocutionary force during the illocutionary phase. Bates' analysis further verified the relationship between linguistic-communicative behavior and social-cognitive behavior described by Piaget's sensorimotor stages. In doing so, she broadened the consideration of pragmatics to include the recognition of nonverbal actions as communicative deeds that are gradually, and increasingly, marked with, or replaced by, verbalizations that are in themselves actions.

To cite only these four contributors is to limit the richness of the development of pragmatics studies in child language. However, the chapters in Section IV of this volume provide a more complete pragmatic perspective, and the reader is encouraged to fully explore these views.

## Assumptions Underlying Pragmatics

Many researchers and theorists have contributed to the pragmatic literature, but clear delineation of the common propositions that underlie the pragmatic perspective in child language is lacking. Until recently, the developing interest area did not require overviewing. In attempting to identify common assumptions, researchers minimized distinctions in order to characterize the general field, thereby masking some of the intricacy and elegance of the theory. In the child pragmatics literature, each view merits careful consideration of its differences. As the field grows and as we seek applications in the clinic and integration into the broader developmental and linguistic contexts, a summary of common assumptions is useful. The assumptions offered here are tentative ones that undoubtedly will be revised and elaborated in the context of future research. Some underlying assumptions have yet to be tested or verified through empirical studies. Four primary assumptions are offered in an order logically related to a discussion of acquisition; the order does not imply the relative importance of the positions.

1. *Communicative language arises from a basis in other behaviors, especially the cognitive skills and social interaction repertoires of the child.* Simply stated, there are prelinguistic patterns of development that predate and are prerequisite to the emergence of language. The pattern of cognitive development characterized by Piaget (1926) in the description of the sensorimotor stages has provided an important theoretical basis for this assumption. The work of Bates (1976) and others (e.g., Bruner, 1968; Greenfield & Smith, 1976) has linked the emergence of communication with particular stages in cognitive development and has identified substages specific to the child's emerging communicative-social repertoire.

Increasingly, children's communication prior to formal language has been the focus of study (Bruner, 1975; Snow & Ferguson, 1977; Greenfield & Smith, 1976). To some extent, the focus on prespeech behavior resulted from the intensive semantic analysis of children's single-word utterances (Bloom, 1973; Nelson, 1973) and the resulting conclusion that communicative intention, if not formal syntactic and semantic knowledge, marks the earliest verbal attempts of children and that these intentions are present prior to representative speech. Some authors, such as Bates (1976), have given maximum credit to the linguistic integrity of gestural, contextually bound communication as a continuous basis for later language. Others, such as Dore (1974), have posited an intermediate set of pragmatic intentions, arguing that communicative intention does not fully develop until verbal language is evident.

In general, although there are differences in characterizing the relationship of early verbal communication to cognition, there is a consensus that the roots of communication are firmly planted in the general cognitive and social abilities of the child. This view is not a new one, but the strength of its proposition and the accumulating data supporting the continuity between prelinguistic and linguistic communication has promoted it as a primary assumption.

2. *Utterances have intentions or forces that define their contextually relevant meanings.* Dore (1974) first offered a model incorporating three aspects of the spoken utterance: force (intention), modality, and proposition (reference). Thus, referential meaning and intentional meaning were distinguished. The intention of an utterance is what the speaker wishes the utterance to do, its supposed effect.[1] Although most prior child language

---

[1] The intent of an utterance and its actual function are not necessarily identical. Function can only be determined by observing the consequences of utterance, which may or may not be those intended. Intention must always be assumed and cannot be empirically proven except by asking a speaker, after the fact, what he or she intended.

work focused on the form (syntax) or referential meaning (semantics), the consideration of intention introduces a new perspective into the analysis. There appears to be considerable overlap among forms, referents, and functions. However, intention is not iconically related to form (with the possible exception of new forms in their earliest usages). Thus, intentional meaning is manifested by the particular use of the utterance to achieve a specific end and may not be perceivable from an examination of the form of the utterance alone. Intention is assumed to exist prior to formalized linguistic means for expressing it, and there is much evidence to support this (e.g., Bruner, 1975).

3. *There are rules underlying the use of intention in conversational discourse*. Ervin-Tripp (1977) has defined the development of pragmatic knowledge as learning to say the right thing at the right time in the right way and has implicitly suggested that there are rules that aid the speaker in selecting appropriately along these three dimensions. Increasing accuracy characterizes the development of communicative competence. Dore (1974) also posited regularities in pragmatic usage and in the selection of lexical-grammatical forms to convey pragmatic intentions. Primary pragmatic functions include declarations, imperatives (request-commands), protests, information seeking, and attention seeking. In addition to these core functions, various authors have identified subsets of pragmatic intentions for children at specific stages of development. There is some variability in number and exact definition of pragmatic functions by individual authors, but the essential elements and distinctions are fairly common.

The rules that govern indication of specific pragmatic intentions are based on the cultural conventions of society. Although the cultural rules may be somewhat indistinct to the casual observer, molecular analyses such as the one reported by Ervin-Tripp and Mitchell-Kernan (1977) and theoretical analyses such as that offered by Halliday (summarized by Kress, 1976) have begun to isolate these rules and their functional effects on language. Because language and context are multilevel, the delineation of rules in other than very general or very specific ways is difficult. Much work in characterizing the cultural and immediate contextual influences in early language remains, and the task of integrating what is known about syntactic systems and semantic systems into the cultural framework and individual communication context is formidable. Although it is common to view the history of child language as somewhat cyclical and faddish, it seems more appropriate to value the intense work on specific areas of syntax and semantics as integral to the understanding of sophisticated, multilevel communication systems. A careful reading of the last 10 years of literature underscores the impression that rarely have researchers concentrated on specific aspects of the system to the exclusion of all others.

Rather, it has been a question of emphasis. To date, however, integration of the syntactic, semantic, and pragmatic systems has been minimal.

In sum, specific rules governing particular aspects of language have been proposed, but the specification of the general cultural rules and their relationship to the specific within-system rules for actualizing the expression of intention is ongoing. The emerging consensus that all aspects of language use, including its formal and functional aspects, are rule governed forms a basis for current and future research.

4. *Meaning is determined by function in context.*[2] The recent emphasis on pragmatics grew, at least in part, from the intensive study of referential meaning. In the course of seeking to define the parameters of conceptual classes and the underlying representational rules, the importance of specific conversational context became apparent. At first, Bloom (1974), Snow (1977), and other researchers relied on context information as a means of verifying semantic classes in child language. It was a short step to considering context as a determiner of meaning. The notion of contextual determinants of meaning did not, of course, arise with the study of child semantics; it had long existed in the anthropological, linguistic, and sociological studies of language (cf. Malinowski, 1923; Whorf, 1956). The immediate use in child language was a rediscovery and an important turning point in the focus of the field.

The relative emphasis on context and speaker intention separate from context varies. However, there seems to be a common acknowledgment of the interactional basis of language development and use and, implicitly, of the conversational context as a determiner of immediate meaning. The more general supposition that common meanings *developed* as the result of consistent use of a form in a specific social context has been posited by Halliday based on previous cultural linguistic work. In recent years, there has been a strong emphasis on parent-child interaction (Shatz, 1978; Snow & Ferguson, 1977) and its general influences in shaping the language of the child. A trend toward considering acquisition as a process of learning contextually defined meanings through interaction with adult speakers seems to be emerging, but such a learning approach currently is not explicitly prescribed.

The assumptions underlying current work in the pragmatics of child language propose that communication arises from the general cognitive and social repertoire of the developing child. Verbal communication is preceded by nonverbal communication and shares a common cognitive basis. Utterances have specific intentions as well as particular form. There

---

[2] From Kress, 1976; derived from Malinowski's definition of meaning as interpreted by Halliday.

are rules that underlie the expression of intention in conversation, and these rules arise from the cultural conventions of the social group. Meaning, in turn, is determined by speaker functions in particular social contexts—it is the actualization of the implicit social conventions, rules for expression, and speaker intentions.

## Processes Underlying Pragmatic Use

Evidence regarding the processes underlying pragmatic use of language is at the same time very rich and very sparse. In many ways, all the previous work in syntax and semantics contributes to current understanding of pragmatic process. If the actualization of intention requires formulation of rule-governed, orderly, representational utterances, then surely many of the detailed analyses of the structural and relational aspects of language are relevant. Similarly, if it is posited that various aspects of pragmatic use are derived from interactions with primary caregivers, then learning processes underpin pragmatics as well. Following this line of logic, it becomes apparent that the study of processes underlying pragmatics could well be the study of all human learning and social behavior—a conclusion that may reintegrate the study of child language into the field of psychology in general and may redefine the term *psycholinguistic* in an ultimately pragmatic way.

An alternative and somewhat more manageable view of processes may focus on interactional strategies as a basis for language learning. In fact, the recent study of pragmatics has analyzed child behavior in dyadic situations, especially mother-child dyads. The parameters of interaction and specific behavior patterns apparent in early mother-child interactions may be indicative of some underlying social and cognitive processes: visual attention, establishment of joint attention, turn taking, application of means-end schemes, differentiation of self from other, and so forth. A plausible list overlaps abundantly with the description of processes outlined by Piaget and considered by Bates, Camaioni and Volterra, Bruner, and others. Again, the discussion of processes returns to the first assumption outlined in the preceding section, that is, that language arises out of a general cognitive-social framework and that processes in language acquisition and pragmatics are identical to those observed in other areas of social and cognitive development.

## Overview of Pragmatics

Pragmatics is a way of describing language. It is a relatively functional approach that recognizes the use of language as action. Increasing evidence supporting the usefulness of this perspective is emerging, and some common assumptions are apparent. A concise taxonomy of the components of the pragmatic system, the rules governing its use, and the processes that characterize its acquisition are beginning to emerge from the descriptive and experimental literature. A full description of the development of pragmatic competence is not yet available, and understanding of pragmatic deficits in special populations is very limited.

## GENERALIZATION

The process of discrimination and generalization may be the most basic mechanism underlying the development of language. From the first days of life, infants discriminate among the aspects of their visual and auditory environments. Newborns detect small variations in acoustic phenomena that are critical to language and communication (Levanthal & Lipsitt, 1964; Stratton & Connolly, 1973). Within a few weeks, they discriminate the characteristics of their mothers' voices (Mills & Melhuish, 1974). By 4 months of age, infants distinguish among many sights and sounds and begin to perceive the relationships between events in the two modalities (Spelke, 1976). Almost as soon as they make clear discriminations among environmental events, infants begin to group this information into functional classes (Berlyne, 1965). The tendency to classify and generalize emerges in the first months of life and continues throughout the acquisition of conceptual, linguistic, and social information.

In general it is rare to see accounts of children's discrimination and generalization patterns outside the infant and experimental analyses of behavior literatures. Few developmental or psycholinguistic accounts of language acquisition discuss the underlying processes that permit rapid acquisition and organization of information. In part this omission seems to have resulted from the general rejection of learning-based models of language which followed Chomsky's (1959) reply to Skinner. Also, most experimental analyses of generalization and discrimination have focused on only one or two specific classes of behavior without giving sufficient attention to the role of these processes in the development of complex systems such as language. The experimental psychologists and behavior analysts who have been primarily interested in these processes have typically limited their investigations to relatively restricted portions of the communication system (articulation and syntax, in particular). As a result, there has been very little integration of experimental analyses of generalization into the language acquisition literature. Until recently, analyses of the processes that underlie learning were not considered relevant to the accounts of child language acquisition. In the emerging pragmatic perspective with its implicit emphasis on the importance of usage, integration of information about the generalization process is necessary in formulating a comprehensive account of acquisition.

Although specific references to generalization and discrimination as processes in children's language acquisition are infrequent, many accounts of child development and of language acquisition describe processes that may be related to, or synonymous with, generalization and discrimination as described by experimental psychologists and behavior analysts. For example, the distinctive features analyses both of phonology (Jakobson, Fant, & Halle, 1951) and of word meaning (Clark-Stewart, 1973) describe discrimination of particular components of the language system and subsequent groupings of these components according to the similarity of their features. Also, some studies in the semantics literature (Anglin, 1977; Bowerman, 1978) describe children's strategies for vocabulary acquisition that point to these underlying processes.

In the following section, the experimental analysis of generalization is briefly overviewed, and suggestions regarding the contribution of this analysis to a comprehensive model of language use are offered. Because generalization and its associated processes have been most frequently studied by behaviorists, much of the discussion presents a behavioral perspective. Whenever possible, relevant psycholinguistic and pragmatic findings have been cited to suggest some congruences between the two perspectives.

## Experimental Analysis of Generalization

There are a variety of definitions for the term *generalization*, ranging from the generic, everyday definition to the highly specific definition used by animal researchers in characterizing generalization gradients. Generalization is both a process and an outcome. In nontechnical terms, it is "an inference from many particulars" (*American Heritage Dictionary of the English Language*, 1969). Psychologists studying human learning typically define generalization as an outcome representing a failure by the organism to discriminate the difference between a positive stimulus (i.e., a stimulus correlated with reinforcement) and a negative stimulus (i.e., a stimulus correlated with periods of extinction; Rilling, 1977). In such technical analyses, generalization is placed at one end of a continuum representing degree of stimulus control, with discrimination at the other end (i.e., tightly controlled). Applied behavior analysts treating dysfunctional behavior have offered a practical definition of generalization: "the occurrence of relevant behavior under different, nontraining conditions without the scheduling of the same events in those conditions as had been scheduled in the training conditions" (Stokes & Baer, 1977, p. 351).

The common thread running through all definitions is that generalization is an extension of a behavior to new circumstances. The type of extension, the degree to which it occurs, and the possible underlying "rules" that govern extension have been of considerable interest to researchers. The great puzzle of human learning centers is how knowledge (or behavior) is acquired without direct experience. The generalization process seems to be the key to understanding that puzzle. To the extent that one is able to document extensions of responding without direct training, one may be able to posit the processes that permit rapid acquisition and productive use of novel responses in unfamiliar circumstances.

## An Overview of Research in Generalization

Certainly, arguments for the critical role of generalization in complex human behavior are not new. Generalization is a familiar research topic for experimental psychologists. Generalization and discrimination were considered extensively in the theories and experiments of early behaviorists (Hull, 1943; Pavlov, 1928; Spence, 1936, 1937; Watson, 1924). Comprehensive theories specifying the development of stimulus control[3] as evidenced by discrimination and generalization were presented by Keller and Schoenfeld (1950), Miller and Dollard (1941), and Skinner (1938). These theoretical speculations were based in the tradition of experimental animal studies and sometimes liberally extended to human verbal behavior. As early as 1925, Esper offered an objective methodology for studying language generalization by humans. Soon after, Wolfe (1934) suggested that many linguistic processes could be explained by a psychological mechanism called generalization, which he defined as "the transfer of a response from one situation in which it has been learned to another in which it has not" (p. 18).

In the 1960s, research on generalization in human behavior recommenced. Two factors spurred this renewed interest. One was the expanding focus on language resulting in part from the publication of Skinner's *Verbal Behavior* (1957) and subsequent replies by Chomsky and other linguists. The second factor was the growing interest in the remediation of

---

[3] Stimulus control refers to the extent to which the value of an antecedent stimulus determines the probability of occurrence of a conditioned response. It is traditionally measured as a change in response probability that results from a change in stimulus value. The greater the change in response probability, the greater the degree of stimulus control with respect to the continuum being studied (Terrace, 1966).

behavior prompted by the emerging behavior modification technology. Measures of generalization were integral to the cause-effect analyses in both areas.

Both basic and applied studies have contributed to analyses of generalization in language learning. Work by Braine (1963), Goldstein (1983), Jenkins and Palermo (1964), Palermo and Eberhart (1968), Sidman (1971), Spradlin, Cotter, and Baxley (1973), Striefel, Wetherby, and Karlan (1976), Whitehurst (1972), and others examined generalization and transfer during acquisition of subunits of natural and miniature linguistic systems. The results of this work documented the formation and use of response classes in language use.

Applied research (see reviews by Garcia & Dehaven, 1974; Harris, 1975; Warren & Rogers-Warren, 1980) has demonstrated that techniques relying on stimulus control and generalization can be used to teach complex language in laboratory and natural settings. Generalization, presumably deriving from the formation of response classes, has been documented in the generative use of elements of morphology (Baer & Guess, 1971, 1973), syntax (Bennett & Ling, 1972; Clark & Sherman, 1975), and conversational speech (Garcia, Guess, & Byrnes, 1973).

Research in teaching language deficient populations has also investigated some stimulus variables affecting generalization. For example, Stokes and Baer's (1977) review of generalization in applied behavior analysis concluded that multiple exemplars of the various stimulus conditions across which generalization is desired may be a necessary condition for generalization. Subsequently, use of multiple training stimuli and multiple trainers were experimentally shown to facilitate acquisition of generalized language skills in moderately retarded (Jeffree, Wheldall, & Mittler, 1973) and severely retarded (Anderson & Spradlin, 1980) adolescents.

Longitudinal observations of severely retarded adolescents and of young language delayed children receiving individualized language training have indicated that generalization to everyday language contexts does not occur until students successfully generalize across less complex, individual stimulus conditions (e.g., objects, trainers, and settings) (Warren, Rogers-Warren, Baer, & Guess, 1980). Conversely, research in stimulus overselectivity with autistic children has demonstrated that incidental stimulus variations may control response and inhibit appropriate generalizations (Rincover & Koegel, 1975).

Results of applied research have also shown that generalization from training to natural environments is a function of the child's complement of language. The degree to which children use language is influenced by their existing repertoires (Hart, 1980). Children with more extensive skills use those skills more frequently than children with smaller repertoires. Generalization is also a function of the environmental opportunities for verbal expression (Hart & Rogers-Warren, 1978; Warren & Rogers-Warren, 1983b). Studies by Hart and Risley (1968, 1980), Rogers-Warren and Warren (1980), and Warren, McQuarter, and Rogers-Warren (1984) have demonstrated that normal and language delayed children's use of newly learned language correlates highly with the frequency of opportunities to talk in a given setting. Generalization has also been shown to be a function of both programmed and natural contingencies of reinforcement (Guess, Keogh, & Sailor, 1978). If the newly trained language is not functional for the child, generalization does not occur. In this case, function is determined by the extent to which language succeeds in mediating the behavior of others in the setting. Finally, generalization is facilitated by the degree of similarity (physical and behavioral) between the training environment and the generalization setting (Rincover & Koegel, 1975). In sum, this research has shown that when developmentally delayed children have something to say (a repertoire), a chance to say it (opportunity), and a reason for saying it (function) in a familiar environment (similar to the one in which the response was first learned), they will generalize newly trained language (Warren & Rogers-Warren, 1985). These ideal conditions for generalization overlap remarkably well with the conditions available to normal children in the context of caregiver-child interactions (Moerk, 1976; Rogers-Warren, Warren, & Baer, 1983).

These findings argue for the critical nature of stimulus control and generalization in the formulation and productive use of a generative language repertoire. Basic research with natural and miniature linguistic systems (Braine, 1963; Wetherby, 1978) has provided an extensive analysis of stimulus and response classes occurring in the syntactic/semantic system. Applied work has shown how environmental variables interact with linguistic information to effect production of specific responses in conversational settings. Together, these experimental studies provide considerable support for the existence and critical role of response class formation, stimulus control, and generalization in language use.

In the following section, stimulus and response generalization are discussed with specific consideration of the parameters of generalization relevant to language and communication.

## Stimulus Generalization

Generalization has two parallel aspects: stimulus generalization and response generalization. Stimulus generalization refers to the production of the same response in the presence of several different, but typically related, stimuli. For example, a child uses the word *cookie* to describe chocolate chip cookies or oatmeal cookies, and he says "cookie" to request a sweet from his grandmother, his mother, and his preschool teacher.

Responding to several different stimuli in the same way promotes the formation of a *stimulus class* and implies that a *stimulus equivalence* has been established. Equivalent stimuli function in the same way; they are exchangeable and substitutable for one another. Equivalent stimuli control common responses with which direct experience has occurred (e.g., training, mother's modeling) and may also control novel responses with which they have not been associated directly but which possess the same conditioned discriminative stimuli (Goldiamond, 1962). However, members of a stimulus class may not be equally appropriate in all situations. Environmental contexts usually serve to specify which member of the class is called for (Goldstein, 1985). Braine (1963) documented syntactically based stimulus classes in natural language.[4] Subsequently, Wetherby (1978), Goldstein (1983), and others have demonstrated how such classes can be acquired through training in a miniature linguistic system.

The analysis of stimulus classes and stimulus equivalences in natural language is complicated because, outside of the laboratory, no stimulus occurs in isolation. A single event is never paired with a single response. Rather, there are *stimulus complexes* that set the occasion for utterances. Context, as discussed by child language researchers, and stimulus complexes described by behaviorists are essentially identical. But, regardless of the terminology, the parameters of context or the relevant stimulus conditions that control responding are not easy to define and measure.

Context is more than who is present, when, with what objects, and the immediate environmental setting. These dimensions are important, but they do not exhaust the range of utterance-external variables that affect the use and interpretation of verbal behavior and that must be considered among the set of potential controlling stimuli. For example, part of the context is language directed to the child and language by the child that precedes an utterance. Aspects of the immediate social relationship between the child and others (e.g., eye contact, body orientation), past history shared by the child and others present (including previous reinforcement history), and numerous other events (occasion, form and content of previous utterances, etc.) are also contextual-stimulus variables. A very general or a very narrow definition of stimulus generalization can avoid the complexities involved in considering the

[4] Braine's work provides an experimental data base for the existence of pivot grammar. Pivot grammar models were later discarded in favor of more semantically based models of early language. Braine's analysis of stimulus and response classes is valid, even though it does not completely explain the use of complex productive language. Comprehensive communication repertoires result from the contributions of several systems: morphologic, syntactic, semantic, and pragmatic. Productive use of any of these systems is based on the processes of stimulus control, discrimination, response class formation, and generalization.

multidimensional context of language. However, such definitions make it impossible to infer[5] the actual stimulus controlling generalization.

The problems involved in defining stimulus classes and inferring patterns of stimulus control are similar to those child language researchers face in analyzing contextual variables. Procedurally, analysis of stimulus control is similar to the methods used during the early 1970s to describe the conceptual knowledge underpinning children's acquisition of vocabulary (Nelson, 1974) and early word combinations (Bowerman, 1976). By observing children's uses of words or word combinations across many contexts and describing the parameters of those contexts, the controlling aspects are inferred based on the co-occurrence of certain variables in the environment and the particular responses being tracked. The task is arduous, not only because stimuli occur in complexes (environments are multifaceted), but also because hierarchies among stimulus variables that control responding can be complex and dynamic. Thus, a mother's preceding utterance (a model) may control the form of child verbalization at 18 months, but not when the child reaches 24 months. Children spontaneously respond to more aspects of the environment and use successively more complex forms as their social and linguistic skills increase. Stimulus classes are not static; they are subject to reorganization and reformulation based on the child's increasing ability to discriminate, increasing knowledge of the world and relationships, and changing reinforcement contingencies.

## Response Generalization

The complement of stimulus generalization is response generalization, the production of several responses to the same stimuli. For example, a child may gesture, utter a word ("cookie"), or take his or her mother by the hand and lead her to the cookie jar as a means of communicating interest in obtaining a cookie. Such groupings of topographically dissimilar responses produced in the presence of a particular stimulus (or a stimulus class) are response classes.

Defining and identifying response classes in child language is complex because language is not a unitary system. It is composed of several interrelated and overlapping systems that cannot be clearly and meaningfully separated from each other. Communication requires discrimination and generalization at the phonological level, in labeling, in producing multiword utterances describable in terms of syntactic or semantic classes,

---

[5] Determining stimulus control is always an inference due to stimulus complexity even in the simplest, most straightforward situations (Sidman, 1979).

in receptive understanding of all aspects of language, and in adapting language to fit the listener, the occasion, and the speaker's immediate behavioral goals. A generative communication repertoire is based on the formation of multiple stimulus and response classes that are dynamic, responsive to changing contingencies, and increase information about the context and the communication system.

The basic discrimination and generalization processes that are essential to initial language learning are continuously applied in language use. The language user must be able to integrate and reconstitute stimulus and response classes as mastery of elementary forms and basic controlling relationships progress and as the immediate social environment dictates. Language use is more than learning which specific stimuli control particular responses and then (forever) acting upon this information. It is learning increasingly complex conditional discriminations for controlling relationships and integrating and reorganizing response classes on the basis of newly learned information and/or environmental contingencies. In short, the process is never static.

At first, a response will be controlled by immediate stimulus variables. With mastery of the response, it will come under the control of more general stimulus variables and/or variables influencing other levels of the communication system. For example, production of sounds is at first learned in isolation and may be controlled by the models and reinforcers available for producing these sounds. For most individuals, once the sound is mastered its production is primarily influenced by variables controlling the larger set to which sounds contribute (i.e., words). On some occasions individual sounds will still be modified by their systemic context (e.g., the sounds that precede it, social contingencies relating to pronunciations of a particular style), but in general sounds will be most affected by contingencies and stimuli not directly associated with their production. Similarly, single words at first will be primarily affected by stimuli related to direct referencing. With acquisition of multiword utterances, syntactic and semantic rules will determine selection of words and order of occurrence. Direct referencing will continue, but it will be modified by the stimuli and contingencies related to the system in which words are embedded. Thus, the particular form of a communicative response will be influenced by stimulus variables controlling all of the subunits of the response and by the social stimuli and contingencies for speaking. Functional contingencies will determine the occurrence of an utterance, its general content, and some aspects of form. Knowledge of form and previous systematic form relationships will impact the exact construction of the utterance.

An analysis of the multiple discriminations and generalizations necessary for a comprehensive communication repertoire is indeed awesome. Consideration of these multiple opportunities suggests a myriad of occasions in which failure to discriminate and/or generalize may result in deficient communication. From the standpoint of language remediation it may not be necessary to fully understand the generalization process, but only what variables can be reliably manipulated to trigger it. At the very least, behavior analysts have made significant progress identifying and studying these variables. Optimistically, we can assume that as technology for triggering the process improves, so will understanding of exactly how these processes work.

## SHARED PERSPECTIVES

Throughout the history of the study of child language, differences, rather than similarities, among points of view have been emphasized. Discussions of differences and shortcomings of various models of language have been productive in many ways. These discussions have prompted researchers to reconsider their data, to reformulate their efforts, and to critically analyze new data and theories. Focusing on differences has presented difficulties, too. First, data and interpretations of information presented from other perspectives are too frequently ignored or discounted without thorough examination of their empirical content. Critical findings may be overlooked when information is dismissed on the basis of the theory from which it arises. Second, no single model or theory is completely developed or completely verified by empirical data. There is overlap among the models of language arising from various theories, but none is complete. Different models may offer a clearer analysis of different portions of the language process. When researchers confine their scholarship to a single perspective, gaps in data and theory may persist. Finally, teaching language deficient individuals is a continuing issue. Although it is important to study normal acquisition, there is great interest, but relatively little urgency, in the analysis of normal development. On the other hand, there is great urgency in the need for more effective procedures to teach language delayed children. Successful, comprehensive interventions will directly affect the prognoses for these children's lives. One of the most important contributions to be gained in emphasizing shared perspectives may be to consolidate the available information about the nature of language and critical processes underlying acquisition in ways that could lead to better solutions to the problems of *what* to teach and *how* to teach it. This practical concern is the foremost reason for emphasizing the perspectives shared by language researchers working in different paradigms. Current scientific and theoretical issues also point to the need to consolidate what is known and what is assumed by various perspectives into a broader, but perhaps more comprehensive, model of language.

The preceding descriptions of work by child language researchers and behavioral and experimental psychologists illustrate a common outcome of parallel, but unintegrated, work conducted by researchers in separate paradigms. Child language researchers have provided an excellent description of what children say, when they say it, and how language is structured syntactically and semantically. Behavioral psychologists have described several processes contributing to learning, use, and generalization of complex behavior. Relatively little integration of analyses of generalization and structural descriptions of children's language has occurred. Most research on generalization has been limited to some subset of the overall communication system; most analyses of children's language have focused on what forms are used and on the order in which these forms are acquired.

The traditional controversy between behaviorists and child linguists has been based on disagreement about the relative innateness of mechanisms for language acquisition. In many ways, this disagreement is not a critical one. Even if the general capacity of language is determined by the physiological structure of the organism, there is still the problem of describing the process by which culturally conveyed information is organized and used. Recent efforts in the area of pragmatics suggest that this issue is becoming increasingly important in the child language field. More important, because understanding of human physiological, neurological, and perceptual processing is insufficient to guide specific intervention efforts (and may never be very helpful in this process anyway), observable aspects of the process, rather than the structural aspects of the organism, are the most readily available avenue for intervention.

Emphasizing shared perspectives and proceeding to propose strategies for teaching language follow a logic laid out by Goldfried (1980) in a discussion of the need for a composite of clinical interventions in the mental health field. Language intervention is in a similar position to that of clinical psychology. Over the last century, many theories of behavior have been proposed. Much research and debate has ensued; yet no single approach has proven to be more appropriate clinically or more theoretically correct than any other (Warren & Rogers-Warren, 1985). Actual clinical practice typically incorporates aspects of several theories, fitting the actual intervention to the specific needs of the client. Goldfried (1980) proposes to emphasize the commonalities among theoretical approaches as a step toward better clinical practice and better training for researchers and clinicians. There is much to be gained by building strategies for intervention that rely on commonalities rather than a theory that reflects only a subset of the empirical and theoretical information available. Clinical strategies are somewhere between a formal theory and everyday techniques. When there is empirical data available, these strategies could be translated into a set of principles for change.

In language intervention, many clinicians already draw on both developmental theory and behavioral techniques to formulate their own strategies for treatment. Clinicians may determine what to teach from their knowledge of developmental sequences but still rely on behavioral techniques to teach this content. Neither set of information suffices without the other; both may be necessary. Emphasizing common perspectives may promote evolution of effective clinical strategies. If such an emphasis facilitates the intervention process and the development of more comprehensive training strategies, it will have served its purpose well.

## Some Areas of Congruence

The essential point of agreement between behavior analysts interested in generalization and child language researchers working in the area of pragmatics is that *language is behavior that controls the behavior of others*. Whether this premise is stated as "verbal behavior is that which mediates the behavior of others" (Skinner, 1957) or whether it is established by defining and characterizing specific types of speech acts (Dore, 1975), the implicit assumptions are similar. From this basic agreement arise several shared tenets about the nature of language and the ideal conditions for acquiring language.

Language has both form and function, and these components are interdependent. There is explicit agreement that language performs specific functions. Language is a means for social interaction; speaking is acting. Language is behavior. There is also agreement that language takes a variety of forms. What is disputed is the exact nature of the interdependency between form and function, and even here there may be grounds for rapprochement. Behavior analysts propose that function is primary. *Verbal behavior* includes gestural, vocal, and written forms: It is *any* behavior that mediates the behavior of others. At first, functions may be expressed without formal linguistic means. Elaborated forms to express functions are acquired when the environment initially reinforces (by complying with the request, for example) the use of simple forms and subsequently credits a demand for more explicit forms. Function does not strictly rely on form, although elaborated forms provide the means by which small differences in function can be expanded.

Pragmatists agree with this view to a certain extent. There is increasing agreement that communicative intent (function) exists prior to a formal means for expressing it. There are a variety of opinions on the degree to which function is assumed to affect form. For example, Halliday (1975) emphasizes the role of cultural consistency in determining the forms used to express particular functions. Searle (1969) and Dore (1975) credit both formal linguistic conventions and cultural context in the selection of forms. However, the relationship between form and function in adult and child language is still to be empirically determined.

There is agreement in both perspectives that form and function are rarely iconic. A single form expresses multiple functions; a single function may be expressed by several forms. Formation of classes of related forms and functions is accomplished via stimulus control, and generalization is viewed from a behavioral perspective. Explanatory analyses other than those focusing on mother input have not yet been offered by pragmatists.

Behaviorists and pragmatists share a perspective of language use that recognizes multiple causation for an utterance. Some of these causes directly affect the function of the utterance; others shape the form. Some aspects of context may affect both form and function. Multiple causation, as described by Skinner,[6] refers to the control of language by numerous stimuli in the environment as well as the speaker's and listener's history of reinforcement.[7] The production of an utterance such as "I like Mom's apple pie" could be prompted by the presence of an apple pie, the preceding utterance by another speaker regarding her favorite apple pie ("I like my husband's apple pie"), the speaker's interest in eating at the moment, his previous history of positive comments and continued conversation resulting from statements regarding his mom's apple pie, and other past and present events. The form of the utterance could be controlled by the form of the preceding utterance, associations between familiar pairs of words (I-like; Mom's-pie) or by previous positive acknowledgment for making personal preference statements in similar contexts.

In a pragmatic perspective, similarly complex causes may account for the form and production of the utterance in this particular context. First, form may result from the specific grammatical and semantic rules known to the speaker. Second, the speaker's intention in uttering the phrase contributes to the selection of the form. And third, expression of intention is determined to some extent by the cultural rules for conversations among speakers of similar status such as those engaged in this conversation.

Two aspects of the form-function relationship are presented differently by pragmatists and behaviorists. First, behaviorists do not consider

---

[6] One frequent misinterpretation of Skinner's theory of verbal behavior is the disregard of his attention to multiple, simultaneous causation and overemphasis on the role of reinforcement. In *Verbal Behavior* (1957), he places a stronger emphasis on stimulus control and generalized reinforcement than on immediate discriminable, specific reinforcement for the form of particular utterances.

[7] The similarities between Skinner's discussion of multiple causation (1957, pp. 227–252) and Ochs' description of context (1979, pp. 1–5) are striking. The terms are used interchangeably in this chapter.

propositions to exist formally outside the context in which language is used. Verbal behavior is a response to the preceding environmental stimuli. The form of an utterance arises from this functional relationship. Although it is possible to describe the content of an utterance as a particular proposition, it is irrelevant to do so. The proposition is implicit in the utterance used in particular contexts and not separable from it.

The pragmatic view, which has its roots in the traditional linguistic perspective, recognizes the propositional content of an utterance and its expression through regularized grammatical conventions. Pragmatists, particularly Dore (1974), maintain that each utterance has a proposition and intention. In general, this difference is one of degree. Behaviorists view form and function as entirely interdependent, and pragmatists view them as somewhat more independent.

Second, pragmatists further separate form from function by characterizing language as a tool for communication of social interaction. Skinner[8] (1957) proposed that language *is* social interaction and therefore should not be characterized as a tool. Given the common view of language as action, this difference seems to be one of degree and may carry fewer implications for joint study of language than it has previously.

The commonalities between behavioral and pragmatic characterizations of language seem to be that (a) language is behavior, (b) communicative actions can take forms other than oral, formal language, but (c) whatever the modality, the system must be used in regularized fashion to be interpretable by other members of the culture, and (d) language has multiple causes and uses. It can be argued that the differences in approach are primarily ones of degree. However, these could end up being profoundly important. For example, it is true that the intent of an utterance and its actual function may often be identical, but they may as often not be. Furthermore, a functional perspective leads one to examine the environmental stimuli controlling speech (including the listener's behavior), while a focus on intent tends to force the researcher to make more and more assumptions about the reasons for the speaker's behavior in the absence of empirical verification. In reality, then, a true rapprochement may be premature.[9] A more useful tack may be to incorporate those general areas

---

[8] There is an important distinction between Skinner and the radical behaviorists who do not accept mediational processes as a part of behavioral theory, on one hand, and other behaviorists past and present who include mediation in the behavioral paradigm, on the other. Behaviorists of the latter group might characterize language as a tool (e.g., Whitehurst & Zimmerman, 1979).

[9] More detailed discussions of the topic of theoretical rapprochement between behavioral and linguistic approaches to language can be found in several sources including Catania (1972), Lee (1981), Pere (1982), Segal (1975), and Whitehurst and Zimmerman (1979).

of agreement into a hybrid model of speech usage that utilizes the study of generalization as its primary test of empirical validity.

## Why Study Generalization?

The study of generalization is the key to understanding how productive speech is acquired, incorporated, and utilized by children. For this reason, its study is also the key to developing optimal intervention strategies. A fundamental premise, then, is that the phenomena of generalization are the most fruitful targets for research by both pragmatists and behaviorists interested in productive language acquisition and use.

The study of generalization from both perspectives is likely to induce a variety of benefits. First, it may provide the empirical basis for resolving the differences between the two approaches and lead to a hybrid approach that more accurately represents the actual processes guiding acquisition and use. A rapprochement of this nature would be guided by empirical data instead of a search for commonalities in the theoretical definitions and concepts represented by the two perspectives. Such a development would have broad implications for the field of child psychology in general.

The study of generalization from each perspective will have a second, perhaps more important, benefit—increased understanding of the handicapped child. Current language intervention efforts represent a "best guess" approach by most therapists (Warren & Rogers-Warren, 1985). Furthermore, these efforts have not been evaluated in terms of lasting generalized language gains. The field of language remediation is dependent on the intensive study of the language generalization process if it is to move forward and become a truly effective therapeutic discipline.

The problem of language acquisition and use is extremely complex, and the study of generalization will have to be equally sophisticated. A multiplicity of factors will likely affect whether generalization occurs. Many of these factors are known and were briefly overviewed earlier in this chapter. What is most needed (descriptively and experimentally) is to show how the generalization process operates *across* the various components of the communication system. One way to consider these operations is to build a model of communication that illustrates their uses at various levels. Thus, the following model of language learning and use is offered based on the shared perspectives of behaviorists and pragmatists. The purpose of the model is to illustrate how generalization might operate within the components of the communication system and how these components might be interfaced into a comprehensive communication repertoire.

# A WORKING MODEL FOR COMMUNICATION

Many models of language acquisition and use have been implicitly and explicitly offered in the language literature. The most common and most problematic deficiency of these models has been the failure to account for the multiple subsystems of language (e.g., phonology, syntax, semantics, pragmatics). When models have addressed more than one subsystem, integration of the components into a comprehensive system has been lacking. Typically, descriptions of the hierarchical organization and underlying processes that permit integration have been absent. These deficiencies are not surprising. The complexity of the linguistic communication system is sufficient to defy description, particularly within the linear confines of language itself. The processes by which language is acquired, selected, and used are more complex than the means humans have for describing them.

To propose a model that adequately addresses all these complexities is outside the scope of this chapter. However, the integration of behavioral and pragmatic approaches into a unitary generalization perspective brings together some information that permits the proposal of a working model of communication. Such a model might have as its goals to show some of the subsystems of the communication system, to provide a framework for relating these systems, and to provide a direction for intervening with deficient populations to facilitate the development of a comprehensive communication repertoire. The primary focus of this working model is to demonstrate what forces contribute to the form of an utterance. In particular, this model might be useful in addressing how form is related to function within conversational contexts.

## A Vector Model of Communication

The productive form of communication, an utterance or a speech act, is determined by four contributing forces: speaker's intention[10] (what function the utterance is to serve in this immediate instance); the interactional context (social, cultural parameters of communication instance; nonlinguistic rules that govern selection of communication form); semantic

---

[10] The term *intention* is used in this context with the full knowledge that it is not acceptable to many behaviorists. However, intention in this context might be construed to mean the function, the reduction of need, a behavior with the purpose of mediating reinforcers, and so forth. It is not assumed that intention arises separately from environmental contingencies or learning history. A behavioral analysis is still assumed to be appropriate, but a shorthand designate was required to facilitate this discussion; thus, *intention* is used throughout this section.

knowledge of the speaker (here, primarily representational or knowledge of word meaning, but strongly related to concept or response class–based knowledge); and syntactic knowledge (use of rules or regularity in combining forms to refer to certain events or intentions).[11] These forces are shown as vectors in Figure 16.1. The vector model borrows from mathematical models in which strength of a force exerted on one object by another is represented by lines of varying lengths corresponding to the relative strength of the force. This model assumes that there is multiple causation for form, but that form primarily arises from function. In this context the development of communicative competence is "coming to say the right things, at the right time, in the right way" (Ervin-Tripp, 1971, p. 233). Right things correspond to speaker intention, and the first step toward competence is realization of intention. This means coming in contact with the basic environmental contingency: Language controls the environment. Intention initially arises from the most basic of human needs: food, warmth, human contact. But quickly, through the natural contingencies of the environment and through the developing perceptual/cognitive system, increasingly discrete needs are discriminated (e.g., preferences for certain types of food, attention from certain persons, access to particular objects or events that are stimulating or reinforcing). In a vector model of communication for a very young child, there will be a strong intention vector and a weak but developing context vector; and minimal force will be exerted by semantic/syntactic knowledge. An example is shown in Figure 16.2.

The contextual vector reflects the child's discrimination and accumulating knowledge of the nonlinguistic factors that must be considered in communication. Early on, these discriminations are quite basic: presence of a listener and knowledge of basic interactional strategies such as establishing eye contact, turn taking, focusing of joint attention. With development, progressively finer discriminations are made: Who is the listener, what is the social context, what knowledge does the listener already share? To say that the speaker has knowledge of these factors does not necessarily imply that the speaker can specify or describe this knowledge. The speaker's behavior is coming under the control of increasingly complex stimulus conditions. Knowledge is reflected in performance that might be explained by attention to certain cultural or social stimuli. All the previous arguments apply regarding the nature of stimulus control and the difficulty in empirically determining what specific aspects of each

---

[11] Again, although somewhat traditional linguistic terms have been used to describe the semantic knowledge, syntactic rules, and context, it could be assumed that the processes associated with acquisition of these types of information can be learning based. Indeed, in previous sections learning accounts have been presented for each type of information incorporated in this model.

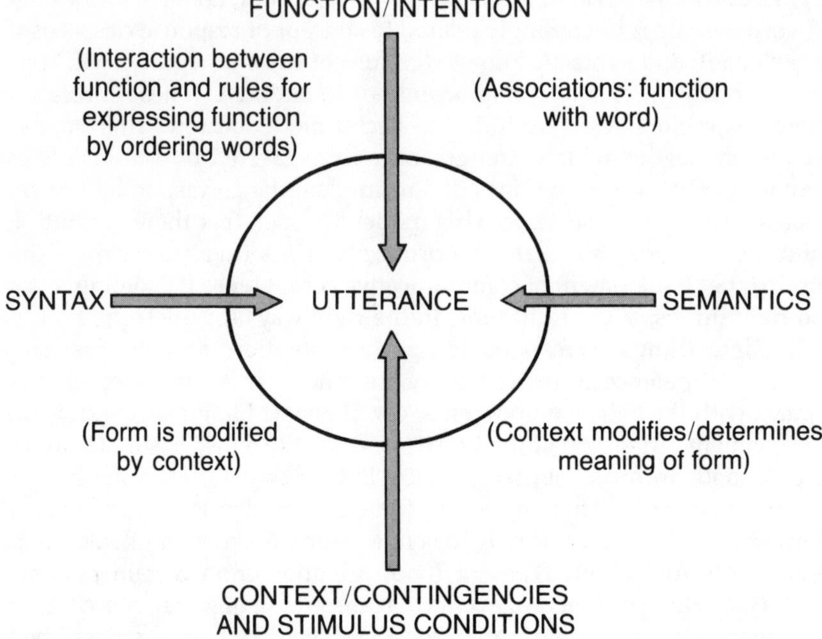


**Figure 16.1.** A changing vector analysis model of language learning and use.

stimulus are controlling the behavior. Early on, the factors that are discriminated (i.e., the contextual stimuli that control the communication act) are probably simpler and fewer than those controlling adult communication. However, the processes underlying the development of stimulus control (discrimination and reinforcement) operate regardless of the complexity of the stimulus event or the number of simultaneous stimuli.

Discrimination of simple stimulus conditions allows the development of basic communication strategies that are compatible with the environmental contingencies and provides a basis for more complex discriminations. The earliest strategies exhibited by the young child evidence knowledge of environmental contingencies and provide a channel or foundation for additional learning. These strategies include attention to novel stimuli, focusing on the listener/speaker, turn taking, imitation, contingent vocalization, joint attention to objects and events, and general attempts to affect behavior of the listener by gesture or establishment of eye contact.

Discrimination of basic environmental conditions and speaker intention can occur without relationship to communication, but it is unlikely

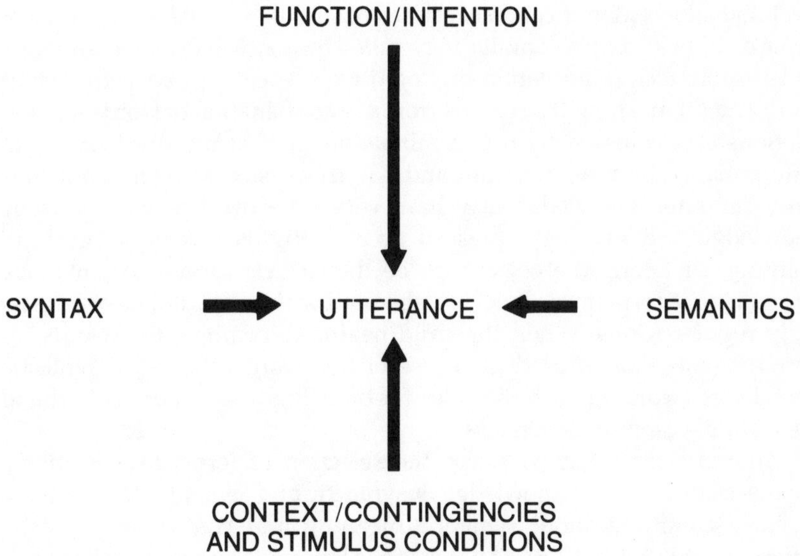


**Figure 16.2.** Vector analysis for communication of a young child or a language deficient individual.

that the reverse is true, at least beyond the earliest stages of communication. Communication without discrimination is, in a sense, possible in the context of caregiver-infant interactions, because adults actively seek to bring the environment into a contingent relationship with whatever early behavior the infants exhibits (Moerk, 1976; Schachter, 1979). The "scaffolding process" (Schachter, 1979) is the caregiver's attempt to make the baby's behavior function to control the environment, a sort of errorless programming device to support learning about how communication can function. The adult assumes an intention for the child and makes the environment work as if that intention had been expressed. For example, the child vocalizes at feeding time, and the mother coming to feed the baby says, "Oh, I bet you're hungry." The child is simultaneously being taught about context, reinforced for expressing intention, and discovering a functional relationship between vocalization and environmental change. Thus, it may be possible that intention (or at least discrimination of intention) is taught by caregivers in the process of arranging the environment to make behavior functional.

The vectors representing syntactic and semantic knowledge may function as a single system but have been shown in these schematics as two sources of input. Semantic knowledge has at least three levels: (a) the ostentatious, pointing level of simple reference; (b) the complex referential level that allows identification of classes of stimuli referred to by the same name or allows a single stimulus to be called by many names (i.e., stimulus and response class formation or, cognitively speaking, concept formation); and (c) meaning that results from the combination of words and the relationship expressed by this combination. It is at the third level that differentiation between semantic and syntactic systems becomes difficult. Early semantic knowledge may have very little overlap with syntactic knowledge and may be expressed nonverbally. For example, gesture, pointing, or taking the object may be the earliest form of ostentatious referencing, a form that is quickly elaborated with vocalizations of increasingly regular forms. When the child begins to combine two words, or perhaps just prior to productive use of two-word utterances, syntactic knowledge (working with the rules for ordering words) begins to shape the form of communication acts.

Intention and context shape the selection of forms to a relatively greater extent than do knowledge of syntactic and semantic conventions. In early communication, semantic meaning and context may not be differentiated (Bates, 1976). The task of the language learner may be one of discriminating and generalizing the relationship between forms and functions. A simplified interpretation of this process is shown in Table 16.1.

Initially, the single form occurs in a single context.[12] The context combined with the form serve to convey a specific function (I). Subsequently, a second form occurs in the same context (II). The first response class may be formed by the child concluding that $\text{Form}_A$ and $\text{Form}_B$ in $\text{Context}_A$ convey the same function (III). For example, both pointing to a cookie and saying "cookie" may result in Daddy providing a cookie when father and child are near the cookie jar (V). If subsequently pointing works to get a cookie from grandmother when she and the child are in the

[12] In this model, the communication system is described only in terms of production, and this is in keeping with current treatment of language development. However, there is certainly a relationship between receptive understanding and productive use of forms and between form and function at the receptive level. Bloom (1974) and others studying language from a semantic viewpoint have argued that some receptive understanding of language precedes production and that receptive language is initially quite context dependent. The processes and relationships described here are posited to work iconically in receptive and productive modes. The productive mode subsumes the receptive mode and exceeds it by adding behaviors necessary for actual production of speech and generation of utterances reflecting semantic, syntactic, and contextual information. The term *occurs* is used in describing this model so as not to limit the analysis to the productive modality. Thus, occurs could possibly refer to production by another speaker (the child learner is then in the receptive mode in forming the relationships described in the model), or it could refer to production by the child, or to some combination of receptive and productive uses.

**TABLE 16.1**

## Formation of Stimulus and Response Classes Based on Form in Context

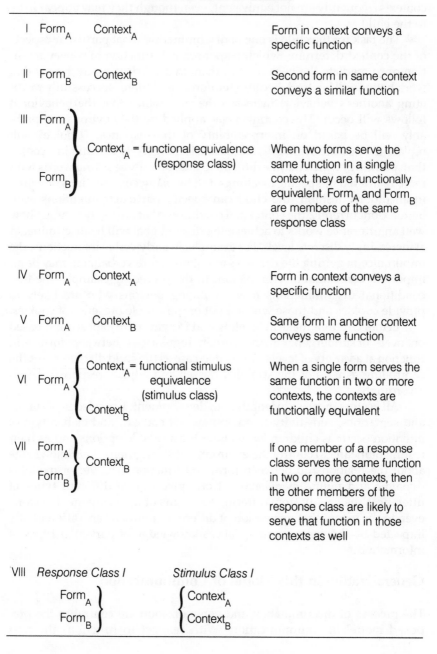

| | Form | Context | Description |
|---|---|---|---|
| I | $Form_A$ | $Context_A$ | Form in context conveys a specific function |
| II | $Form_B$ | $Context_B$ | Second form in same context conveys a similar function |
| III | $Form_A$ } $Form_B$ | $Context_A$ = functional equivalence (response class) | When two forms serve the same function in a single context, they are functionally equivalent. $Form_A$ and $Form_B$ are members of the same response class |
| IV | $Form_A$ | $Context_A$ | Form in context conveys a specific function |
| V | $Form_A$ | $Context_B$ | Same form in another context conveys same function |
| VI | $Form_A$ | { $Context_A$ = functional stimulus equivalence (stimulus class) $Context_B$ | When a single form serves the same function in two or more contexts, the contexts are functionally equivalent |
| VII | $Form_A$ } $Form_B$ | $Context_B$ | If one member of a response class serves the same function in two or more contexts, then the other members of the response class are likely to serve that function in those contexts as well |
| VIII | *Response Class I*: $Form_A$ } $Form_B$ | *Stimulus Class I*: { $Context_A$ $Context_B$ | |

grocery store (VI), it would seem likely that the child correctly concluded that saying "cookie" would work equally well. The child responds to two contextual stimuli as if they are equivalent, and function (requesting cookies) may be conveyed by the use of either form (VII). Of course, contexts frequently are not equivalent, even though they may appear to be to the child.

The task for the child is one of discriminating what particular aspects of the context determine which responses will function to convey intention or to mediate the behavior of others in a particular way. Forms that work better will be used, because reinforcement (here, successfully mediating another's behavior) increases the probability that the behavior it follows will occur. The contingencies applied by the environment probably will be based on interpretability of the response. "Cookie" will replace the gesture eventually, because it is more likely to result in a cookie than pointing, which may be difficult to interpret. By selecting words with more restricted or specific meanings and by using combinations of words in an orderly fashion, the child can specify particular intentions even better. Concurrently, the contextual conditions that are likely to affect how well an utterance works to achieve the desired goal will be discriminated at increasingly discrete levels. For example, in early verbal interactions, the importance of getting the listener's attention before verbalizing may be an important contextual discrimination. In the preceding example, the first conditional discriminations may be among persons who are likely to provide cookies and those who are not or the simple presence of cookies.

Errors children make in labeling and in syntax are logical ones, based on over- or undergeneralizing certain regularities between form and function at a variety of levels. Errors decrease as the child discriminates the controlling aspects of the stimulus classes and adjusts response classes accordingly.

All vectors increase in length with development. Knowledge of syntax and semantics, sensitivity to environmental context, and elaboration of intention occur as children learn about the available options and as their testing of means to control the environment strengthens their knowledge about the relationship between form and function. The vector model is dynamic and multidimensional. At any given point different types of utterances may result from differing strengths of the component vectors, even to the extent that expression of different intentions are differentially impacted by the context and speaker's knowledge of particular types of information.

## Generalization in this Model of Communication

The process of discrimination and generalization are central to the proposed model of communication. With respect to function, the first generalization is to successfully mediate the behavior of various people, in a range of settings, on different occasions. Acquisition of culturally standard forms plays an important role in the generalization process, because standardized forms work in all kinds of places, with many different people, and express a variety of ideas.

In addition to across-setting and event generalization, there are several types of within-system generalization and transfer that characterize language learning and use.

***Cross Modal Transfer.*** Cross modal transfer is essential within each level of the language system. Cross modal transfer basically describes the relationship between receptive and productive language. Forms heard (e.g., modeled) become a part of the child's productive repertoire through this transfer process. Children must acquire both receptive and productive skills to use language viably. Both modes are essential in conversations and in learning new forms from the environment. In terms of economy in learning, cross modal transfer is a necessary process.

***Class Formation.*** Language use is based on formation of stimulus and response classes. At every level of the communication system, response classes are the key to generative usage. Vocabulary learning often is construed as acquisition of relatively simple associations. However, response and stimulus class formation is integral even at this level. For example, mastery of the label "cup" implies that the label can be applied to every cup encountered. The actual association is not simply between one object *cup* and the word "cup," but between a general class of stimuli (all fitting the criterion of *cup*) and the word "cup." Building vocabulary links stimulus classes and response classes. For the class of stimuli *cup*, there will not be just one word but several (mug, cup, teacup, coffee cup, etc.) that may describe all or some members of the class. Further, in the flow of conversational speech, indefinite referents (it, that, those, this) become immediate and temporary members of the response class that maps the stimulus class *cup*.

At another level, "cup" is a member of the syntactic class of nouns that can occur in certain slots within sentential structure and that can serve particular semantic functions (agent or object, but not action or complement). The utterance "cup" can belong to several functional classes depending upon the immediate stimulus conditions and the individual history of use. "Cup" can be used to request a cup, to answer a question (What is this?), and so forth. Membership in a response class is separate from form: The same form may be a member of many functional response classes.

***Application of Basic Processes.*** The basic processes essential to initial language learning are continuously applied in language use. To maintain maximally functional communication, the language user must be able to integrate and reconstitute stimulus and response classes as mastery of elemental forms and basic controlling relationships progresses and as the immediate social environment dictates. Language use is much more than learning which specific stimuli control particular responses and then (forever) acting upon this information. It is learning increasingly complex conditional discriminations for controlling relationships and integrating and reorganizing response classes on the basis of newly learned information and/or environmental contingencies.

At first, a response is controlled by immediate stimulus variables. With mastery of the response, it comes under the control of more general stimulus variables and/or variables influencing other levels of the communication system. For example, production of sounds is at first learned in isolation and may be controlled by the models and reinforcers available for producing these sounds. For most individuals once the sound is mastered its production is primarily influenced by variables controlling the larger set to which sounds contribute (words). On some occasions individual sounds will still be modified by their systemic context (e.g., the sounds that precede it, social contingencies relating to pronunciations of a particular style), but in general, sounds will be most affected by contingencies and stimuli not directly associated with their production. Similarly, single words at first will be primarily affected by stimuli related to direct referencing. With acquisition of multiword utterances, syntactic and semantic rules will affect selection of words and order of occurrence. Direct referencing will continue, but it will be modified by the stimuli and contingencies related to the system in which words are embedded. Thus, the particular form of a communicative response will be influenced by stimulus variables controlling all of the subunits of the response and by the social stimuli and contingencies for speaking. Functional contingencies will determine the occurrence of an utterance, its general content, and some aspects of form. Knowledge of form and previous systematic form relationships will impact the exact construction of the utterance.

## Acquisition of Language

Communication is shaped by a number of forces: intention, knowledge of vocabulary, syntax, semantics, pragmatic context, and also a host of listener skill variables. At first, young children communicate only in response to the most predominant force: their own needs or intentions. First communicative intentions are straightforward. Intentions are easily conveyed to a listener, and communicative acts with minimal formal properties are functional in mediating the behavior of the listener. As attention, discrimination, and generalization emerge as processes in learning, children refine their communication attempts by utilizing increasingly complex formal means for expressing increasingly complex or specific intentions. The role of the listener—or, more accurately, the co-operator—in a communicative interchange is critical. The co-operator determines the functionality of the communication attempts of the child. If the child communicates to the co-operator, the co-operator responds as the child intended, and the communication attempt is functional. The exact same communication attempt may be functional or not depending on the response of the co-operator.

The role of primary caregiver in early language acquisition is one of making informal communication attempts functional for the language learning child. In the context of these attempts, caregivers give specific information about more formal means (vocabulary, syntax, etc.) that could increase the probability of children's communication attempts being functional in a wider range of circumstances and especially with less familiar listeners. Modeling and expansions of child utterances are critical to children's learning of formal means for expressing communicative intentions. Probably, the timing of modeling and expansions is important. The temporal proximity of modeling with demonstration of the contingent relationships between formal verbalizations and consequences maximizes the child's attention to more elaborate formal means and to the relationship between forms and functions.

Organization of information about the formal and functional properties of language depends on discrimination among the components of each system and the development of stimulus and response classes. Global, relatively primitive generalizations such as generalization across people and settings are necessary but not sufficient for acquiring comprehensive communication repertoires. Learning the syntactic and semantic systems relies on acquiring sequentially finer differentiations and classifications among the units of each system while simultaneously building hierarchies within these classifications. Generative use of multiple forms to express a variety of functions depends on the establishment of functional equivalences between form and function classes.

In the hierarchical organization among subsystems of language, pragmatic or context variables take precedence over formal variables. The exact social context affects the topography of the communication act more than any other force unless specific conditional contingencies are directed toward the particular form of the utterance (e.g., a mother prompting her child to say a particular word or phrase: Say "amb*u*lance" not "ambliance"). Because of the referential and relational nature of linguistic forms, a communication act is always impacted by the nonsocial aspects of the context (e.g., topic of the conversation). Rules for ordering sounds and words and expressing relationships are almost implicit in adult communication. That is, after the acquisition period, these rules are so thoroughly learned and practiced that the speaker uses them automatically.

Both children and caregivers follow this hierarchy during the children's language learning. Both focus on function of the utterance, but they attend to formal aspects of communication sequentially until all are acquired with some degree of competence. When babies begin to vocalize, both caregivers and children engage in sound play. During the period of first words, modeling new words and imitating them is a common format for interaction. Later, mothers expand child utterances to resemble adult syntactic and semantic strings. Throughout the acquisition period, there is a match in mother and child focus on forms, but always the functional contingencies for language are primary. Teaching and learning of forms always occurs in the context of communication acts.

## Summary

The proposed model of communication arises from previous models of communication formally and informally posited by behaviorists and pragmatists. The model is grounded in the commonalities between these two perspectives: Language has both form and function, and form and function are interdependent. Function is primary, because communication is a social exchange in which the speaker seeks to mediate the behavior of the listener. The behavioral paradigm contributes to this model an explanation of the processes that underlie language learning. These underlying processes are discrimination and generalization, the two ends of the stimulus control continuum.

# IMPLICATIONS

This chapter has pointed out some congruencies between a behavioral approach to language and recent communication theory and research offered from a pragmatic perspective. The similarities in approach are more general than specific, but there is definitely the possibility of some rapprochement between the two areas. If such rapprochement is to occur, it is likely to be in the arena of a specific research problem rather than in the reconciliation of theoretical differences. We propose that one meeting point may be in research on generalization.

Generalization is fundamental to the language learning process. Generalization is the process that links the structural and pragmatic levels of language. Although studies of generalization have traditionally been the realm of behaviorists, such a course of study is not incompatible with a pragmatic approach to language, because it focuses on the conditions under which language is used to fulfill particular functions. Conditional and functional analyses of language learning, particularly if focused on the social context for language, should be of interest to both behaviorists and pragmatists. Furthermore, rapprochement becomes a possibility with a shared data base. (In the more abstract realm of theory, agreement is less likely.) A conditional analysis of language learning, use, and generalization requires observation of language in contexts. The process of generalization becomes observable through longitudinal tracking of input to the child (either in training with the handicapped or in parent-child interactions with normal children) and child use of the newly learned language in naturalistic and probe situations.

For behaviorists and pragmatists to achieve an arena for rapprochement, a common data base, two critical changes are required. Behaviorists must look at language use in natural settings; pragmatists must link their observations of input to children with their observations of child use. Both must focus on topography of the communicative behavior and the conditions under which communication occurs. Both analyses must bring to the task a functional perspective on use, although the manifestations of this perspective will be slightly different. Compatible data, data specifying the conditions under which communication skills are learned and used, are sufficient for linking the two disciplines; pragmatists and behaviorists need not pursue identical problems with identical methods to facilitate rapprochement.

In this chapter a model of language learning and use has been presented that integrates four vectors of language use into a single analysis. The process by which these vectors or contributing forces are linked in daily communication is generalization. Hence, the focal process for study in the development of children's language is generalization. In the following section, the implications of this model and its focus on generalization are discussed in terms of an emerging theory of language, research, and remedial training.

## An Emerging Theory of Language

The proposed model broadens and integrates behavioral and pragmatic perspectives on language. There are two resulting implications for a theory of language development. First, an adequate theory of language must account for structure, intention, and function as an integrated unit while also reflecting the separate contributions of each subcomponent of the language system to the overall form and use of language. Repeatedly, analyses of single subcomponents (syntax, semantics, social use) of the

interactions between children and caregivers (e.g., Bijou & Baer, 1965; Mowrer, 1954). The linear analysis in which stimulus and response events are arranged in chained temporal sequences (e.g., Skinner, 1957) has proven to be an insufficient model to deal with the multiple stimuli and response events that constitute communication. These problems do not represent limitations in the behavioral paradigm as much as its incomplete analysis in basic language research. Research on response class formation and stimulus equivalency are especially relevant to the proposed communication model, but this research must be integrated and broadened to extend to natural settings. The analysis of stimulus control implicit in this research must be multivariate. Analyses of natural settings (Wahler & Fox, 1981) must be brought into the equation as well. Understanding how response classes are formed and how they are used is of fundamental importance to understanding language generalization.

During the past 15 years, applied behavioral research on language intervention has had a considerable effect on clinical procedures used in remediation (Warren & Rogers-Warren, 1985) especially with very low functioning and autistic persons (Guess, 1980). Analyses of generalization resulting from this research have amplified the question, "What controls generalization?" and have contributed to an embryonic technology for programming generalization (Stokes & Baer, 1977).

In general, applied behavior analysis research on language generalization has been narrowly focused. An unduly large proportion of this work has addressed acquisition and generalization of referent labels, an aspect of language learning that persons with severe mental retardation generally master. Analyses of other aspects of language are rare in recent years, and few descriptions of environmental conditions affecting either acquisition or generalization have been forthcoming. Typically, generalization measures have been restricted, usually including only the occurrence of trained forms under somewhat different stimulus conditions (e.g., generalization across trainers, settings, and single stimuli). "Recombinatory generalization," or generalization across responses and response classes as a basis for complex language use, has not been intensively studied in recent years. Furthermore, the common stimulus-response training approach in most behavioral language research may be inherently biased against generalization and functional usage because of the intense emphasis on discrimination during the training phase. Because methods undoubtedly affect the results when analyzing generalization, training formats must be considered as independent variables in the analysis of generalization. The analysis must be a conditional one; under a specific set of training conditions, generalization occurs to a specific set of nontraining conditions. Both extrasystemic (generalization across environmental settings) and intrasystemic (generalization across stimulus-response classes, which constitute formal language) must be analyzed in this conditional framework.

Applied behavioral research in many respects has been unduly content oriented, reflecting the 1960s influence of psycholinguists on the subject matter addressed by behavioral researchers (Pere, 1982). However, several examples of "process oriented" research have been published recently, including the work on milieu teaching strategies (Hart, 1985; Hart & Rogers-Warren, 1978). This process oriented research suggests a renewed interest in the "how" rather than the "what" of language acquisition.

In contrast, research on child pragmatics has a relatively brief, mainly descriptive history. Most research to date has been concerned with the development of reliable taxonomies of pragmatic functions. Several taxonomies have been offered (e.g., Coggins & Carpenter, 1981; Dore, 1975; Moerk, 1976), but their usefulness in research is largely untested. Implicit in this issue of taxonomy is a lingering confusion over "intent" versus "function." Intention and function have often been used interchangeably, or the distinctions made between them have further confused the more basic question of function (Frances, 1979). Actual function cannot be determined by the structure of an utterance, and it cannot be assumed a priori. Function must be determined by observing the actual consequences of the communicative event (Skinner, 1957). The need for a more behavioral focus (i.e., focused on actual behaviors and their consequences rather than assumed intention) in pragmatic research would resolve many of the methodological difficulties that currently make interpretation of data difficult.

Pragmatists have often dealt with the naturalistic aspects of language use more adequately than behaviorists; however, they have used a less rigorous experimental method in their investigations. The need to establish and employ clear standards for naturalistic investigations is paramount. Methodological advances must interface with the resolution of the definitional difference between intention and function and should be accompanied by the development of a taxonomy of consequences for behaviors as a means of defining actual functions of language in naturalistic settings.

## Intervention

Despite the implicitly functional approach of behavior analysis, the first generation of language remediation programs derived from a behavioral perspective were not implicitly functional. The procedures used in these programs were offshoots of the operant infrahuman experimental paradigm. A basic (implicit) assumption was that human speech could be shaped in the same way the behavior of rats is shaped to press a bar. Furthermore, the content trained in many of these programs was limited and sometimes inappropriate for eliciting natural reinforcers in a child's normal day-to-day environment. Not surprisingly, the generalization and maintenance resulting from these initial training models apparently has been limited (Warren & Rogers-Warren, 1980).[13]

One of the most positive effects of the developing emphasis on pragmatics has been to call into question the way in which language is trained. If one takes a pragmatically oriented approach to intervention, then the goal of training becomes teaching the child to communicate appropriately in a variety of situations. In contrast, a syntactic focus emphasizes how to say things; a semantic perspective emphasizes the conceptual underpinnings of grammar. A pragmatic perspective potentially incorporates both syntax and semantics into a training model that focuses first and foremost on use in context. Words and sentences are taught in a context that makes them functional. Reinforcement is defined in terms of the natural consequences for an utterance. If a child asks a question, he or she gets an answer (not an M&M); if a child requests a ball, he or she gets a ball (not a token). The child specifies the reinforcer with utterances and, thus, a truly functional relationship is maintained between what the child says and what happens as a result.

The location and agent of training may change, too. The therapist may relinquish the primary role in training because he or she cannot supply a range of functional reinforcers nor easily maintain a close communicative match with the child with sufficient frequency to accelerate the child's communication (MacDonald, 1985). The child's parent and/or classroom teachers may become primary trainers, with the therapist acting as parent trainer and consultant. Training ideally occurs throughout the day in many appropriate settings. Training "trials" or episodes are initiated by the child. The parent cues the child's interests to teach new language. Intervention techniques mimic normal mother-child interaction. Parents and teachers may use one or more "process" oriented training techniques (e.g., incidental teaching, mand-model techniques, time delay, contingent imitation, etc.) taught by a therapist.

The content of training varies also. A rigid sequence of training forms is not allowed. Training targets are determined by the therapist and parent or teacher on the basis of the child's observed communication skills. A developmental sequence may be followed, but the primary emphasis is on maintaining a "communicative match" between parent (or teacher) and

---

13 We use the term *apparently* because generalization has usually been measured in a limited way. When generalization is measured more broadly, certain limitations of this training model may be evident (e.g., Warren & Rogers-Warren, 1983a, 1983b).

child. In facilitative matching the parent requires and supports slightly more complex speech than the child typically uses. Studies of normal development suggest that this is one of the fundamental processes by which mothers naturally teach language to their children (Snow & Ferguson, 1977). There is also evidence from studies of language generalization suggesting that generalization from training to the child's day-to-day communication occurs most readily when there is correspondence between the level of training and the child's current linguistic level (Warren & Rogers-Warren, 1983b; Warren, Rogers-Warren, & Buchanan, 1981).

The model of training just described is one widely supported in the current language intervention literature (cf. MacDonald, 1985; McLean & Snyder-McLean, 1978; Warren & Rogers-Warrren, 1985), and there is a modest research base to support some of its premises (e.g., Halle, Marshall, & Spradlin, 1979; Hart & Risley, 1968, 1975, 1980). However, many of its premises are experimentally untested, especially with severely handicapped learners and as a sole intervention method with even moderately handicapped students. The temptation to abandon structured training for naturalistic teaching strategies is considerable, but potentially unwise.

Although these pragmatic approaches are essentially correct, they have not yet addressed the critical problem in language intervention: how to teach a student with a history of failure to attend to the contextual variables that control language usage. Children have serious language deficits because they cannot learn communication skills adequately from the natural environment and typical communicative interactions. Relying on existing processes as the sole means of intervention is unlikely to be sufficient to remediate their delays, because these interactions provide insufficient support for the acquisition of more sophisticated language. Potentially, a pragmatic or naturalistic approach can work, but only if the method, goals, and outcomes are clearly specified and carefully applied.

Although the method of intervention may vary, it can be no less rigorous than traditional one-to-one training. Training must occur with regularity, data must be kept on the child's acquisition, and generalization to other settings must be analyzed. Rigid behavior modification programs in the past may have produced limited generalization, but they consistently verified that the child did learn the forms of communication in a limited setting. Primary acquisition during training is the naturalistic approach to training as well. Acquisition of both linguistic structure and pragmatic use are critical to adequate communication. A marriage, rather than substitution, of the two approaches is appropriate.

Two particular challenges are to be faced in building a pragmatically oriented intervention program. One challenge is to develop specific teaching techniques that can be reliably trained and that consistently produce gains in child communicative competence. The other is to develop a data system that verifies the application of the teaching procedures and child learning.

Parents and teachers are ideal language instructors in many ways, but they are also untrained as clinicians and committed to a myriad of other tasks. It is an empirical question whether teachers and parents can deliver sufficient "incidental" training to handicapped children to accelerate their language development. In this instance, a simple experimental demonstration is not sufficient. A longitudinal applied analysis, in real families and real classrooms that have similar staffing patterns and demands applied to ordinary settings, is critical before a primarily parent or teacher based model of language intervention can be promoted.

Because of multiple communication deficits, many children will continue to require instruction in specific aspects of structure and phonology. This instruction, when paired with naturalistic teaching methods, may prove to be the most effective approach. Our understanding of the importance of the social bases of language does not eliminate the processing difficulties of handicapped children nor preclude individual training. There are no easy ways to teach comprehensive communication skills to severely impaired students, and our recent discoveries have added to, not decreased, our concerns.

The proposed model of communication may provide a prototype of therapy. All four aspects of communication must be addressed. For some language delayed children, naturalistic training may be sufficient; for severely handicapped children, multiple sources of input (one-to-one training, contextual training, parent based facilitation) are needed. A program that interfaces structural knowledge and pragmatic use with training that emphasizes generalization is not yet developed. Certainly, it is the prototype to which we should be directing our efforts.

Determining if the proposed intervention approach is more effective than previous approaches will require an extensive analysis of generalization. The proposed communication model is offered as a general guide for analyzing generalizations. Specific measures will have to be developed to assess specific outcomes within this model.

## SUMMARY

In this chapter we have reviewed the pragmatic perspective and the behavioral perspective on language. We have noted where these perspectives overlap and where they do not. We have proposed that these approaches can be unified into a hybrid model through the study of language generalization, and we have suggested a model to guide this research. Finally, we have presented some implications of this broadened perspective for theory, research, and intervention. Clearly, pragmatists and behaviorists interested in language both have a great deal to gain from studying each other's theory and research. For the pragmatists, behaviorists offer a way to solve the intervention versus function problem. This solution is implicit in the proposed model of communication. Intention is not overlooked, it is merely definable in a more functional manner. For behavior analysts, pragmatists offer many suggestions for dealing with the shortcomings of the operant stimulus-response training model, which, despite the inherent functional nature of the overall behavioral approach, has not yet resulted in a fully functional training model.

## REFERENCES

Anderson, S. R., & Spradlin, J. E. (1980). The generalized effects of productive labeling training involving common object classes. *Journal of the Association of the Severely Handicapped, 5*, 143–157.

Anglin, J. M. (1977). *Word, object and conceptual development*. New York: W. W. Norton.

Austin, J. L. (1962). *How to do things with words*. London: Oxford University Press.

Baer, D. M., & Guess, D. (1971). Receptive training of adjectival inflections in mental retardates. *Journal of Applied Behavior Analysis, 4*, 129–139.

Baer, D. M., & Guess, D. (1973). Teaching productive noun suffixes to severely retarded children. *American Journal of Mental Deficiency, 77*, 498–505.

Bandura, A. (1977). *Social learning theory*. Englewood Cliffs, NJ: Prentice-Hall.

Bates, E. *Language and context*. (1976). New York: Academic Press.

Bates, E., Camaioni, L., & Volterra, V. (1979). The acquisition of performatives prior to speech. In E. Ochs & B. Schieffelin (Eds.), *Developmental pragmatics* (pp. 111–129). New York: Academic Press.

Bennett, C. W., & Ling, D. (1972). Teaching a complex verbal response to a hearing impaired girl. *Journal of Applied Behavior Analysis, 5*, 321–327.

Berlyne, D. E. (1965). *Structure and direction in thinking*. New York: John Wiley.

Bijou, S. W., & Baer, D. M. (1965). *Child development I: A systematic and empirical theory*. Englewood Cliffs, NJ: Prentice-Hall.

Bloom, L. (1973). *One word at a time: The use of single word utterances before syntax*. The Hague: Mouton.

Bloom, L. (1974). Talking, understanding, and thinking. In R. L. Schiefelbusch & L. L. Lloyd (Eds.), *Language perspectives—Acquisition, retardation, and intervention* (pp. 285–311). Austin, TX: PRO-ED.

Bowerman, M. F. (1976). Semantic factors in the acquisition of rules for word use and sentence construction. In D. Morehead & A. Morehead (Eds.), *Normal and deficient language development* (pp. 99–179). Austin, TX: PRO-ED.

Bowerman, M. (1978). Semantic and syntactic development: A review of what, when and how in language acquisition. In R. L. Schiefelbusch (Ed.), *Bases of language intervention* (pp. 97–189). Austin, TX: PRO-ED.

Braine, M. D. S. (1963). The ontogeny of English phrase structure: The first phase. Reprinted from *Language, 39*, 1–13.

Bruner, J. S. (1968). The course of cognitive growth. In N. S. Endler, L. R. Boulter, & H. Osser (Eds.), *Contemporary issues in developmental psychology* (pp. 36–69). New York: Holt, Rinehart and Winston.

Bruner, J. W. (1975). The ontogenesis of speech acts. *Journal of Child Language, 2*, 1–19.

Catania, A. C. (1972). Chomsky's formal analysis of natural languages: A behavioral translation. *Behaviorism, 1*, 1–15.

Chomsky, N. (1959). Verbal behavior by B. F. Skinner. *Language, 35*, 25–58.

Clark, H. B., & Sherman, J. A. (1975). Teaching generative use of sentence answers. *Journal of Applied Behavior Analysis, 8*, 321–330.

Clark-Stewart, K. A. (1973). Interactions between mothers and their young children: Characteristics and consequences. *SRCD Monograph, 38*(153).

Coggins, T. E., & Carpenter, R. (1981). The communication intention inventory: A system for observing and coding children's early intentional communication. *Applied Psycholinguistics, 2*, 235–252.

deLaguna, G. (1927). *Speech: Its function and development*. Bloomington, IN: Indiana University Press.

Dore, J. (1974). A pragmatic description of early language development. *Journal of Psycholinguistic Research, 3*, 343–350.

Dore, J. (1975) Holophrases, speech acts and language universals. *Journal of Child Language, 2*, 21–40.

Ervin-Tripp, S. (1971). Social backgrounds and verbal skills. In R. Huxley & E. Ingram (Eds.), *Language acquisition: Models and methods* (pp. 230–251). New York: Academic Press.

Ervin-Tripp, S. (1977). Wait for me, roller skate! In S. Ervin-Tripp & C. Mitchell-Kernan (Eds.), *Child discourse* (pp. 165–188). New York: Academic Press.

Esper, E. (1925). A technique for the experimental investigation of associative interference in artificial linguistic material. *Language Monographs, 1*, 1–34.

Fodor, J. A. (1980). The mind-body problem. *Scientific American, 243*, 114–123.

Frances, H. (1979). What does the child mean? A critique of the 'functional' approach to language acquisition. *Journal of Child Language, 6*, 201–210.

Garcia, E., & DeHaven, E. D. (1974). Use of operant techniques in the establishment and generalization of language: A review and analysis. *American Journal of Mental Deficiency, 79*, 169–178.

Garcia, E., Guess, D., & Byrnes, J. (1973). Development of syntax in a retarded girl using procedures of imitation, reinforcement, and modeling. *Journal of Applied Behavior Analysis, 6*, 299–310.

Goldfried, M. R. (1980). Toward the delineation of therapeutic change principles. *American Psychologist, 35*, 991–999.

Goldiamond, I. (1962). The maintenance of ongoing fluent verbal behavior and stuttering. *Mathetics, 1*, 57–95.

Goldstein, H. (1983). Training generative repertoires within agent-action-object miniature linguistic systems with children. *Journal of Speech and Hearing Research, 26*, 76–89.

Goldstein, H. (1985). Enhancing language generalization using matrix and stimulus equivalence training. In S. F. Warren & A. K. Rogers-Warren (Eds.), *Teaching functional language* (pp. 225–249). Austin, TX: PRO-ED.

Greenfield, P. M., & J. H. (1976). *The structure of communication in early language development*. New York: Academic Press.

Guess, D. (1980). Methods in communication instruction for severely handicapped persons. In W. Sailor, B. Wilcox, & L. Brown (Eds.), *Methods of instruction for severely handicapped students*. Baltimore: Brooks.

Guess, D., Keogh, W., & Sailor, W. (1978). Generalization of speech and language behavior. In R. L. Schiefelbusch (Ed.), *Bases of language intervention* (pp. 373–395). Austin, TX: PRO-ED.

Halle, J. W., Marshall, A. M., & Spradlin, J. E. (1979). Time delay: A technique to increase language use and facilitate generalization in retarded children. *Journal of Applied Behavior Analysis, 12*, 431–439.

Halliday, M. A. K. (1975). *Learning how to mean*. New York: Elsevier.

Harris, S. L. (1975). Teaching language to nonverbal children—with emphasis on problems of generalization. *Psychological Record, 82*, 565–580.

Hart, B. (1980). Pragmatics and language development. In B. B. Lahey & A. E. Kazdin (Eds.), *Advances in clinical child psychology* (Vol. 3, pp. 106–143). New York: Plenum Press.

Hart, B. (1985). Naturalistic language training strategies. In. S. F. Warren & A. K. Rogers-Warren (Eds.), *Teaching functional language* (pp. 63–88). Austin, TX: PRO-ED.

Hart, B. M., & Risley, T. R. (1968). Establishing the use of descriptive adjectives in the spontaneous speech of disadvantaged preschool children. *Journal of Applied Behavior Analysis, 1*, 109–120.

Hart, B., & Risley, T. R. (1975). Incidental teaching of language in the preschool. *Journal of Applied Behavior Analysis, 8*, 411–420.

Hart, B., & Risley, T. R. (1980). In vivo language training: Unanticipated and general effects. *Journal of Applied Behavior Analysis, 13*, 407–432.

Hart, B., & Rogers-Warren, A. (1978). Milieu language training. In R. L. Schiefelbusch (Ed.), *Language intervention strategies* (pp. 193–235). Austin, TX: PRO-ED.

Hilgard, E. R., & Bower, G. H. (1975). *Theories of learning*. Englewood Cliffs, NJ: Prentice-Hall.

Hull, C. L. (1943). *Principles of behavior*. New York: Appleton-Century-Crofts.

Jakobson, R., Fant, G., & Halle, M. (1951). *Preliminaries to speech analysis: The distinctive features and their correlates*. Cambridge, MA: MIT Press.

Jeffree, D., Wheldall, K., & Mittler, P. (1973). Facilitating two-word utterances in two Down's syndrome boys. *American Journal of Mental Deficiency, 78*, 117–122.

Jenkins, J. J., & Palermo, D. S. (1964). Mediation processes and the acquisition of linguistic structure. In U. Bellugi & R. Brown (Eds.), *The acquisition of language*. Monograph of the Society for Research in Child Development, *29*.

Keller, F. S., & Schoenfeld, W. N. (1950). *Principles of psychology: A systematic text in the science of behavior*. New York: Appleton-Century-Crofts.

Kress, G. (1976). *Halliday: System and function in language*. London: Oxford University Press.

Lee, V. L. (1981). Terminological and conceptual revisions in the experimental analysis of language development: Why? *Behaviorism, 9*, 25–55.

Levanthal, A., & Lipsitt, L. P. (1964). Adaptation, pitch discrimination, and sound localization in the neonate. *Child Development, 35*, 759–767.

MacDonald, J. M. (1985). Language through conversation: A model for intervention with the severely language delayed. In. S. F. Warren & A. K. Rogers-Warren (Eds.), *Teaching functional language* (pp. 89–122). Austin, TX: PRO-ED.

McLean, J. E., & Snyder-McLean, L. K. (1978). *A transactional approach to early language training*. Columbus, OH: Charles E. Merrill.

Malinowksi, B. (1923). The problem of meaning in primitive language. In C. K. Ogden & I. A. Richards (Eds.), *The meaning of meaning* (pp. 101–143). New York: Harcourt, Brace & World.

Miller, N. E., & Dollard, J. (1941). *Social learning and imitation*. New Haven, CT: Yale University Press.

Mills, M., & Melhuish, E. (1974). Recognition of mother's voice in early infancy. *Nature, 252*, 123–124.

Moerk, E. L. (1976). Processes of language teaching and training in the interactions of mother-child dyads. *Child Development, 47*, 1064–1078.

Moerk, E. (1977). *Pragmatic and semantic aspects of early language development*. Austin, TX: PRO-ED.

Morris, C. (1938). Foundations of the theory of signs. In *International encyclopedia of unified science* (Vol. 1, pp. 216–229). Chicago: University of Chicago Press.

Mowrer, O. H. (1954). The psychologist looks at language. *American Psychologist, 9*, 660–694.

Nelson, K. (1973). Structure and strategy in learning to talk. *Society for Research in Child Development Monographs, 38*, 1–68.

Nelson, K. (1974). Concept, word, and sentence: Interrelations in acquisition and development. *Psychological Review, 81*, 267–285.

Ochs, E. (1979). Introduction: What child language can contribute to pragmatics. In E. Ochs & B. B. Schieffelin (Eds.), *Developmental pragmatics* (pp. 1–17). New York: Academic Press.

Palermo, D. S., & Eberhart, V. L. (1968). On the learning of morphological rules: An experimental analogy. *Journal of Verbal Learning and Verbal Behavior, 7*, 337–344.

Pavlov, I. P. (1928). *Lectures on conditioned reflexes*. New York: International Publishers.

Pere, J. (1982). Can linguistics contribute to the study of verbal behavior? *The Behavior Analyst, 5*, 9–21.

Piaget, J. (1926). *The language and thought of the child*. New York: Harcourt & Brace.

Ratner, N., & Bruner, J. (1978). Games, social exchange and the acquisition of language. *Journal of Child Language, 5*, 391–401.

Reitman, W. R. (1964). Information processing models in psychology. *Science, 144*, 1192–1198.

Rilling, M. (1977). Stimulus control and inhibitory processes. In W. K. Hoenig & J. E. R. Staddon (Eds.), *Handbook of operant behavior*. Englewood Cliffs, NJ: Prentice-Hall.

Rincover, A., & Koegel, R. L. (1975). Setting generality and stimulus control in autistic children. *Journal of Applied Behavior Analysis, 8*, 235–246.

Rogers-Warren, A., & Warren, S. F. (1980). Mands for verbalization: Facilitating the display of newly taught language. *Behavior Modification*, *4*, 361–382.

Rogers-Warren, A., Warren, S. F., & Baer, D. M. (1983). Interactional bases of language learning. In K. Kernan, R. Edgerton, & M. Begab (Eds.), *Impact of specific settings on the development and behavior of retarded persons*. Baltimore: University Park Press.

Schacter, F. F. (1979). *Everyday mother talk to toddlers*. New York: Academic Press.

Searle, J. R. (1969). *Speech acts: An essay in the philosophy of language*. New York: Cambridge University Press.

Segal, E. F. (1975). Psycholinguistics discovers the operant. *Journal of the Experimental Analysis of Behavior*, *23*, 149–158.

Shatz, M. (1978). Children's comprehension of their mothers' question-directives. *Journal of Child Language*, *5*, 39–46.

Sidman, M. (1971). Reading and auditory-visual equivalences. *Journal of Speech and Hearing Research*, *14*, 5–17.

Sidman, M. (1979). Remarks. *Behaviorism*, *7*, 123–125.

Sidman, M., & Tailby, W. (1984). Conditional discrimination vs. matching to sample: An expansion of the testing paradigm. *Journal of the Experimental Analysis of Behavior*, *37*, 5–23.

Skinner, B. F. (1938). *The behavior of organisms: An experimental analysis*. New York: Appleton-Century-Crofts.

Skinner, B. F. (1953). *Science and human behavior*. New York: Macmillan.

Skinner, B. F. (1957). *Verbal behavior*. New York: Appleton-Century-Crofts.

Snow, C. E. (1977). The development of conversation between mothers and babies. *Journal of Child Language*, *4*, 1–22.

Snow, C., & Ferguson, C. (Eds.). (1977). *Talking to children: Language input and acquisition*. New York: Cambridge University Press.

Spelke, E. (1976). Infants' intermodal perception of events. *Cognitive Psychology*, *8*, 553–560.

Spence, K. W. (1936). The nature of discrimination learning in animals. *Psychological Review*, *43*, 427–449.

Spence, K. W. (1937). The differential response in animals to stimuli varying within a single dimension. *Psychological Review*, *44*, 430–444.

Spradlin, J. E., Cotter, V. W., & Baxley, N. (1973). Establishing a conditional discrimination without training: A study of transfer with retarded adolescents. *American Journal of Mental Deficiency*, *77*, 556–566.

Spradlin, J. E., Dixon, M. H., Marquesen, V., & Paul, L. (in press). Classes and receptive labels. In J. E. Spradlin & K. F. Ruder (Eds.), *Issues in receptive language and generalization*. American Speech, Language and Hearing Monograph.

Stokes, T. F., & Baer, D. M. (1977). An implicit technology of generalization. *Journal of Applied Behavior Analysis*, *10*, 349–367.

Stratton, P. M., & Connolly, K. (1973). Discrimination by newborns of the intensity, frequency and temporal characteristics of auditory stimuli. *British Journal of Psychology*, *64*, 219–232.

Striefel, S., Wetherby, B., & Karlan, G. F. (1976) Establishing generalized verb-noun instruction-following skills in retarded children. *Journal of Experimental Child Psychology*, *22*, 247–260.

Terrace, H. S. (1966). Stimulus control. In W. K. Honig (Ed.), *Operant behavior: Areas of research and application* (pp. 271–344). New York: Appleton-Century-Crofts.

Wahler, R. G., & Fox, J. J. (1981). Setting events in applied behavior analysis: Toward a conceptual and methodological analysis. *Journal of Applied Behavior Analysis, 14*, 327–338.

Warren, S. F., McQuarter, R. J., & Rogers-Warren, A. K. (1984). The effects of mands and models on the speech of unresponsive socially isolate children. *Journal of Speech and Hearing Disorders, 47*, 42–52.

Warren, S. F., & Rogers-Warren, A. (1980). Current perspectives in language remediation: A special monograph. *Education and Treatment of Children, 5*, 133–153.

Warren, S. F., & Rogers-Warren, A. K. (1983a). Setting variables affecting the display of trained noun referents by retarded children. In K. Kernan, M. Begab, & R. Edgerton (Eds.), *Environments and behavior* (pp. 123–151). Austin, TX: PRO-ED.

Warren, S. F., & Rogers-Warren, A. K. (1983b). A longitudinal analysis of language generalization among adolescents with severely handicapping conditions. *Journal of the Association for the Severely Handicapped, 8*, 18–32.

Warren, S. F., & Rogers-Warren, A. K. (Eds.). (1985). *Teaching functional language*. Austin, TX: PRO-ED.

Warren, S. F., Rogers-Warren, A. K., Baer, D. M., & Guess, D. (1980). The assessment and facilitation of language generalization. In W. Sailor, B. Wilcox, & L. Brown (Eds.), *Instructional design for the severely handicapped* (pp. 227–258). Baltimore: Brooks Publishers.

Warren, S. F., Rogers-Warren, A. K., & Buchanan, B. (1981, April). *A longitudinal analysis of comprehensive language training: Generalization to the real world*. Paper presented at the biannual meeting of the Society for Research in Child Development, Boston.

Watson, J. B. (1924). *Psychology from the standpoint of a behaviorist* (2nd ed.). Philadelphia: J. B. Lippincott.

Wetherby, B. (1978). Miniature languages and the functional analysis of verbal behavior. In R. L. Schiefelbusch (Ed.), *Bases of language intervention* (pp. 397–448). Austin, TX: PRO-ED.

Whitehurst, G. J., Novak, G., & Zorn, G. A. (1972). Delayed speech studied in the home. *Developmental Psychology, 2*, 169–177.

Whitehurst, G. J., & Zimmerman, B. J. (1979). *The functions of language and cognition*. New York: Academic Press.

Whorf, B. L. (1956). *Language, thought and reality*. Cambridge, MA: MIT Press.

Wittgenstein, L. (1953). *Philosophical investigations*. New York: Macmillan.

Wolfe, J. B. (1934). The effect of delayed reward upon learning in the white rat. *Journal of Comparative Psychology, 17*, 1–21.

# Author Index



An "f" after a page number denotes footnoted material.

# *Subject Index*